Pain Research

METHODS IN MOLECULAR MEDICINE™

John M. Walker, SERIES EDITOR

METHODS IN MOLECULAR MEDICINE™

Pain Research

Methods and Protocols

Edited by

Z. David Luo, MD, PhD

Department of Anesthesiology,
University of California Irvine Medical Center,
Orange, CA

HUMANA PRESS ✳ TOTOWA, NEW JERSEY

© 2004 Humana Press Inc.
999 Riverview Drive, Suite 208
Totowa, New Jersey 07512

humanapress.com

This publication is printed on acid-free paper. ∞
ANSI Z39.48-1984 (American Standards Institute) Permanence of Paper for Printed Library Materials.

Production Editor: Robin B. Weisberg.
Cover design by Patricia F. Cleary.

Printed in the United States of America. 10 9 8 7 6 5 4 3 2 1

1-59259-770-X (E-ISBN)

Library of Congress Cataloging-in-Publication Data

Pain research : methods and protocols / edited by David Z. Luo.
    p. ; cm. -- (Methods in molecular medicine, ISSN 1543-1894 ; 99)

Includes bibliographical references and index.
  ISBN 1-58829-103-0 (alk. paper)
  1. Pain--Animal models--Laboratory manuals.
  [DNLM: 1. Pain--physiopathology--Laboratory Manuals. 2. Animal
Experimentation--Laboratory Manuals. 3. Mice--Laboratory Manuals. 4. Models,
Animal--Laboratory Manuals .5. Neural Pathways--physiopathology--Laboratory
Manuals. 6. Rats--Laboratory Manuals. 7. Signal Transduction--physiology--Laboratory
Manuals. WL 25 P144 2004] I. Luo, David Z. II. Series.
  RB127.P344 2004
  616'.0472--dc22

                                                                  2003025346

Contents

Contributors

LIA G. ABRAHAMS • *Department of Neuroscience, University of Minnesota, Minneapolis, MN*

JEFFREY W. ALLEN • *Department of Anesthesiology, University of California San Diego, La Jolla, CA*

ANTON BITTNER • *Pharmaceutical Research & Development, Johnson & Johnson, San Diego, CA*

THOMAS H. BURKEY • *Department of Pharmacology and Toxicology, Indiana University School of Medicine, Indianapolis, IN*

NIGEL A. CALCUTT • *Department of Pathology, University of California San Diego, La Jolla, CA*

DAVID CAIN • *Department of Oral Science, University of Minnesota, Minneapolis, MN*

SUSAN CARLTON • *Department of Anatomy and Neurosciences, University of Texas Medical Branch, Galveston, TX*

SANDRA R. CHAPLAN • *Pharmaceutical Research & Development, Johnson & Johnson , San Diego, CA*

JIN MO CHUNG • *Marine Biomedical Institute and Department of Anatomy and Neurosciences, University of Texas Medical Branch, Galveston, TX*

KYUNGSOON CHUNG • *Marine Biomedical Institute and Department of Anatomy and Neurosciences, University of Texas Medical Branch, Galveston, TX*

ANTHONY H. DICKENSON • *Department of Pharmacology, University College London, London, UK*

ANDRÉE DIERICH • *Institut de Génétique et de Biologie Moléculaire et Cellulaire, Illkirch, France*

GUOPING FENG • *Department of Neurobiology, Duke University Medical Center, Durham, NC*

WILLARD M. FREEMAN • *Department of Behavioral Neuroscience, Oregon Health and Science University, Portland, OR*

JIMMY GROSS • *Department of Neurobiology, Duke University Medical Center, Durham, NC*

HONG QING GUO • *Pharmaceutical Research & Development, Johnson & Johnson, San Diego, CA*

EMILIANO S. HIGUERA • *Department of Anesthesiology, University of California San Diego, LaJolla, CA*

CYNTHIA M. HINGTGEN • *Departments of Neurology, Pharmacology and Toxicology, Indiana University School of Medicine, Indianapolis, IN*

KOICHI IWATA • *Department of Physiology, Nihon University, School of Dentistry, Osaka, Japan*

LUC JASMIN • *Department of Neurological Surgery, University of California San Francisco, San Francisco, CA*

FREDRIK KAMME • *Pharmaceutical Research & Development, Johnson & Johnson, San Diego, CA*

BRIGITTE L. KIEFFER • *Institut de Génétique et de Biologie Moléculaire et Cellulaire, Illkirch, France*

HEE KEE KIM • *Marine Biomedical Institute and Department of Anatomy and Neurosciences, University of Texas Medical Branch, Galveston, TX*

THIES LINDENLAUB • *Neurologische Klinik, Universitätskliniken des Saarlandes, Hamburg, Germany*

JING LU • *Department of Neurobiology, Duke University Medical Center, Durham, NC*

LIN LUO • *Pharmaceutical Research & Development, Johnson & Johnson, San Diego, CA*

Z. DAVID LUO • *Departments of Anesthesiology and Pharmacology, University of California Irvine, Irvine, CA*

SHELLE A. MALKMUS • *Department of Anesthesiology, University of California San Diego, La Jolla, CA*

STEVEN F. MAIER • *Department of Psychology and Center for Neuroscience, University of Colorado, Boulder, CO*

MARTIN MARSALA • *Department of Anesthesiology, University of California San Diego, La Jolla, CA*

YUJI MASUDA • *Division of Oral and Maxillofacial Biology, Institute of Oral Science, Matsumoto Dental University, Nagano, Japan*

BERNHARD MEURERS • *Pharmaceutical Research & Development, Johnson & Johnson, San Diego, CA*

ERIN D. MILLIGAN • *Department of Psychology and Center for Neuroscience, University of Colorado, Boulder, CO*

PETER T. OHARA • *Department of Anatomy, University of California San Francisco, San Francisco, CA*

KE REN • *Department of Biomedical Sciences, University of Maryland Dental School, Baltimore, Maryland*

VIRGINIA S. SEYBOLD • *Department of Neuroscience, University of Minnesota, Minneapolis, MN*

MARIA SCHÄFERS • *Department of Anesthesiology, University of California San Diego, La Jolla, CA*

CLAUDIA SOMMER • *Neurologische Klinik der Universität Würzburg, Würzburg, Germany*

LOUISE C. STANFA • *Department of Pharmacology, University College London, London, UK*

DA-THAO TRAN • *Pharmaceutical Research and Development, Johnson & Johnson, San Diego, CA*

MICHAEL R. VASKO • *Departments of Anesthesia, Pharmacology and Toxicology, Indiana University School of Medicine, Indianapolis, IN*

KENT E. VRANA • *Center for the Neurobiological Investigation of Drug Abuse and Neurobehavioral Study of Alcohol; Department of Physiology and Pharmacology, Wake Forest University School of Medicine, Winston-Salem, NC*

STEPHEN J. WALKER • *Center for the Neurobiological Investigation of Drug Abuse and Neurobehavioral Study of Alcohol; Department of Physiology and Pharmacology, Wake Forest University School of Medicine, Winston-Salem, NC*

JACKSON WAN • *Pharmaceutical Research & Development, Johnson & Johnson, San Diego, CA*

LINDA R. WATKINS • *Department of Psychology & Center for Neuroscience, University of Colorado, Boulder, CO*

KARIN WESTLUND • *Department of Anatomy and Neurosciences, University of Texas Medical Branch, Galveston, TX*

TRAVIS J. WORST • *Center for the Neurobiological Investigation of Drug Abuse and Neurobehavioral Study of Alcohol; Department of Physiology and Pharmacology, Wake Forest University School of Medicine, Winston-Salem, NC*

TONY L. YAKSH • *Department of Anesthesiology, University of California San Diego, La Jolla, CA*

JINGXUE YU • *Pharmaceutical Research & Development, Johnson & Johnson, San Diego, CA*

JESSICA ZHU • *Pharmaceutical Research & Development, Johnson & Johnson, San Diego, CA*

1

Mechanistic Dissection of Pain

From DNA to Animal Models

Z. David Luo

1. Introduction

The detrimental effects of pain to our society are overwhelming and affect many different aspects of the quality of our daily life. In addition to physical, spiritual, emotional, and social suffering, it has been estimated that pain costs $55 billion annually in loss of productivity in the United States alone (1). Over the past decades, pain treatment has relied mainly on empirical approaches and symptom relief, and most long-term treatments with pain medications are associated with adverse side effects, usually intolerable and sometimes life-threatening. Except for a few newly developed agents, target-derived, specific agents for pain treatment are not available because the cellular mechanisms underlying pain states are poorly understood. With the increase in the life span of human beings and the survival rates of patients with pain-inducing disorders as the consequences of rapid advancements in disease prevention, diagnosis, and therapeutic interventions, the demands of mechanism-based pain medications for improving quality of life are rapidly increasing. Thus, studying the mechanisms of nociception and searching for potential targets for specific pain therapies have become two of the top priorities on the agendas of increasing numbers of research and health organizations as well as pharmaceutical companies. This increasing demand is reflected by the constant yearly increase in the number of research publications related to the topic of "pain" in peer review journals for the past decades (Fig. 1). It is predicted that this trend will continue for at least the foreseeable future.

The complexity of pain transduction is now appreciated to be due, at least in part, the result of the following factors: (1) The molecular basis underlying pain states derived from different pathological conditions differs, even though some of these pain states may display similar behavioral endpoints. (2) With few

From: *Methods in Molecular Medicine, Vol. 99: Pain Research: Methods and Protocols*
Edited by: Z. D. Luo © Humana Press Inc., Totowa, NJ

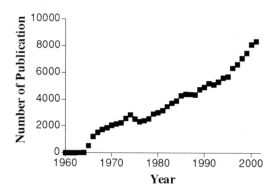

Fig. 1. Number of annual publications from the past 42 yr retrieved from PubMed using the key word "pain."

exceptions, such as familial hemiplegic migraine *(2)* and congenital insensitivity to pain with anhidrosis *(3)* in which mutations in a single gene have been identified and thought to be responsible for the disorders, it is now believed that pain transmission is a polygenic issue involving altered expression/modification of multiple, rather than single, factors/mediators in sensory pathways *(4,5)* and it is the unique interactions of these factors/mediators that underlie the pathogenesis of different pain states. (3) Individual vulnerability to pain is affected by social, environmental, gender, age, and genetic factors *(6–8)*. Therefore, it is difficult to find a "magic pain pill" that can be used to treat different pain conditions, and our goals to develop effective and specific pain medicines have to rely on our better understanding in the molecular basis of different pain states.

2. Methodologies in Pain Research
2.1. Preparations Using Animal Models

Over the past decades, a large body of evidence from behavioral pharmacology and electrophysiology studies in animal models has provided important information to define the pathophysiology and pharmacology of systems involved in pain transmission. Animal models are also good for predictions of drug efficacy and toxicity in humans. The concept that pain states derived from different pathologies have distinct underlying mechanisms makes these animal models great assets in pain research. New animal pain models are continuously being developed, leading to a constant expansion of systemic tools to characterize the pathophysiological and pharmacological aspects of various pain states. These systemic approaches continue to be the bridges connecting preclinical research to the final stages of development and evaluation of analgesic drugs and other pain interventions. In addition, combining animal pain models with genetically modified animals has become an important approach in studying the contribution of specific genes in nociception. Although each animal model has its advantages and limitations on the characterization of a particular pain state, detailed descriptions of all animal models for pain study easily can occupy an entire book volume. Unfortunately, with the intention of a broad coverage in methods and protocols of pain research, only limited numbers of animal models representing different types of pain-inducing conditions are included in this volume.

In addition to pathophysiology and behavioral pharmacology studies in animal models, characterization of neurotransmission in vivo such as regulation of neuraxial excitatory and inhibitory tone in a defined model provides another level of understanding in the neurobiochemistry of sensory pathways mediating the behavioral hypersensitivity to different stimuli. In this regard, intrathecal catheterization in research animals is widely used in pain research for accessing and delivering compounds into the intrathecal space, and collecting cerebral spinal fluid samples for biochemical analyses. This allows the characterization of spinal mechanisms of nociception and spinal-cord actions of different drugs, including their pharmacodynamics and pharmacokinetics. We are so fortunate that detailed information about spinal catheterization and sampling is well-covered in chapters of "Intrathecal Catheterization and Drug Delivery" by S. Malkmus and Dr. T. Yaksh and "Spinal Microdialyses" by Dr. M. Marsala, respectively.

The structural integrity and electrophysiological properties of sensory neurons, associated axons, and postsynaptic spinal dorsal-horn neurons are functionally important components in maintaining normal sensation and in pain transduction. Briefly, sensory neurons in dorsal root ganglia (DRG) are pseudounipolar neurons with a single process extending from the cell body that bifurcates into two functionally distinct branches: the peripheral and central branches. The peripheral branch innervates tissue and organs, whereas the central branch terminates in the spinal cord, where it forms synapses with spinal neurons. Sensory processing involves the collection of sensory information by the peripheral terminals, also called afferent fibers, from innervated tissue or organs and the generation of nerve impulses that propagate first into first-order DRG neurons, then to the spinal dorsal horn through the central branches, where neurotransmitters and modulators are released. These released biochemical signals then activate the postsynaptic, secondary dorsal-horn neurons, where sensory information is processed locally or referred to the brain.

Some specific features of sensory neurons are important in nociception processing. Different neurons and their associated fibers have different sensitivities to various stimulation, including that to innocuous and noxious levels of thermal, mechanical, and chemical stimuli; they synthesize and release different neurotransmitters and/or peptides under various conditions; and they are sensitive to growth factors for survival and responsive to various changes at the peripheral side, including inflammatory cytokines and nerve injury. These unique features of sensory neurons and their connections with spinal dorsal-horn neurons, also heterogeneous, permit the discrimination of various sensations at different anatomical levels along the sensory pathway.

Early studies by Erlanger and Gasser *(9,10)* established that stimulation of peripheral terminals of sensory neurons activates different afferent fibers with distinct conduction velocity. The conduction velocity correlates positively with the cross-sectional diameter of the fibers, including myelinated A and unmyelinated C fibers. The A fibers can be subdivided into α, β, δ with a decreasing order of axonal diameter and conduction velocity. The C fibers are the smallest in diameter and slowest in conduction. Early correlative studies between human evoked sensory experiences and selective blocking of conduction of subsets of afferent fibers have indicated that these fibers differ in sensory modalities. The larger-diameter fibers are mainly associated with proprioceptive stimulation, whereas the small myelinated and unmyelinated fibers are important in sensing temperature changes and noxious stimulation *(11)*.

Sensory processing also differs among DRG neurons that can be divided into subgroups with different sizes (small, medium, and large; or small and large only) corresponding to, in general, the order of their afferent sizes. In addition, DRG neurons are known to express neurotransmitters differentially, e.g., neuropeptides are found primarily in small DRG neurons. Furthermore, under various pathological conditions associated with chronic pain, such as nerve injury and peripheral inflammation, DRG neurons undergo dynamic changes, including altered gene expression and modulation of functional proteins such as membrane receptors, ion channels, and molecules important in intracellular signaling pathways. These biochemical, functional diversities and plasticity of DRG neurons, thus, are important regulatory components in responses to various stimuli, because they modulate the neuronal circuits in the spinal dorsal horn through presynaptic release of neurotransmitter or modulators.

Sensory processing is also regulated in the spinal dorsal horn, where neurons with cutaneous receptive fields form mono- or poly-synapses with afferent fibers in a stereotypical manner and have different response thresholds to various stimuli. Briefly, low-threshold neurons respond mainly to light touch or innocuous temperature on the receptive field, whereas high-threshold neurons respond mainly to noxious stimulation. Some neurons in the spinal dorsal horn have a wide dynamic range in responding to different strength of stimulation. Even though different types of dorsal-horn neurons have distinctive distributions and synaptic interactions with afferents in the spinal cord, there is a certain degree of convergence in the inputs to some of these neurons. The best example is the poly-synaptic interaction of wide dynamic neurons with excitatory inputs from terminals of afferents as well as inhibitory inputs from interneurons so that low-intensity stimulation can activate the inhibitory tone and reduce the neuronal response to high-intensity stimulation. This is the Gate Control Theory proposed by Drs. Melzack and Wall in 1965 *(12)*. Finally, the spinal sensory circuits are regulated by descending modulations, both excitatory and inhibitory, from structures in the upper central nervous system, including brainstem, hypothalamus, and cortex.

Taken together, sensation is a complex, interactive, and integrated process that requires the functional integrity of each component in the sensory pathway. Under most circumstances, changes in the excitability of these entities, either through long-term changes in gene expression or short-term modulation through interactions with injury factors and neurotransmitters, are the driving force of pain sensation. Thus, identification of neurons responsive to various stimuli along the pathway and altered electrophysiological properties in these neurons and associated fibers are critical in understanding the mechanisms of pain transduction. Detailed protocols related to these techniques are covered in the following chapters: "Anatomical Identification of Neurons Responsive to Nociceptive Stimuli" by Drs. L. Jasmin and P. Ohara; "Trigeminal Neuronal Recording in Animal Models of Orofacial Pain" by Dr. K. Iwata and his colleagues; "In Vivo Electrophysiology of Dorsal Horn Neurons" by Drs. L. Stanfa and A. Dickenson; and "Single Fiber Recording: In Vivo and In Vitro Preparations" by Drs. M. Schafers and D. Cain, respectively.

2.2. In Vitro Studies

As a complementary approach to in vivo studies, where integrated pathophysiological questions related to sensory processing can be investigated, in vitro studies using primary cultured cells from spinal cord and DRG allow us to gain molecular insights into sensory neuron excitability and neurotransmission regulation in a well-defined system. In addition, these in vitro systems allow us to assess precisely the dose-dependent effects and stereospecificity of agents on a biological system related to nociception without the pharmacokinetic complications of drug absorption, distribution, and biotransformation. Examples of using cultured spinal cord or DRG neurons in pain-relevant investigations are numerous, including, but not limited to: electrophysiological studies in neuronal excitability and channel kinetics, regulation of intracellular signaling pathways and neurotransmitter release by pain-inducing agents or irritants, sterospecificity and binding affinity evaluations of new compounds interacting with pain-related target sites. The advantages and limitations, and detailed protocols of these culture systems are well-described in the following chapters: "Isolation and Culture of Sensory Neurons from the Dorsal Root Ganglia of Embryonic or Adult Rats" by Dr. M. Vasko and his colleagues, and "Primary Cultures of Neonatal Rat Spinal Cord" by Dr. V. Seybold and L. Abrahams.

2.3. Molecular Investigations

Although studies using primary cultures and then animal models are the ultimate choices for characterization of pain-transduction pathways as well as pharmacological evaluation of drug specificity, efficacy, and safety, the capacity and speed of discovery using these means in identifying potential pain relevant targets are limited by the availability and specificity of the pharmacological tools and the fact that only one or few target molecules can be studied at a time. These limitations are now overcome by the rapid advance of molecular biology techniques that permits not only the rapid screening of potential targets for pain therapies, but also the extension of our knowledge in pain transduction to the molecular level, even to within a single cell type. These molecular approaches include gene-chip microarray analysis and proteomics that allow detection in an unbiased manner of potential changes in tissue from a defined pathophysiological condition at the mRNA and protein level, respectively, up to thousands of targets in one experiment. Furthermore, the ability of observing co-regulated molecules related to known functional pathways under a defined condition may provide important clues for interaction of orchestral proteins in pain transduction; therefore providing an additional advantage of these techniques. Currently, the use of commercially available gene chips, designed for either global gene-expression profiling or exploring specific pathways, are rapidly increasing owing to improvement in affordability and the availability of core facilities in most major research institutions and pharmaceutical companies. The chapter, "Functional Genomic Analysis in Pain Research Using Hybridization Arrays" by Dr. S. Walker and his colleagues illustrates the details as well as advantages and limitations of gene-chip assays. The chapter, "Semi-Quantitative Real-Time PCR for Pain Research" by Drs. H. Guo and S. Chaplan describes a sensitive method in validating gene chip data and measuring changes in mRNA levels rapidly.

Ideally, we need not only the power of massive data acquisition and parallel analyses of microarray assays, but also the specificity of these detections. This is extremely important in study of pain mechanisms because DRG and spinal-cord neurons are heterogeneous, and differ in their cell morphology, electrophysiology, biochemistry, and responses to various stimuli *(13)*. Furthermore, a large body of evidence from recent studies has indicated that non-neuronal cells in the spinal cord and DRG also contribute to pain transduction *(14)*, and painful stimuli induce changes not only in neurons, but also in non-neuronal cells in these tissues. Therefore, cell type-specific regulation and interactions may form the basis of plasticity mediating various pain states. Thus, detecting changes in a defined cell type in response to a pain-inducing condition will be a preferred experimental condition. This "dream" of experimental design is now achievable by combining the microarray analysis with the technique of laser capture microdissection that allows single-cell dissections and collections *(15)*. This technique and the subsequence protocols for RNA amplification are described in details in the chapter "Single-Cell Laser Capture Microdissection and RNA Amplification" by Dr. F. Kamme and his colleagues.

One of the limitations in gene-chip analysis is that detected changes at the mRNA level in a pain-inducing condition do not necessary reflect changes at the level of protein, the ultimate entity involved in cell functions. Very often, these changes may derive from the process of protein translation and posttranslational modifications such as phosphorylation/dephosphorylation that play crucial roles in cell-excitability regulation. Thus, the emerging proteomic techniques have been adapting rapidly. It is predicted that high-throughput detection of these changes can be accomplished in individual laboratories or core facilities in research institutions as a result of rapid improvements of the proteomic techniques and their affordability. More importantly, the functional implications of these changes now can be characterized using emerging high-throughput techniques for functional expression profiling, including the latest addition of Planar-Array-Based voltage clamp *(16)*. Although these exciting and cutting-edge techniques of high-throughput proteomics and functional expression profiling are major breakthroughs in the discovery phase for pain and other clinically relevant targets, most of these techniques are still under validation, and the associated high cost is still a limitation in their application in individual laboratories, at least at the present time. Thus, detailed methods of these techniques are beyond the scope of this volume.

Ultimately, functional characterization of potential target genes, their encoding proteins, underlying pathways, and pathopharmacology of a disease state, such as nociception, has to rely on studies performed in a well-integrated in vivo system, the animal models. The most commonly used practice in defining the functional roles of a given protein in a pain state is the gain- or loss-of-function analyses after in vivo treatment with pharmacological agonists or antagonists, respectively, designed to act on or block their respective functional receptors, such as membrane proteins and intracellular signaling molecules. In some cases, the loss of function can be achieved by treating the animals with neutralizing antibodies *(17,18)* to block or sequester target proteins. Although these approaches are convenient, reversible, and relatively economical, their applications are often limited by the availability and specificity of the available agents, especially for studies involved a functional protein with multiple isoforms or subtypes, a common biological phenomenon as indicated by a rapidly increased numbers of genes with alternatively spliced variants identified. Some novel approaches, including synthetic fusion protein approach *(19)* and the toxin-mediated target protein knockout approach *(20)*, may provide improved specificity. However, loss of function in these approaches is irreversible, thus, hindering investigations of reversibility and developmental regulation of the target proteins.

Alternatively, the loss of function of a particular gene can be studied by chemical knockdown of the transcript of a given gene. Techniques used to knockdown mRNA and thus prevent production of functional proteins include applications of antisense oligonucleotides *(21,22)*, peptide nucleic acid *(23)*, and the latest addition of small interfering RNA (siRNA) technique *(24–26)*. The siRNA technique is especially attractive because its specificity, potency, and long-lasting effects *(24,27)*. These chemical knockdown approaches are powerful in defining gene functions in biological research, and have a great potential in therapeutic applications upon further characterizations.

Finally, the contribution of potential target genes to nociception can be studied by examining altered phenotypes in pain models generated from either transgenic mice that overexpress a target gene and its encoding protein, or gene-targeted mice that carry a null gene and lack the functional protein. Thus, the gain or loss of function, respectively, in responses to different stimuli in these genetically modified mice would suggest a functional role of the gene product in nociception. Just like other techniques, these genetically modified mouse approaches are not without limitations. For example, embryonic lethality of the disrupted gene would prevent functional and behavioral analysis at a later stage of development. The complete knockout approach is irreversible and not for a specific target site or tissue, thus, genetic and developmental defects may interfere with phenotype analysis. In addition, the targeted-gene deficiency may result in a compensatory adaptation that leads to secondary phenotype or covers up the phenotype of the targeted gene. Thanks to the advancement in molecular biology techniques, these limitations can be overcome at different degree by combinations with tissue or cell type-specific *(28,29)* and inducible promoters *(28,30–32)*, allowing gene targeting in a spatial and temporal controlled manner. It is predicted that the use of these techniques in combination with different pain models will increase dramatically in pain research to characterize the molecular basis of nociception in the postgenomic era. We are so fortunate to have the methodologies of these techniques described in details in the chapters "Generation of Transgenic Mice" by Dr. G. Feng and his colleagues and "Knockout Mouse Models in Pain Research" by Drs. A. Dierich and B. Kieffer.

3. Conclusions

Although in vivo studies using animal models and in vitro studies using isolated tissue and cells provide a solid foundation in our understanding of behavioral pharmacology, electrophysiology, and biochemistry of nociception processing, the rapid development of molecular biology techniques enables us to study pain-transduction mechanisms in a more specific, in-depth, and rapid manner. However, each technique has its advantages and limitations. Because each pain state is likely to be a multimechanism disorder involving interactions of multiple mediators/modulations in a defined pathway, the ultimate discovery of these specific pathways and potential targets for specific pain medications has to rely on a multidisciplinary approach. One obvious example is the challenge that we are facing in the postgenomic era: the functional characterization of a large pool of rapidly identified potential molecular targets after gene microarray and proteomic analyses. In addition to in vitro high-throughput functional analysis in isolated biological systems, the discovery of contributory roles of these molecular targets to pain transduction, and the evaluation of mechanism-based, target-specific pain medications have to be done in well-integrated biological systems, the animal models.

References

1. Katz, N. (2002) The impact of pain management on quality of life. *J. Pain Sympt. Manage* **24,** S38–47.
2. Ophoff, R. A., Terwindt, G. M., Vergouwe, M. N., et al. (1996) Familial hemiplegic migraine and episodic ataxia type-2 are caused by mutations in the Ca^{2+} channel gene CACNL1A4. *Cell* **87,** 543–552.
3. Indo, Y., Tsuruta, M., Hayashida, Y., et al. (1996) Mutations in the TRKA/NGF receptor gene in patients with congenital insensitivity to pain with anhidrosis. *Nat Genet* **13,** 485–488.
4. Mogil, J. S., Yu, L., and Basbaum, A. I. (2000) Pain genes?: natural variation and transgenic mutants. *Ann. Rev. Neurosci.* **23,** 777–811.
5. Woolf, C. J. and Decosterd, I. (1999) Implications of recent advances in the understanding of pain pathophysiology for the assessment of pain in patients. *Pain* **Suppl 6,** S141–147.
6. Edwards, P. W., Zeichner, A., Kuczmierczyk, A. R., and Boczkowski, J. (1985) Familial pain models: the relationship between family history of pain and current pain experience. *Pain* **21,** 379–384.
7. Zatzick, D. F. and Dimsdale, J. E. (1990) Cultural variations in response to painful stimuli. *Psychosom. Med.* **52,** 544–557.
8. Bachiocco, V., Scesi, M., Morselli, A. M., and Carli, G. (1993) Individual pain history and familial pain tolerance models: relationships to post-surgical pain. *Clin. J. Pain* **9,** 266–271.
9. Erlanger, J., and Gasser, H. S. (1924) The compound nature of the action current of nerve as disclosed by the cathode ray oscillograph. *American Journal of Physiology* **70,** 624–666
10. Erlanger, J., and Gasser, H. S. (1930) The action potential in fibers of slow conduction in spinal roots and somatic nerves. *Americal Journal of Physiology* **92,** 43–82
11. Perl, E. R. (1992) Function of Dorsal Root Ganglion Neurons: An Overview. in *Sensory Neurons: Diversity, Development, and Plasticity* (Scott, S. A., ed), Oxford University Press, New York, pp. 3–23,
12. Melzack, R., and Wall, P. D. (1965) Pain mechanisms: a new theory. *Science* **150,** 971–979
13. Lawson, S. N. (1992) Morphological and biochemical cell types of sensory neurons. in *Sensory Neurons: Diversity, development, and plasticity* (Scott, S. A., ed), Oxford University Press, New York, pp. 27–59,
14. Watkins, L. R., and Maier, S. F. (2002) Beyond neurons: evidence that immune and glial cells contribute to pathological pain states. *Physiol Rev* **82,** 981–1011
15. Emmert-Buck, M. R., Bonner, R. F., Smith, P. D., Chuaqui, R. F., Zhuang, Z., Goldstein, S. R., Weiss, R. A., and Liotta, L. A. (1996) Laser capture microdissection [see comments]. *Science* **274,** 998–1001
16. Kiss, L., Bennett, P. B., Uebele, V. N., Koblan, K. S., Kane, S. A., Neagle, B., and Schroeder, K. (2003) Hig throughput ion-channel pharmacology: Planar-Array-Based voltage clamp. *ASSAY and Drug Development Technologies* **1,** 127
17. Safieh-Garabedian, B., Poole, S., Allchorne, A., Winter, J., and Woolf, C. J. (1995) Contribution of interleukin-1 beta to the inflammation-induced increase in nerve

growth factor levels and inflammatory hyperalgesia. *British Journal of Pharmacology* **115**, 1265–1275

18. Lewin, G. R., Rueff, A., and Mendell, L. M. (1994) Peripheral and central mechanisms of NGF-induced hyperalgesia. *European Journal of Neuroscience* **6**, 1903–1912

19. McMahon, S. B., Bennett, D. L., Priestley, J. V., and Shelton, D. L. (1995) The biological effects of endogenous nerve growth factor on adult sensory neurons revealed by a trkA-IgG fusion molecule [see comments]. *Nature Medicine* **1**, 774–780

20. Mantyh, P. W., Rogers, S. D., Honore, P., Allen, B. J., Ghilardi, J. R., Li, J., Daughters, R. S., Lappi, D. A., Wiley, R. G., and Simone, D. A. (1997) Inhibition of hyperalgesia by ablation of lamina I spinal neurons expressing the substance P receptor [see comments]. *Science* **278**, 275–279

21. Lönnberg, H., and Vuorio, E. (1996) Towards genomic drug therapy with antisense oligonucleotides. *Annals of Medicine* **28**, 511–522

22. Crooke, S. T. (1998) Antisense therapeutics. *Biotechnology and Genetic Engineering Reviews* **15**, 121–157

23. Nielsen, P. E., Egholm, M., and Buchardt, O. (1994) Peptide nucleic acid (PNA). A DNA mimic with a peptide backbone. *Bioconjugate Chemistry* **5**, 3–7

24. Fire, A., Xu, S., Montgomery, M. K., Kostas, S. A., Driver, S. E., and Mello, C. C. (1998) Potent and specific genetic interference by double-stranded RNA in Caenorhabditis elegans. *Nature (London)* **391**, 806–811.

25. Sharp, P. A. (2001) RNA interference—2001. *Genes Dev* **15**, 485–490.

26. Bosher, J. M., and Labouesse, M. (2000) RNA interference: genetic wand and genetic watchdog. *Nat Cell Biol* **2**, E31–36.

27. Yang, D., Buchholz, F., Huang, Z., et al. (2002) Short RNA duplexes produced by hydrolysis with Escherichia coli RNase III mediate effective RNA interference in mammalian cells. *Proc. Natl. Acad. Sci. USA* **99**, 9942–9947.

28. Orban, P. C., Chui, D., and Marth, J. D. (1992) Tissue- and site-specific DNA recombination in transgenic mice. *Proc. Natl. Acad. Sci. USA* **89**, 6861–6865.

29. Katarova, Z., Mugnaini, E., Sekerkova, G., et al. (1998) Regulation of cell-type specific expression of lacZ by the 5-′flanking region of mouse GAD67 gene in the central nervous system of transgenic mice. *Europ. J. Neurosci.* **10**, 989–999.

30. Lakso, M., Sauer, B., Mosinger, B., Jr., et al. (1992) Targeted oncogene activation by site-specific recombination in transgenic mice. *Proc. Natl. Acad. Sci. USA* **89**, 6232–6236.

31. Kühn, R., Schwenk, F., Aguet, M., and Rajewsky, K. (1995) Inducible gene targeting in mice. *Science* **269**, 1427–1429.

32. Sauer, B. and Henderson, N. (1988) Site-specific DNA recombination in mammalian cells by the Cre recombinase of bacteriophage P1. *Proc. Natl. Acad. Sci. USA* **85**, 5166–5170.

2

Assessment of Acute Thermal Nociception in Laboratory Animals

Jeffrey W. Allen and Tony L. Yaksh

Summary

Models of acute nociception using a thermal stimulus are widely employed as screening methods for nociceptive properties of new drug compounds. In this chapter, detailed descriptions for conducting of two of the most commonly used models; the hot plate test and the "Hargreaves test," are described. These models are applicable to both rats and mice and have the advantage of allowing repeated and multiple testing using a single animal because the stimulus is transitory and produces no tissue damage. Additionally, a modification of these models using a skin-twitch reflex that is applicable to large laboratory animals such a dogs or sheep is described. Guidance concerning potential confounding variable are discussed, as are tips for reducing variably among testing sessions.

Key Words: Thermal; nociception; pain; c-fibers; rodents; dogs; hot plate; Hargreaves; skin twitch.

1. Introduction

The acute application of a high-intensity thermal stimulus to the skin is one of the most commonly used models to assess nociceptive processing as an assay to screen for the analgesic activity of a drug or physiological manipulation. In principle, the manipulation serves to activate high-threshold sensory fibers that innervate the skin. These axons transduce temperatures that are in the range of those that produce escape behavior when applied to the skin, with the frequency of discharge proportional to the intensity of the stimulus to which the skin is exposed *(1)*. Such afferent traffic correspondingly activates dorsal-horn neurons located in the superficial spinal lamina, which project in the contralateral ventro-lateral tracts to supraspinal sites where they serve to activate neurons in the medulla, mesencephalon, and thalamus *(2)*. The application of such stimuli

From: *Methods in Molecular Medicine, Vol. 99: Pain Research: Methods and Protocols*
Edited by: Z. D. Luo © Humana Press Inc., Totowa, NJ

evokes a behavioral response that displays several defining characteristics: (1) the escape response evoked by such a focal noxious stimulus is organized somatotopically, e.g., a stimulus applied to the foot will initiate a withdrawal of that foot; and (2) the response latency varies inversely with the intensity of the stimulus *(3,4)*. Drugs or physiological manipulations that diminish the frequency of the evoked discharge or diminish the activity of spinal neurons activated by that input will accordingly increase the response latency *(5)*. If the experimental treatment has no effect on motor function and an increase in latency is observed, then the treatment is said to be antinociceptive or analgesic. Conversely, if a treatment, such as an inflammation of the paw, serves to decrease the response latency, it is said to induce hyperalgesia *(6)*.

The assessment of the acute response of the animal to a strong thermal stimulus is typically accomplished by allowing the animal to stand on a heated metal plate (hot-plate test) *(7)*, placing a heated probe on the skin *(8)*, or placing the tail in heated water (tail-flick immersion test) *(9)*. More recently, these tests have been adapted in which an indirect thermal stimulus is applied to the paw using a heat source such as a focused high-intensity light bulb *(10)*. In this chapter, we will specifically describe the use of a paw thermal escape evoked by: (1) placing the animal on a thermally regulated surface (hot plate); and (2) application of a radiant stimulus to the paw, referred to as the Hargreaves test, both of which are suitable for rodents (mice and rats). In addition, we will describe a skin-twitch reflex test applicable to large animals that was initially performed in spinalized dogs *(8,11,12)*. Protocols for both the hot plate and Hargreaves tests herein will be presented for rats, and experimental adjustments for differences with other species such as mice will be included as appropriate (*see* **Note 1**).

2. Materials

2.1. Hot Plate Test

1. Animals: 150–400 g rats. As in all behavioral testing models, animals should undergo several episodes of adaptation to handling and exposure to the test environment. This includes transporting the animal to the test room, placing the animal in the test device, and returning the animal to the home cage.
2. Testing Chamber: Hot-plate apparatus consisting of a Plexiglass enclosure without a bottom placed on the surface of a thermally controlled metal plate as seen in **Fig. 1**.
   a. The plexiglass enclosure is typically about 30 cm high and 15 cm in diameter. These chamber sizes are approximate and are suitable for animals of approx 250 g. Smaller chamber sizes may be employed for proportionately smaller animals. The chamber size should be selected to provide just enough room for the animal to assume a normal crouching posture and sufficient height to prevent the animal to readily escape by jumping. The thermal surface must be of a size that extends beyond the edge of the plexiglass chamber. It must provide for a temperature that is uniform across its surface from edge

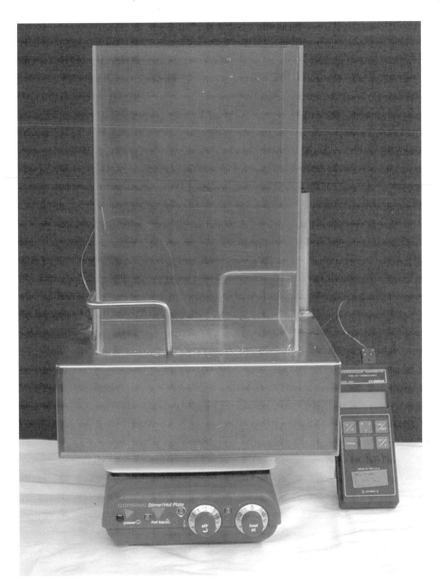

Fig. 1. Picture showing a hot-plate system. The metal water bath is placed on top of a stirring hot plate, which has been modified to have a proportional feedback circuit driven by a temperature probe affixed to the metal surface, which constitutes the floor of the thermal escape chamber. A stirring bar is mounted inside of the water bath to ensure uniform mixing and the side filling tube is present to ensure that the chamber is always full to prevent air bubbles inside the water bath.

to edge and be able to maintain the nominal surface temperature to within 1% of the target temperature.

   b. Units often employ a water bath with a metal (testing) surface that possesses the desired controlling parameters. The water bath under the testing surface typically requires active circulation of the water bath to avoid hot spots. The temperature control must be governed by the actual measured temperature of the hot-plate surface upon which the animal will be placed.

   c. Various commercial hot-plate apparatuses are available, typically offering a range of automation including built in timers and digital output (Columbus Instruments, Columbus, OH; San Diego Instruments, Inc., San Diego, CA; TSE, Technical & Scientific Equipment GmbH, Bad Homburg, Germany).

   d. Test environment should be selected as to minimize extraneous noise and traffic. The area should avoid direct drafts from air conditioning or direct sunlight. Mice and rat testing should be carried out in separate rooms to minimize the presence of species-specific odors.

3. 1-cc Syringe with 26 G needle for subcutaneous (sc) or intraperitoneal (ip) drug delivery.
4. Stopwatch or timer for assessing response latency to the nearest 0.1 s.
5. Test article, plus vehicle if appropriate.

2.2. Hargreaves Test

1. Animals: 150–400 g rats.
2. Testing chamber: Thermal nociception testing devices derived from the description by Hargreaves et al. *(10)* are commercially available from a number of sources. The system shown in **Fig. 2** is available from University of California-San Diego (Department of Anesthesiology, Attn. Mr. George Ozaki, 9500 Gilman drive, La Jolla CA 92093-0818). A similar device is also available from Ugo Basile (Biological Research Apparatus, Via G. Borghi 43, 21025 Comerio VA, Italy).
3. Test environment issues should be considered as noted for the hot-plate model.
4. 1-cc Syringe with 26 G needle for sc or ip drug delivery.
5. Stopwatch/timer.
6. Test article, plus vehicle.

2.3. Thermally Evoked Skin Twitch

1. Animals: Purpose-bred beagle dogs (8–16 kg).
2. Testing apparatus: Thermally conductive brass probe with an area of approx 1.2 cm^2 connected to a heated circulating water bath at 62.5°C. See **Fig. 3** for a typical skin-twitch testing unit including an automated timer.
3. Sling for immobilization during testing.
4. 1–3 cc Syringe with 23 G needle for sc or intramuscular (im) drug delivery.
5. Stopwatch or timer.
6. Test article, plus vehicle if appropriate.

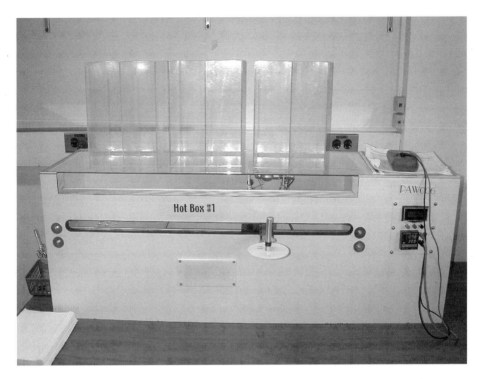

Fig. 2. A Hargreaves-type device prepared to permit concurrent testing of six rats. Note the presence of a Voltmeter on the instrument used for tracking changes in stimulus intensity over time.

3. Methods

3.1. Hot-Plate Test

1. Preheat the hot plate to the selected target temperature, typically 52.5°C (55°C for mice). The targeted temperature should be additionally measured periodically (at the beginning of each day) with a calibrated standard. Records of stability should be maintained with the daily experimental log.

2. For testing, the animal is placed on the hot plate and the timer is started immediately. On the observation of the criterion behavior (*see* **Note 2**), the timer is stopped and the animal is immediately removed from the testing apparatus and placed back in its cage. If the animal does not respond within a criterion time ("cut-off time," *see* **Note 2b**), the animal is removed from the testing apparatus to prevent tissue injury and is assigned the maximal cutoff time. Following each test, the surface of the hot plate should be cleansed of any urine and feces.

3. Test sequence typically involves one or two pretreatment baseline response measures at approx 15-min intervals (T = –30, –15 min), delivery of the test article

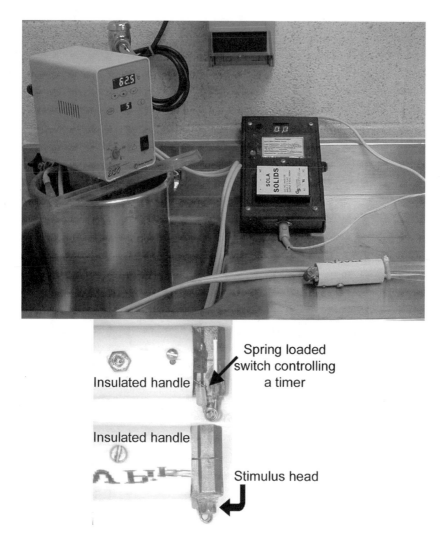

Fig. 3. Example of a canine skin-twitch device consisting of a circulating water bath at 62.5°C connected to a stimulus probe. The stimulus probe is also connected to a timing device that provides an alarm if the cut-off time is reached prior to a response.

(T = 0) and then testing at preselected intervals thereafter. A typical test time interval would be T = +1, 30, 60, 120, and 180 min. Particular timing will depend on the anticipated time of onset and duration of the test article. See **Notes 3–5** concerning data collection and analysis.

4. Suggested drug volume and pretreatment times are listed in **Table 1.**

Table 1
Guideline for Volumes and Pretreatment Times for Drug Dosing in the Hot-Plate and Hargreaves Tests in Rats

Route	Suggested Volumes	Pretreatment Time
Oral	10 mL/kg	30 min
Subcutaneous	1 mL/kg	15–30 min
Intrapertioneal	4 mL/kg	15–30 min
Intravenous	1 mL/kg	10 min
Intrathecal	10 μL + 10 μL flush	10 min

3.2. Hargreaves Test Using a Thermal Paw Stimulator

1. The use of radiant-heat devices requires daily assessment of thermal intensity. Different devices may require different protocols. Typically, it will involve two components: (i) Checking the current and voltage delivered to the heating lamp; and (ii) checking the temperature heating curve of the stimulus using a standard temperature probe (thermister or thermocouple) that has a rapid response time (typically $T_{1/2}$ of < 2 s).

   a. As the lamp output will diminish with age, these assessments should be logged daily for apparent shifts over time. Practically, the calibration of the system in the beginning will be accomplished by defining the response latencies in different groups of animals with different stimulus currents and correlating this with the measured heating curve.

   b. Different stimulus systems will display different heating curves vs current relationships and the initial calibration with naïve groups of animals is critical.

   c. Some devices can readily and repeatably alter stimulus currents and hence heating curves. Having multiple stimulus intensities are useful for reliably producing different response latencies by adjusting stimulus intensities.

2. Animals should be acclimatized to the testing apparatus on the day of testing for approx 30 min. Placing a paper towel underneath the animal during this time prevents urine and feces from accumulating of the glass surface. It is important to keep the surface of the glass clean and dry because if water is present on the surface, the thermal transfer characteristics to the paw will be altered.

3. After acclimatization has occurred, rats will display some exploratory behavior such as rearing. At this time remove the paper towels by sliding them from underneath the rat. They will be disturbed briefly but will quickly stop exploratory behavior. Baseline latencies are obtained by moving the light source under the plantar surface of the hind paw as shown in **Figs. 4** and **5**. The stimulus lamp and timer are simultaneously activated by pressing the Start button. **Note 6** discusses response analysis and reporting.

4. Test sequence typically involves one or two pretreatment baseline response measures at approx 15-min intervals (T = –30, –15 min), delivery of the test article

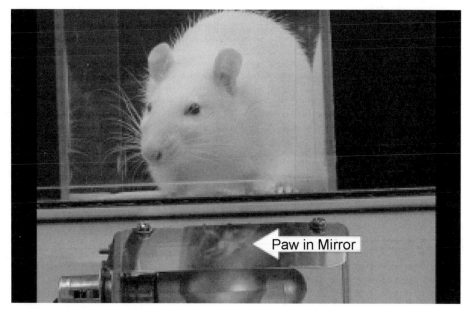

Fig. 4. A rat in a modified Hargreaves box (UCSD Anesthesiology). The plantar surface of the rear paw is visible in the mirror used to position the focused light source.

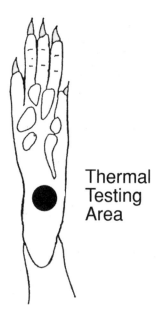

Fig. 5. The area represented by the black circle is the target for the focused light beam in the Hargreaves test. Inconsistent placement of the light beam will introduce variability in the results owing to differences in skin thickness throughout the paw.

(T = 0), and then testing at preselected intervals thereafter. A typical test time interval would be T = +15, 30, 60, 120, and 180 min. Particular timing will depend on the anticipated time of onset and duration of the test article. See **Notes 3–5** concerning data collection and analysis.

5. If the animal does not respond within a criterion time ("cut-off time"; *see* **Note 6b**), the animal is removed from the testing apparatus to prevent tissue injury and is assigned the maximal cutoff time. Following each test, the surface of the testing box should be cleansed of any urine and feces.

6. Animals are returned to their cages on an hourly basis to their cage to permit feeding and drinking. They are returned to the test chamber 15 min prior to testing. Re-acclimatization for the 120- and 180-min testing points should require less than 15 min.

3.3. Skin-Twitch Latency in Beagle Dogs

1. Dogs are placed in a sling of appropriate size to minimize movement. It is convenient to place the sling on a table so that the people testing the animal can test in a standing posture. Significant physical restraint is not usually necessary once dogs have been acclimated to the handling, the sling, and testing environment.

2. An area of approx 2 × 3 cm is shaved bilaterally in the lower dorsal T12-L3 region, just off midline and rostral to a line drawn between the pelvic crests.

3. The probe is gently placed within the shaved area on one side until a brief "twitch" is seen localized to the area of probe placement. The probe should be removed immediately following visualization of the response and the latency time is recorded. The maximal time of contact between the probe and skin is 6 s to prevent thermal damage to the skin. If no twitch is present within this time-frame, the probe is removed and a latency of 6 s is recorded. The testing is then repeated on the contralateral side. The sequence is generally repeated only three times per testing interval to prevent tissue damage. Note that different regions within the shaved area should be used for testing so that repeated heating of a small area is avoided. The lowest latency times for the left and right side are averaged to provide a single latency for each time point. *See* **Note 7** for further tips concerning maximizing skin-twitch probability.

4. The observed response is a brisk local contraction of the underlying cutaneous musculature within approx 3 s. On occasion, a dog may display a similar brisk response almost contiguously with the touching of the probe (e.g., latency < 1 s). This is a confounder that reflects the activation of low-threshold, tactile afferents (also referred to as a "flea or fly flick").

5. As with other thermal testing protocols, the predetermined testing intervals are chosen on the basis of the anticipated pharmacokinetics of the test agent.

4. Notes

1. In the United States, animal studies are undertaken with a protocol approved by the Institutional Animal Care and Use Committee (IACUC). In the absence of other surgical or treatment requirement, these acute stimulation models are considered to

be minimally intrusive or stressful. As described, the animal has complete control over the application of the stimulus. Withdrawal or escape will terminate the stimulus. Comparable studies involving acute escape are routinely performed in humans for somatosensory testing procedures and are uniformly considered to be ethical *(13)*.

2. Hot Plate.

   a. Selection of criterion response. Observation of induced behavior after placing the rat on the thermal surface reveals one or more behaviors appearing in the following sequence: (i) grooming with the fore paws; (ii) an increase in ambulatory activity; (iii) rapidly repeated elevations of either hind paw ("foot stomping"); (iv) licking of the hind paw; (v) agitated behavior; and (vi) jumping. Convention has typically focused on the licking of the hind paw to indicate the criterion response. On occasion, an animal will not lick, but show either jumping or evident agitation. It is important that the same end point be used throughout the study. However, if jumping is seen, that must be taken as an endpoint because clearly it is evidence of escape. Similarly, a high level of agitation (frantic ambulation around the hot-plate surface or vocalization), although less desirable and definitive, must also be taken as a termination endpoint. In these cases where an alternate endpoint is employed, that should be part of the data record (e.g., 12J or 12A, indicating jump or agitation at 12 s as the endpoint).

   b. Selection of criterion cut-off time. The purpose of the cutoff time is to prevent significant injury. As the test-surface temperature is increased, typically the shorter the baseline response latency and the shorter the time the animal can be allowed to remain on the surface without paw injury (oedema, erythema, or blistering). It is important to avoid injury with repeated testing to avoid creating a sensitized skin surface that will confound drug effects. In general, with a 52.5 ± 0.5°C surface, repeated testing may be carried out by convention with a 40-s response cut-off for a rat and 30-s response cut-off for a mouse. Selection of a cut-off time should be undertaken as part of the calibration of any test system.

   c. Criterion response behaviors. Determining which one of the possible behaviors will be quantified, e.g., the paw lick or jump, should be done prior to testing; this behavior should be used consistently throughout the study. Selection of the behavior may be influenced by drug side effects; for example, morphine increases motor activity in mice, thus paw lick would be a more appropriate measure.

3. Data for hot plate, Hargreaves test, and thermal skin twitch may be expressed as mean and SEM of the response latency in seconds. Alternately, these data may be expressed as percent maximum possible effect (%MPE). This is calculated using the formula below

$$\%MPE = [(\text{latency–baseline})/(\text{cutoff–baseline})] \times 100$$

4. The use of the MPE has several advantages. (a) It allows the researcher to normalize the results for each animal with respect to its own control. It is assumed that the baseline differences between animals in a given treatment are distributed randomly

and this normalization procedure will reduce between-animal variations. On the other hand, if there are systematic differences in baseline (secondary to other treatments, strain differences, or differences in the experimental apparatus calibrations), then the normalization procedure will be essentially misleading. In such cases, raw response latencies should be part of the discussion of the data set. (b) If one has generated a dose-response curve using several doses, the dose of the test article that produces a 50% maximal effect (ED_{50}) can be calculated to compare the relative potency of different drugs.

5. Careful and systematic assessment of motor and sensory function using either a functional observation battery (FOB) is suggested when testing drugs that may alter motor function or may be either sedative or stimulants. For example, a rat treated with a neuroleptic such as the dopamine D2 antagonist haloperidol or with high doses of stimulants such as amphetamine may be unable to lick the hind paw or jump when placed on the hot plate, but this does not mean that these compounds have analgesic efficacy. These drugs have simply disrupted motor function by causing akinesia in the case of the haloperidol or stereotypy in the case of amphetamine.

6. Hargreaves model
   a. The criterion response is the abrupt withdrawal of the stimulated hind paw. Upon withdrawal of the paw, the stimulus and timer are terminated. The latency time is recorded and the opposite hind paw in similarly tested. If either hind paw is normal, then the response latencies for the two paws are averaged to obtain a single value for each paw.
   b. Selection of criterion cut-off time. As described for the hot plate, the purpose of the cutoff time is to prevent significant injury. It is important to avoid injury with repeated testing to avoid creating a sensitized skin surface, which will confound drug effects. Selection of a cutoff time should be undertaken as part of the calibration of any test system. Usually, a 20-s cut-off time is chosen for a rat and a 15-s cut-off time is chosen for a mouse.
   c. The above description has been for the assessment of acute nociception. The model is expanded readily to consider the effects of treatments that serve to produce hyperalgesia. For example, injection of an irritant such as carrageenan ([λ]-Carrageenan, Sigma Chemical Company, St. Louis, MO) into the dorsum of the paw will result in a progressive appearance of inflammation over 2–3 h. The paw becomes edematous and swollen. Testing the thermal escape latency of the inflamed paw will show that its response latencies are much reduced as compared with the noninjected paw *(14,15)*. This enhanced behavioral responsiveness reflects both a local peripheral sensitization, such that the afferent fires vigorously in response to a modest stimulus, and a central sensitization, in which there is an exaggerated response to afferent input *(16,17)*.

7. Thermal Skin Twitch.
   a. It should be noted that there can be significant variability between dogs with latencies, ranging from 1 s to greater than 6 s. In general, with a 62.5°C probe, repeated testing may be carried out by convention with a 6-s response cut-off. It is our routine practice to screen dogs and exclude animals with latency greater

than 6 s after three acclimatization sessions. Additionally, it is important to verify that the twitch truly is thermally evoked, and not owing to tactile cues or hypersensitivity. This can be accomplished easily by applying an equally sized and thermally neutral stimulus, such as an unsharpened pencil, to the testing area.

b. Dogs are allowed to acclimatize for at least three testing sessions prior to collection of baseline data. Most dogs readily acclimatize to standing in the sling for the duration necessary for nociceptive testing. When anxious, some dogs will often display a very minor whole body shaking, during which time the twitch reflex in inhibited.

Thermal nociception assays of some sort are a common feature of many experimental laboratories studying the perception of pain, including both laboratory animals and humans subjects. They provide rapid and reliable models to assess the effects of physical or pharmacological treatments on the perception of acute pain.

References

1. Treede, R. D., Meyer, R. A., Raja, S. N., and Campbell, J. N. (1992) Peripheral and central mechanisms of cutaneous hyperalgesia. *Prog. Neurobiol.* **38,** 397–421.
2. Willis, W. D. and Westlund, K. N. (1997) Neuroanatomy of the pain system and of the pathways that modulate pain. *J. Clin. Neurophysiol.* **14,** 2–31.
3. Tsuruoka, M., Matsui, A., and Matsui, Y. (1988) Quantitative relationship between the stimulus intensity and the response magnitude in the tail flick reflex. *Physiol. Behav.* **43,** 79–83.
4. Dirig, D. M. and Yaksh, T. L. (1995) Differential right shifts in the dose-response curve for intrathecal morphine and sufentanil as a function of stimulus intensity. *Pain* **62,** 321–328.
5. Le Bars, D., Gozariu, M., and Cadden, S. W. (2001) Animal models of nociception. *Pharmacol. Rev.* **53,** 597–652.
6. Yaksh TL. Preclinical models of nociception, in *Anesthesia: Biologic Foundations* (Yaksh, T. L., Lynch III, C., Zapol, W. M., et al., eds.). Lippincott-Raven Publishers, Philadelphia, pp. 685–718.
7. D'Amour, F. E. and Smith, D. L. (1941) A method for determining loss of pain sensation. *J. Phamacol. Exp. Ther.* **72,** 74–79.
8. Martin, W. R., Eades, C. G., Fraser, H. F., and Winkler, A. (1964) Use of hindlimb reflexes of the chronic spinal dog for comparing analgesics. *J. Pharmacol. Exp. Ther.* **144,** 8–11.
9. Janssen, P. A. J., Niemegeers, C. J. E., and Dony, J. G. H. (1963) The inhibitory effect of fentanyl and other morphine like analgesics on the warm water induced tail withdrawal reflex in the rat. *Arzneimittelforsch* **13,** 502–507.
10. Hargreaves, K., Dubner, R., Brown, F., Flores, C., and Joris, J. (1988) A new and sensitive method for measuring thermal nociception in cutaneous hyperalgesia. *Pain* **32,** 77–88.
11. Sabbe, M. B., Grafe, M. R., Mjanger, E., et al. (1994) Spinal delivery of sufentanil, alfentanil, and morphine in dogs. Physiologic and toxicologic investigations. *Anesthesiology* **81,** 899–920.

12. Yaksh, T. L. (ed.) (1999) *Spinal Drug Delivery.* Elsevier Science, New York, NY.
13. Defrin, R., Ohry, A., Blumen, N., and Urca, G. (2002) Sensory determinants of thermal pain. *Brain* **125,** 501–510.
14. Dirig, D. M., Isakson, P. C., and Yaksh, T. L. (1998) Effect of COX-1 and COX-2 inhibition on induction and maintenance of carrageenan-evoked thermal hyperalgesia in rats. *J. Pharmacol. Exp. Ther.* **285,** 1031–1037.
15. Hurley, R. W., Chatterjea, D., Rose Feng, M., et al. (2002) Gabapentin and pregabalin can interact synergistically with naproxen to produce antihyperalgesia. *Anesthesiology* **97,** 1263–1273.
16. Yaksh, T. L., Hua, X.-Y., Kalcheva, I., et al. (1999) The spinal biology in humans and animals of pain states generated by persistent small afferent input. *Proc. Natl. Acad. Sci. USA* **96,** 7680–7686.
17. Yaksh, T. L. (1999) Spinal systems and pain processing, development of novel analgesic drugs with mechanistically defined models. *Trends Pharmacol. Sci.* **20,** 329–337.

3

Tissue Injury Models of Persistent Nociception in Rats

Jeffrey W. Allen and Tony L. Yaksh

Summary

The purpose of this chapter is to provide guidance to the novice investigator as to two models of ongoing nociception in rats. The models described herein are the formalin test, in which an irritant is injected subcutaneously into a dorsal paw and the numbers of flinches produced over 60 min are counted, and a mild burn model that produces a transitory primary and secondary thermal and mechanical hyperalgesia lasting approx 90 min. These models allow assessment of spinal sensitization, which may be an important factor when considering plasticity associated with human pain states. Detailed protocols using both manual and automated counting for the formalin test are included, as are methods concerning data analysis.

Key Words: Persistent pain; nociception; burn; formalin; spinal sensitization; plasticity; rats.

1. Introduction

Pain conditions in humans are often the result of some type of tissue injury, e.g., postsurgical pain, burns, arthritis, or minor trauma. Following such tissue injury or inflammation, the observer will report an ongoing spontaneous aching pain as well as areas at the injury and surrounding the site where an otherwise modestly aversive stimulus will be reported as painful (primary hyperalgesia), whereas light touch at adjacent uninjured sites will be reported as aversive (secondary tactile allodynia). Current thinking indicates that this ongoing pain state, which persists after the initial injury, and the exaggerated pain response reflects two components: a peripheral and a central sensitization. In the periphery, inflammation leads to release of active factors, which initiates activities in sensory C-fibers and sensitizes these nerve endings so that a moderate stimulus initiates a high level of sensory activity. Within the central nervous system (CNS), it is understood that ongoing small afferent

From: *Methods in Molecular Medicine, Vol. 99: Pain Research: Methods and Protocols*
Edited by: Z. D. Luo © Humana Press Inc., Totowa, NJ

input leads to a complex biochemical cascade that serves to sensitize spinal neurons such that for any given input, there is a progressively enhanced output. This spinal output signals the nature of the peripheral stimulus, and accordingly the sensitization leads to an enhanced signal, indicating a greater pain state for any given stimulus *(1)*.

Given the distinct mechanistic components, animal models of nociception that parallel the events seen with tissue injury have been developed. Such models are in contrast of those in which the response of a normal animal to an acute, high-intensity stimulus is assessed (e.g., as in the hot plate or tail flick) in the absence of tissue and central sensitization. This section describes two models involving nociceptive sensitization after tissue injury: (1) the formalin test *(2)*, which produces robust spinal sensitization; and (2) a thermal injury (mild burn) model *(3)*, which produces a primary hyperalgesia and a secondary tactile allodynia. The formalin test has the advantage of being relatively simple with a high degree of reproducibility. Its underlying mechanisms suggest a central sensitization based on the appreciation that formalin results in an initial burst of activity followed by a low level of long ongoing afferent traffic *(4)*. This afferent patterning of activity leads to a central sensitization *(1,5)*.

The technical limitations of the formalin model are that animals can only be used once and that, if performed manually, it can be labor-intensive. In contrast, the thermal injury model appears to provide a model that possess behavioral components of both peripheral and central sensitization that reproduce the syndrome commonly seen in humans, e.g., sensitization with mild thermal injury *(6,7)*. In addition, this model can be used to follow the time-course of drug action with repeated testing in the same animal.

2. Materials

2.1. Formalin Test

1. Animals: 150–400 g rats. Strain and sex do not generally have a major impact of the formalin test; however, pilot studies and appropriate controls are suggested when comparing rats of different strains, sexes, or even vendors (*see* **Note 1**).
2. 5% Formalin: Dilute 10% neutral buffered formalin with and equal volume of 0.9% saline. This should be prepared fresh each day. Note that "10% formalin" actually contains 4% formaldehyde plus 1% methanol as a stabilizer, and thus 5% formalin solution actually contains 2% formaldehyde. The 10% formalin nomenclature is a remnant from the use of a 10% dilution of 37–40% formaldehyde stock solutions used in tissue preservation (*See* **Note 1**).
3. 1-cc syringe with 26-G needle for subcutaneous (sc) or intraperitoneal (ip) drug delivery.
4. 50- or 100-μL Hamilton glass syringe with a 0.5-in 30-G needle for formalin injections.
5. Stopwatch or timer.

6. Mirror.
7. Clear plexiglass container such as a shoebox cage with lid or a clear cylinder. If a cylinder is used it must be of an appropriate diameter to allow the animal to comfortably turn around and tall enough to prevent escape. We generally use cylinders with a radius of approx 10 cm and a height of approx 30 cm.
8. Hand-held counter for tallying flinches.
9. An automated system has been developed that allows simultaneous quantification of flinching of the injected paw in four animals *(8)*. This is accomplished by attaching a lightweight metal band to the hind paw of the rat prior to formalin injection, and using an electromagnetic loop antenna combined with customized analysis software. Methods for this system will be discussed only briefly.

2.2. Mild Burn Model

1. Animals: 275–350 g rats. Strain and sex should not have a major impact in this mild burn model; however, as suggested previously, pilot studies and appropriate controls should be performed when comparing rats of different strains, sexes, or even vendors.
2. Hot plate and thermister.
3. Sand pouch weighing 10 g.
4. Timer or stopwatch.
5. Volatile anesthetic such as halothane or isoflurane. Use of a calibrated anesthetic vaporizer is highly recommended. However if this equipment is unavailable rats may be anesthetized in a chamber containing using halothane or isoflurane. See **Table 1** *(9)* for suggested amounts of halothane and isoflurane for different size induction chambers. Once anesthetized, anesthesia can be maintained by using a gauze pad dampened with the anesthetic in a plastic 50-mL conical tube that is placed over the face of the rat. It this method is used, great care must be taken to assure a proper plane of anesthesia. The depth of anesthesia of the animal can be maintained by applying or removing the conical tube from the face of the rat as necessary.
6. Paw thermal stimulation testing apparatus (Hargreaves apparatus) (*see* Chapter 2).
7. Mechanical threshold testing apparatus including von Frey filaments (*see* Chapter 4).

3. Methods

3.1. Formalin Test

1. Rats should be acclimated to the testing chamber for 30 min. Placing a mirror behind the chamber aids in viewing flinches. If the automated system is used, a metal band should be glued to the ventral surface of the right hind paw as seen in **Fig. 1.**
2. A Hamilton type syringe with 5% formalin and a 30-G needle should be prepared. A new needle should be used for each injection.
3. For injection of formalin, the rats can be briefly immobilized by placing them in a commercially available restraint cone, or more simply by placing them in a hand towel and gently rolling them in the towel. This allows immobilization yet free access to the hind limbs.

Table 1
Recommended Volumes of Anesthetic for Induction of Anesthesia

Concentration of anesthetic	Internal volume of anesthetic chamber (mL)				
	1000	2000	3000	4000	5000
Halothane*					
1%	0.04	0.09	0.13	0.18	0.22
2%	0.09	0.18	0.26	0.35	0.44
3%	0.13	0.26	0.40	0.53	0.66
4%	0.18	0.35	0.53	0.71	0.88
5%	0.22	0.44	0.66	0.88	1.10
Isoflurane*					
1%	0.05	0.10	0.15	0.20	0.26
2%	0.10	0.20	0.31	0.41	0.51
3%	0.15	0.31	0.46	0.61	0.77
4%	0.20	0.41	0.61	0.82	1.02
5%	0.26	0.51	0.77	1.02	1.28

* Volume given in mL. Calculations at 20°C and 760 mmHg. (Adapted with permission from **ref. 9.**)

4. The right hind paw is held dorsal side up and 50 μL of formalin is injected subcutaneously in the area noted in **Fig. 1.** This is most easily accomplished by placing the syringe parallel to the surface of the paw and inserting the needle bevel side up at an angle of approx 20 degrees. A "bubble" of formalin should be visible immediately following injection. If this is not seen, then it is likely that the injection is in the structures of the paw, suggesting that the angle of insertion was too great. If large amounts of formalin immediately leak out from the injection site, it is likely that the injection is intradermal, suggesting that the angle of insertion of the needle was too small.

5. Rats are placed in the testing chamber and flinches are counted and tallied at 1-min intervals for a total of 60 min. If using the ANA system, up to four rats can be placed in the testing chambers for data acquisition. A typical response curve is shown in **Fig. 2** highlighting the two distinct phases (I and II) seen following formalin injection. *See* **Notes 2–8** for discussion of factors such as flinch determination, inter- and intraobserver considerations, and data analysis.

6. The animals are sacrificed immediately following the 60-min observations.

3.2. Focal Thermal Injury

1. Baseline paw withdrawal thresholds to mechanical stimuli are obtained using von Frey filaments either as described in this volume (*see* Chapter 4) or as described by Chaplan et al. (*10*). The testing areas for mechanical thresholds are noted in **Fig. 3.** A cut-off value of 15 g is normally used and only rats with thresholds greater than 10 g are considered "normal" and used in studies.

DORSUM **PLANTAR**

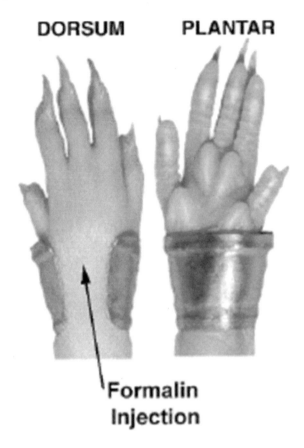

Formalin Injection

Fig. 1. Illustration of placement of formalin in the dorsal aspect of a rat paw. Localization of the metal band is also illustrated for use with the ANA system. (Adapted with permission from ref. **8.**)

2. Baseline paw withdrawal threshold to thermal stimuli is determined as noted in Chapter 2.
3. Following collection of baseline mechanical and thermal threshold data, the rat is briefly anesthetized and a well-defined focal thermal injury is produced on the plantar area of the hind paw. See **Fig. 3** for depiction of area of thermal injury and primary and secondary hyperalgesia. The injury is induced by placing the hind paw on a $52 \pm 1°C$ hot plate for 45 s. To assure constant pressure, and thus a consistent injury, a 10-g sand pouch is place on the dorsum of the paw. A more detailed discussion of the focal nature of the injury is found in **Note 9.**
4. Experimental drugs are usually given intrathecally 5 min prior to injury induction for pretreatments or 30 min after injury for posttreatment.

Allen and Yaksh

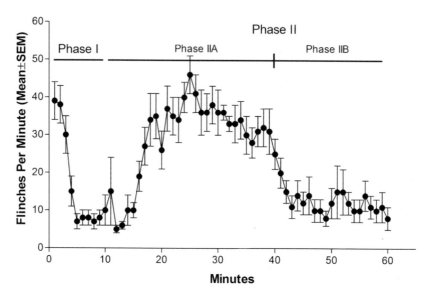

Fig. 2. Representative graph of typical flinching profiles as measured per minute with an automated detector.

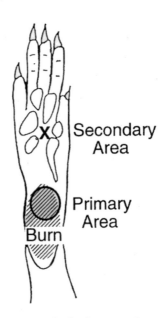

Fig. 3. Diagram of injury area and of primary and secondary hyperalgesia testing. The extent of injury is noted by the hatched area of a hind paw. Mechanical withdrawal thresholds (secondary hyperalgesia) are tested in the area noted by the X, whereas thermal thresholds (primary hyperalgesia) are tested in the area noted by the circle. (Adapted with permission from ref. *3.*)

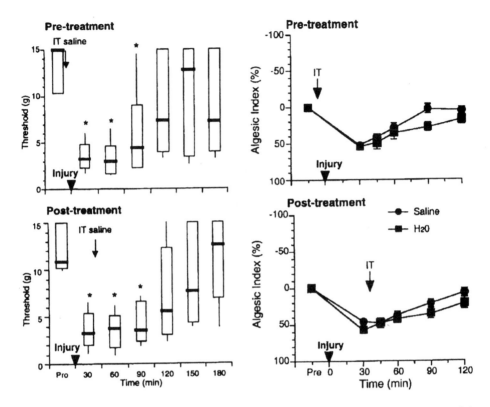

Fig. 4. Time course of mechanical (left) and thermal (right) hyperalgesia in the mild burn model. (Adapted with permission from ref. *3.*)

5. Thermal threshold testing of the primary area is conducted at 30, 45, 60, 90, and 120 min after the injury. Mechanical thresholds are assessed every 30 min for 3 h. Typical results are displayed in **Fig. 4.** For further consideration of data analysis, please see **Note 10.**

6. Rats may undergo the burn procedure up to three times. Within 3 d any injury should have been completely recovered and the animal may be re-tested using the contralateral hind paw. Re-testing on the ipsilateral paw should be done with at least 7 d between sessions.

4. Notes

1. Because of issues related to intergroup variation, each group of drug-treated animals requires concurrent animals receiving control vehicle. These represent the control animals.

2. Injection of formalin into the hind paw produces a characteristic biphasic response as noted in **Fig. 2.** In Phase I (0–9 min) a large amount of flinching

occurs immediately after injection, which is followed by a quiescent period. After the brief quiescent period, flinching resumes and persists for approximately an additional 50 min (Phase II).

3. Data analysis consists of summing the number of flinches measured during a given time interval. Typically, for individual animal analysis, the data are presented as Phase I and Phase II. Phase II can be further broken down into Phase IIA (11–39 min) and Phase IIB (40–60 min) as shown in **Fig. 2.** The respective data are then accumulated for each treatment group and expressed as a mean and standard error. Previous work has indicated that the data are normally distributed *(8)*. To normalize the flinching data across groups, data from the drug-treated group are divided by the mean of the respective Phase I and II values obtained from the corresponding vehicle control group. In this manner, where a dose–response curve has been created, the dose of drug required to produce a 50% reduction in the flinching behavior can be calculated.

4. In performing the formalin test with manual counting, the skill and consistency of the observer is essential for reproducible results. Defining the basic flinch is straightforward but subject to observer's judgment. What constitutes a "flinch" must be consistent from day-to-day. Once skilled, it is possible to observe multiple animals, theoretically up to four, by staggering dosing/viewing time by 1 min.

5. Although the present discussion employs flinch counts, other forms of quantifying the formalin response have been to employ weighted scoring procedures that consider the time spent in guarding, paw elevation, or grooming *(11–13)*. Although useful, the number of animals that can be concurrently followed is limited by such complex assessments. Specific efforts to perform multiple sampling have indicated the ability to follow a number of animals without loss of precision *(14)*. In any case, such detailed behavioral analysis requires an extensive training effort for each observer to ensure interobserver reliability.

6. The present study describes the use of 50 μL/5% formalin. Lower concentrations can be employed to produce a less robust flinching behavior that may prove more sensitive to different drug classes *(15,16)*.

7. The models as described are employed in the rat. However, automated procedures (S. Malkmus and T.L. Yaksh, unpublished results) and behavioral assessments may be employed in the mouse *(17)*.

8. When instituting the formalin model, as with any complex behavioral task, detailed attention to training is important. Considerable attention must be paid to consistency over time. Validation of the model by completing dose–response curves with a variety of standard compounds, including representative opiates and NMDA antagonists, is necessary *(8)*.

9. This model produces an area of primary thermal hyperalgesia and secondary tactile hyperalgesia generally lasting for 90 min *(3,18*; **Fig. 4)**. A vital aspect of this model is the degree and reproducibility of the thermal injury. A thermister should always be used to assure proper temperature of the hot plate. Following the thermal injury, there should be an erythema localized to the heel and not the distal area of the paw or toes. Animals should be checked daily following the injury to assure that no

ongoing injury is present. If blistering should occur, the injury is too severe and the animal should be excluded. In our experience, this occurs in less than 1% of animals tested. It should be noted that up to 5–10% of normal animals may display baseline mechanical thresholds less than 10 g and thus need to be excluded from these studies.

10. Examination of the distribution of the response data for the thermal injury models has indicated that the data are not normally distributed. Accordingly, data may be most clearly presented by showing the median and quartile data for the raw escape latencies. Nonparametric statistics is most useful in these analyses *(18)*. Alternately, data obtained from the thermal injury model can be presented by computing the analgesic index (AI) using the following formula.

$$AI = [(\text{baseline value} - \text{postinjury value})/\text{baseline value}] \times 100$$

Although more labor-intensive than acute nociception models, we believe these tissue-injury models are vital for proper screening of potential analgesic compounds in that they more closely parallel the final human condition for which the drugs are destined.

References

1. Yaksh, T. L., Hua, X. Y., Kalcheva, I., et al. (1999) The spinal biology in humans and animals of pain states generated by persistent small afferent input. *Proc. Natl. Acad. Sci. USA* **96,** 7680–7686.
2. Dubuisson, D. and Dennis, S. G. (1977) The formalin test: a quantitative study of the analgesic effects of morphine, meperidine, and brain stem stimulation in rats and cats. *Pain* **4,** 161–174.
3. Nozaki-Taguchi, N. and Yaksh, T. L. (2002) Pharmacology of spinal glutamatergic receptors in post-thermal injury-evoked tactile allodynia and thermal hyperalgesia. *Anesthesiology* **96,** 617–626.
4. Puig, S. and Sorkin, L. S. (1996) Formalin-evoked activity in identified primary afferent fibers: systemic lidocaine suppresses phase-2 activity. *Pain* **64,** 345–355.
5. Porro, C. A. and Cavazzuti, M. (1993) Spatial and temporal aspects of spinal cord and brainstem activation in the formalin pain model. *Prog. Neurobiol.* **41,** 565–607.
6. Reeh, P. W. and Petho, G. (2000) Nociceptor excitation by thermal sensitization— a hypothesis. *Prog. Brain Res.* **129,** 39–50.
7. Dirks. J., Petersen, K. L., Rowbotham, M. C., and Dahl, J. B. (2002) Gabapentin suppresses cutaneous hyperalgesia following heat-capsaicin sensitization. *Anesthesiology* **97,** 102–107.
8. Yaksh, T. L., Ozaki, G., McCumber, D., et al. (2001) An automated flinch detecting system for use in the formalin nociceptive bioassay. *J. Appl. Physiol.* **90,** 2386–2403.
9. Brunson, D. B. (1997) Pharmacology of inhalation anesthetics, in *Anesthesia and Analgesia in Laboratory Animals* (Benson, G. J., Kohn, D. F., White, W. J., and Wixson, S. K., eds.), Academic Press, San Diego, CA, p. 32.
10. Chaplan, S. R., Bach, F. W., Pogrel, J. W., et al. (1994) Quantitative assessment of tactile allodynia in the rat paw. *J. Neurosci. Methods* **53,** 55–63.

11. Wheeler-Aceto, H. and Cowan, A. (1991) Standardization of the rat paw formalin test for the evaluation of analgesics. *Psychopharmacology (Berl.)* **104,** 35–44.
12. Coderre T. J., Fundytus, M. E., McKenna, J. E., et al. (1993) The formalin test: a validation of the weighted-scores method of behavioural pain rating. *Pain* **54,** 43–50.
13. Abbott, F. V., Franklin, K. B., and Westbrook, R. F. (1995) The formalin test: scoring properties of the first and second phases of the pain response in rats. *Pain* **60,** 91–102.
14. Abbott, F. V., Ocvirk, R., Najafee, R., and Franklin, K. B. (1999) Improving the efficiency of the formalin test. *Pain* **83,** 561–569.
15. Aloisi, A. M., Albonetti, M. E., and Carli, G. (1995) Behavioural effects of different intensities of formalin pain in rats. *Physiol. Behav.* **58,** 603–610.
16. Poon, A. and Sawynok J. (1995) Antinociception by adenosine analogs and an adenosine kinase inhibitor: dependence on formalin concentration. *Eur. J. Pharmacol.* **286,** 177–1784.
17. Saddi, G. and Abbott, F. V. (2000) The formalin test in the mouse: a parametric analysis of scoring properties. *Pain* **89,** 53–63.
18. Nozaki-Taguchi, N. and Yaksh, T. L. (1998) A novel model of primary and secondary hyperalgesia after mild thermal injury in the rat. *Neurosci. Lett.* **254,** 25–28.

4

Segmental Spinal Nerve Ligation Model of Neuropathic Pain

Jin Mo Chung, Hee Kee Kim, and Kyungsoon Chung

Summary

Since its introduction in 1992, the spinal nerve ligation (SNL) model of neuropathic pain has been widely used for various investigative works on neuropathic pain mechanisms as well as in screening tests for the development of new analgesic drugs. This model was developed by tightly ligating one (L5) or two (L5 and L6) segmental spinal nerves in the rat. The operation results in long-lasting behavioral signs of mechanical allodynia, heat hyperalgesia, cold allodynia, and ongoing pain. In the process of widespread usage, however, many different variations of the SNL model have been produced, either intentionally or unintentionally, by different investigators. Although the factors that cause these variations themselves are interesting and important topics to be studied, the pain mechanisms involved in these variations are likely different from the original model. Therefore, this chapter describes, in detail, the method for producing the spinal nerve ligation model that will minimally induce potential factors that may contribute to these variations. It is hoped that this description will help many investigators to produce a consistent animal model with uniform pathophysiological mechanisms.

Key Words: Animal model; mechanical allodynia; pain model; peripheral nerve injury; peripheral neuropathy.

1. Introduction

We first described the method of segmental spinal nerve ligation (SNL) in the rat for use as an animal model of neuropathic pain in 1992 *(1)*. Since then, this model has been used widely for various investigative studies on pain mechanisms and as a testing tool for the discovery of analgesic drugs. Although this method has been widely used, there are other scientists who may want to learn the technique as well as some current users who do not know the proper technique in some aspects of the method. Therefore, we decided to describe, in detail, the method of SNL. We are emphasizing several points that we believe are a common source of induced variability of data.

From: *Methods in Molecular Medicine, Vol. 99: Pain Research: Methods and Protocols*
Edited by: Z. D. Luo © Humana Press Inc., Totowa, NJ

2. Materials

1. Animals. We normally purchase young (*see* **Note 1**) adult male (*see* **Note 2**) Sprague-Dawley (*see* **Note 3**) rats weighing 150–175 g from a single vendor (see **Note 3** for further description). The animals are housed in groups of three to four in plastic cages with soft bedding (*see* **Note 4**) at the University Animal Care facility with a 12/12 h reversed light–dark cycle (light from 8 PM to 8 AM and dark from 8 AM to 8 PM) (*see* **Note 5**). Animals are given free access to food (*see* **Note 6**) and water. The rats are normally kept for about 1 wk under these conditions before surgery.
2. Anesthesia. Rats are anesthetized with either inhalation gas (halothane) or intraperitoneal (ip) injection of sodium pentobarbital (*see* **Note 7**).
3. Surgical tools. Routine surgical tools for rodents are used. These include a scalpel, a small pair of scissors with blunt tips, several pairs of forceps, a small tissue retractor, a small bone scraper, a hook or curved forceps, and a small rongeur (*see* **Note 8**). A dissecting microscope with a long focal distance (15 cm) is used.

3. Methods

3.1. Surgical Preparation

Animals are anesthetized as described earlier and the hair on their backs is clipped. Each animal is then placed on a surgical platform in a prone position, and the limbs are fixed with masking tape. Under sterile conditions, a longitudinal incision (about 3 cm in length and 5 mm lateral from the midline) is made at the lower lumbar and sacral levels (from the caudal part of the L5 vertebra to the first sacral vertebra), exposing the paraspinal muscles on the left. The location of the incision is determined by the position of the L5 spinous process, which is located at the level (rostro-caudally) of the rostral end of the iliac crest. We found that operating on the left side was more convenient than the right side for most right-handed persons. Using small scissors with blunt tips, the paraspinal muscles are isolated and removed, from the level of the L5 spinous process to the sacrum. This opens up the space ventrolateral to the articular processes, dorsal to the L6 transverse process, and medial to the ileum. Connective tissues and remaining muscles are removed by a small scraper, after which one should be able to see bony structures, as in **Fig. 1**.

Under a dissecting microscope, a small rongeur (*see* **Note 8**) is used to remove the L6 transverse process, which is covering the ventral rami of the L4 and L5 spinal nerves. Access to the L5 spinal nerve is easier after removing the transverse process very close to the body of the vertebrae. One should be very careful when removing the transverse process because the L4 and L5 spinal nerves run just underneath the process. One can normally visualize the ventral rami (*see* **Note 9**) of the L4 and L5 spinal nerves (a thin sheet of connective tissue may cover them in some animals) once the L6 transverse process is carefully removed. The L4

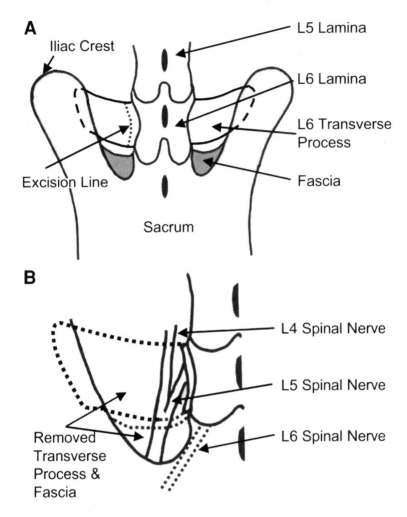

Fig. 1. Schematic diagram showing the dorsal view of the bony structures at the lower lumbar and sacral levels. (**A**) A lower magnification of bony structures after removal of paraspinal muscles. (**B**) A higher magnification of the left side after removal of the L6 transverse process and fascia.

spinal nerve usually runs more laterally (or ventrally in some animals) than the L5 and these two nerves join distally (**Fig. 1**), but there is a great deal of individual variability where these two nerves join. Thus, the L4 and L5 spinal nerves need to be separated in some animals to make the L5 spinal nerve accessible for ligation. It is of great importance not to damage the L4 nerve during this process because we find that even slight damage to the L4 spinal nerve invariably results in a much-reduced mechanical sensitivity of the foot (*see* **Subheading 3.2.**). Damage to the L4 spinal nerve can occur with a seemingly mild mechanical trauma (excessive touch, gentle stretch, or slight entrapment within the epineurial sheet). If an extensive manipulation of the L4 spinal nerve is required to separate it from the L5 spinal nerve, it may be safer to discard the animal rather than taking a chance of damaging the L4 nerve. Once enough length of the L5 spinal nerve is freed from the adjacent structure, a piece of 6-0 silk thread is placed around the L5 spinal nerve and the nerve is tightly ligated to interrupt all axons in the nerve (*see* **Note 10**). Another option would be to cut the spinal nerve just distal to the ligation to make sure all fibers are interrupted.

If it is desired, the L6 spinal nerve can also be ligated (*see* **Note 11**). The L6 spinal nerve runs underneath the sacrum and is not visible without chipping away a part of the sacrum (**Fig. 1**). Because chipped sacrum bleed a lot, our usual method is to approach L6 blindly without chipping the sacrum. This approach necessitates the investigator being familiar with the position of the L6 spinal nerve prior to the operation. To ligate the L6 spinal nerve, it is also necessary to remove a sheet of the fascia joining sacrum to ileum. After carefully removing the fascia, we place a small glass hook underneath the sacrum and gently pull the L6 spinal nerve out into the paravertebral space and ligate it tightly with 6-0 silk thread.

On completion of the operation, which normally takes about 10 min (after some experience), hemostasis is confirmed and the muscles are sutured in layers using silk thread and the skin is closed with metal clips, anesthesia is then discontinued. Normally, antibiotics are not necessary if sterile conditions are maintained. However, antibiotics may be applied systemically or locally right after the surgery. Animals are then placed in a new cage with warm bedding until they completely recover from anesthesia.

3.2. Behavioral Outcome of Surgery

Successful surgery should result in several behavioral outcomes indicative of neuropathic pain. Because the procedures of behavioral testing for neuropathic pain in the rat are common in all models presented in multiple chapters in this book, we will simply point out several expected behavioral outcomes, especially those aspects that are specific to the SNL model. Detailed methods of behavioral testing procedures can also be found in earlier publications (*1–3*).

3.2.1. Motor Deficit

Successfully operated animals normally do not show any motor deficits beyond a mild inversion of the foot with slightly ventroflexed toes. The most common and obvious motor deficit of unsuccessfully operated animals is dragging the hindlimb of the operated side, a sign of paralyzed proximal muscles.

This invariably indicates damage to the L4 spinal nerve because this nerve innervates many proximal muscles of the hindlimb. Because most behavioral tests for neuropathic pain are based on foot withdrawal responses to external stimuli, rats with a damaged L4 nerve may not show neuropathic pain behaviors due, in part, to their inability to withdraw the foot because of paralyzed proximal muscles. Although these animals may show some improvement of motor function over several days, neuropathic pain behaviors may not necessarily be restored, presumably due to permanent damage to some sensory fibers in the L4 nerve.

3.2.2. Mechanical Allodynia

A successfully operated rat shows various behavioral signs of neuropathic pain such as ongoing pain, heat hyperalgesia, and mechanical as well as cold allodynia. Because the SNL model shows a particularly robust sign of mechanical allodynia, one can use the degree of hypersensitivity of the foot to gauge the success of the operation. Mechanical sensitivity is quantified either by measuring response frequency to mechanical stimuli applied with von Frey filaments *(1,4)* or by determining the mechanical threshold *(3,5)*. Another way of testing mechanical allodynia is to measure the frequency of foot withdrawals to stimulation with cotton-tip applicators (Q-tips), which is a technique commonly used in clinics to test touch sensation. **Figure 2** shows these three allodynia indices in a group of spinal nerve ligated rats along with a sham-operated group (*see* **Note 12**). A successful surgical operation will result in a clear sign of mechanical allodynia demonstrated by: (1) lowering the foot withdrawal threshold below the normal nociceptor activation threshold (below 1. 4 g [**6**]), (2) frequent foot withdrawals to mechanical stimulation at a strength below the normal nociceptor activation threshold, or (3) frequent foot withdrawals by obviously innocuous stimulations. On the other hand, sham-operation should not produce any significant changes in mechanical threshold. A significant lowering of the threshold following sham-operation invariably indicates that the surgery induced damage and/or inflammation to the nerve and is thus an unsuccessful operation because it introduced unknown factors.

Another important factor that influences the sign of mechanical allodynia is the exact spot on the paw where the mechanical stimulation is applied. To stimulate a clinical situation where the most intensely painful area is attended, it is logical to measure the threshold at the most sensitive area in the rat. The most sensitive area of the paw after ligation of the L5 or both the L5 and L6 spinal nerves is the base of the third or fourth toe *(7)*. The most sensitive spot of the paw after SNL is confined to a small area and does not vary much between rats, presumably due to stereotyped denervation of the foot by the surgical procedure. **Figure 3** shows the average values of mechanical thresholds

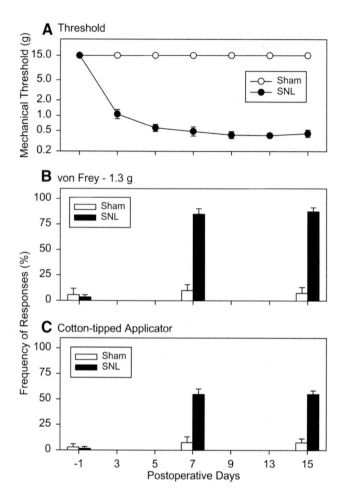

at three different locations on the paw, measured when the sign of mechanical allodynia was fully developed after L5 ligation (at postoperative wk 1). When measuring from the most sensitive area, the threshold is usually well below the 1 g range, whereas the threshold ranges from 2 to 3 g if one measures it by stimulating the mid-plantar area.

4. Notes

1. We usually use young adult rats (6–7 wk old) for two reasons. First, we find it is easier to operate on young rats (softer bones, etc.). Second, young rats show more robust neuropathic pain behaviors *(8)*, although why young rats show more robust behaviors is unclear. It is possible that the pain generator mechanisms are stronger in

Fig. 2. An example of the outcome of a successful operation showing signs of mechanical allodynia. The left L5 spinal nerve was ligated in a group of 8 Wistar Furth rats and sham surgery was conducted in another 8 rats. (**A**) Changes in the mechanical threshold of the paw for 50% foot withdrawals determined by the up–down method of Dixon (*16*). The thresholds are expressed in a logarithmic scale because the Dixon method (tested von Frey filaments section, the calculation formula, etc.) is established under the assumption of logarithmic sensory perception. The thresholds decrease to well below the 1 g level within a few days after the operation and this level is maintained for a long time. The thresholds of sham-operated rats are maintained at a 15 g level, which is the cut-off point of the threshold determination method. (**B**) Changes in frequency of foot withdrawals to stimulation of the paw with a von Frey filament (1.3 g bending force). The von Frey filament was applied five times and the number of foot withdrawals was counted. Rats with spinal nerve ligation responded to almost every von Frey filament application, whereas sham-operated rats rarely responded. (**C**) Changes in frequency of foot withdrawals to stimulation of the paw with a cotton-tipped applicator. The applicator was touched to the paw and twisted 90° to ensure good contact with the skin. The cotton-tipped applicator was applied five times and the number of foot withdrawals was counted. Rats with spinal nerve ligation responded about half the time to the stimulations, whereas sham-operated rats rarely responded.

young rats and/or young rats may simply have more lively behavioral expressions. Whatever the reason, young rats are both more convenient and more practical.

2. We normally use male rats because behaviors of female rats may be influenced, in part, by estrous cycles. Although that in itself is an interesting topic, it adds an extra experimental variable and we wish to eliminate as many variables as possible in our experimental conditions.

3. The strain of rats is an important variable. Different strains of rats show not only different levels of neuropathic pain behaviors (*9*), but also different degrees of adrenergic dependency of these behaviors (*10*). In addition, different levels of pain behaviors can also be seen in different substrains of Sprague-Dawley rats obtained from different suppliers (*9*). For this reason, we normally purchase rats from a single source. Even so, we still experience a batch difference of animal behaviors occasionally. This batch difference is presumably due to the fact that Sprague-Dawley is an out-bred strain and different batches may have different genetic factors.

4. We keep our rats on soft bedding, such as Tek-Fresh paper bedding. Because the rats are allodynic, we worry that hard bedding, such as corncobs or sanichips, may stress the animals due to excessive stimulation of the mechanically sensitive foot.

5. We keep our rats in reverse light–dark cycles. This is because we want to test rats during their active period, which is during the dark cycle. In addition, we are testing animals in a room illuminated by red-colored darkroom lighting.

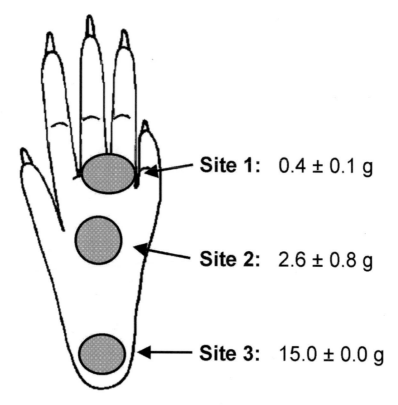

Site 1: 0.4 ± 0.1 g

Site 2: 2.6 ± 0.8 g

Site 3: 15.0 ± 0.0 g

Fig. 3. Mechanical sensitivity of three different sites of the paw after L5 spinal nerve ligation. The L5 spinal nerve was ligated in nine rats. After behavioral signs for mechanical allodynia was fully developed (1 wk after the operation), the mechanical thresholds of the paw for 50% foot withdrawals were determined at three different sites. The lowest threshold is obtained by stimulating the base of the third and fourth toes (site 1). The middle of the paw (site 2) had much higher threshold and the heel of the paw (site 3) was not responsive at all. Because the base of the third and fourth toes is the most sensitive site, this is the area that should be stimulated for threshold testing after spinal nerve ligation.

6. Another unexpected but potentially important factor influencing neuropathic pain behaviors is diet. Shir et al. *(11)* found that rats fed with a high soybean diet produced much diminished levels of neuropathic pain behaviors. Therefore, one should avoid feeding the rat a high soybean diet if one wants to produce a robust experimental neuropathic pain model.
7. We normally anesthetize rats using a mixture of halothane (2% for induction and 1% for maintenance) and a 2:1 flow ratio of N_2O and O_2. We sometimes use halothane (3% for induction and 1.5–2% for maintenance) in air or oxygen gas.

The advantages of gas anesthesia include: (1) the level of anesthesia can be adjusted quickly and easily, and (2) animals recover quickly (within 5–10 min) after the operation. We have also successfully used sodium pentobarbital (Nembutal, 50 mg/kg) anesthesia in the past. However, one should avoid using ketamine. Pretreatment of animals with ketamine is known to impede the development of neuropathic pain behaviors *(12–14)*, presumably by interfering with central sensitization because ketamine is an *N*-methyl-D-aspartic acid receptor blocker.

8. Although all surgical tools are important, the use of the right size rongeur is particularly important for successful operation. The L4 and L5 spinal nerves merge together distally shortly after they exit from the vertebrate and the L6 transverse process covers dorsally the entire portion of the L5 spinal nerve before it joins with the L4. To expose the L5 spinal nerve enough length to ligate, it is necessary to either separate the L5 spinal nerve from the merged L4/L5 bundle at the distal part or to remove the L6 transverse process as close to the vertebrate as possible and expose the most proximal part of the L5 nerve that has not joined the L4. Because the former approach usually damages the L4 spinal nerve, the latter approach is desirable. A rongeur with a curved and pointed tip works best to remove the L6 transverse process cleanly because the working space is small and deep. We tried several different kinds and decided to use a rongeur from Fine Science Tools (part no. 16021-14). A rongeur from other companies with a similar configuration should work as well. Nevertheless, this is the most important step in the operation and failure at this stage commonly results in damage to the L4 spinal nerve. Consequences of L4 spinal nerve damage include: (1) dragging the foot because of damage to the motor nerve innervating the proximal muscles of the leg, (2) development of neuropathic pain behaviors in sham-operated rats, or (3) development of a less clear sign of mechanical allodynia with higher mechanical thresholds (e.g., much higher than 1 g).

9. The dorsal ramus of the L5 spinal nerve is located proximal to the ligation site. Although we usually do not ligate it, most of its innervation is invariably interrupted by removal of the paraspinal muscles.

10. How tightly should the nerve be ligated? The object of tight ligation is to axotomize all fibers within the nerve and prevent the injured axons from regenerating, which may contribute to a delay in recovery. Sometimes the nerve can be accidentally severed in the process of tight ligation, however, we have not noticed a significant difference in behaviors between cutting and ligating the spinal nerve, at least during the short postoperative periods (1–2 wk) *(15)*. In addition, the nerve can be sectioned distal to the ligation to ensure a complete axotomy.

11. The L6 spinal nerve contains a small number of afferent fibers innervating the hindlimb. Why then, do we ligate this nerve? Our empirical reason is that adding the L6 produces a somewhat larger behavioral response than ligating the L5 spinal nerve alone *(1)*. The reason for this is, presumably, that a larger number of injured afferents (regardless of their origin) produce more ectopic discharges, which in turn produces stronger central sensitization.

12. Sham surgery should be done completely. For example, every step in the sham surgery is done in the same way as the ligation surgery up to the point of the actual ligation of the nerve. As the final step, we place silk thread around the L5 nerve and then remove it without actually ligating the nerve.

Acknowledgments

This work was supported by NIH Grants NS 31860 and NS 11255.

References

1. Kim, S. H. and Chung, J. M. (1992) An experimental model for peripheral neuropathy produced by segmental spinal nerve ligation in the rat. *Pain* **50,** 355–363.
2. Choi, Y., Yoon, Y. W., Na, H. S., et al. (1994) Behavioral signs of ongoing pain and cold allodynia in a rat model of neuropathic pain. *Pain* **59,** 369–376.
3. Chaplan, S. R., Bach, F. W., Pogrel, J. W., et al. (1994) Quantitative assessment of tactile allodynia in the rat paw. *J. Neurosci. Methods* **53,** 55–63.
4. Kim, S. H. and Chung, J. M. (1991) Sympathectomy alleviates mechanical allodynia in an experimental animal model for neuropathy in the rat. *Neurosci. Lett.* **134,** 131–134.
5. Park, S. K., Chung, K., and Chung, J. M. (2000) Effects of purinergic and adrenergic antagonists in a rat model of painful peripheral neuropathy. *Pain* **87,** 171–179.
6. Leem, J. W., Willis, W. D., and Chung, J. M. (1993) Cutaneous sensory receptors in the rat foot. *J. Neurophysiol.* **69,** 1684–1699.
7. Xie, J., Yoon, Y. W., Yom, S. S., and Chung, J. M. (1995) Norepinephrine rekindles mechanical allodynia in sympathectomized neuropathic rat. *Analgesia* **1,** 107–113.
8. Chung, J. M., Choi, Y., Yoon, Y. W., and Na, H. S. (1995) Effects of age on behavioral signs of neuropathic pain in an experimental rat model. *Neurosci. Lett.* **183,** 54–57.
9. Yoon, Y. W., Lee, D. H., Lee, B. H., et al. (1999) Different strains and substrains of rats show different levels of neuropathic pain behaviors. *Exp. Brain Res.* **129,** 167–171.
10. Lee, D. H., Chung, K., and Chung, J. M. (1997) Strain differences in adrenergic sensitivity of neuropathic pain behaviors in an experimental rat model. *NeuroReport* **8,** 3453–3456.
11. Shir, Y., Ratner, A., Raja, S. N., Campbell, J. N., and Seltzer, Z. (1998) Neuropathic pain following partial nerve injury in rats is suppressed by dietary soy. *Neurosci. Lett.* **240,** 73–76.
12. Burton, A. W., Lee, D. H., Saab, C., and Chung, J. M. (1999) Preemptive intrathecal ketamine injection produces a long-lasting decrease in neuropathic pain behaviors in a rat model. *Reg Anesth. Pain Med.* **24,** 208–213.
13. Mao, J., Price, D. D., Mayer, D. J., et al. (1992) Intrathecal MK-801 and local nerve anesthesia synergistically reduce nociceptive behaviors in rats with experimental peripheral mononeuropathy. *Brain Res.* **576,** 254–262.

14. Mao, J., Price, D. D., Hayes, R. L., et al. (1993) Intrathecal treatment with dextror-phan or ketamine potently reduces pain-related behaviors in a rat model of periph-eral mononeuropathy. *Brain Res.* **605,** 164–168.
15. Sheen, K. and Chung, J. M. (1993) Signs of neuropathic pain depend on signals from injured nerve fibers in a rat model. *Brain Res.* **610,** 62–68.
16. Dixon, W. J. (1980) Efficient analysis of experimental observations. *Ann. Rev. Phar. Tox.* **20,** 441–462.

5

Partial Sciatic Nerve Transection

Thies Lindenlaub and Claudia Sommer

Summary

Partial sciatic nerve transection (PST) of the sciatic nerve of rats and mice is described as a model of painful neuropathy. The rationale for developing this model was to establish a simple partial nerve injury without application of foreign material. In contrast to the frequently used model of chronic constriction injury (CCI), PST allows to relate animal behavior and drug effects to endoneurial changes, undisturbed by major epineurial inflammation. PST is easy to perform in rats and mice and leads to reproducible pain-related behavior for 5 wk or longer.

Key Words: Partial sciatic nerve transection (PST); chronic constriction injury (CCI); neuropathy; hyperalgesia; pain-related behavior.

1. Introduction

Animal models of partial nerve injury have been proven to be of great value for the analysis of mechanisms of neuropathic pain and for the assessment of new drugs. In particular, the model of chronic constriction injury (CCI) of the sciatic nerve, described by Bennett and Xie in 1988 *(1)* in the rat, has been used in many experimental paradigms because it is reliable and easy to reproduce. We have used CCI in the rat in a number of experiments, specifically to study cytokine expression in the injured nerve and the potential of cytokine antagonists in the treatment of neuropathic pain *(2,3)*. We furthermore adapted the CCI model to the mouse, in order to be able to compare different genetic strains and knockout mice *(4,5)*.

One point of criticism when using CCI for studies of cytokines or other inflammatory mediators has been the presence of "foreign" material, the ligatures, around the nerve. These ligatures lead to extensive epineurial cellular infiltration, mostly by macrophages, i.e., an epineurial inflammatory reaction. Thus CCI is a combined model of nerve injury and epineurial inflammation. The

From: *Methods in Molecular Medicine, Vol. 99: Pain Research: Methods and Protocols*
Edited by: Z. D. Luo © Humana Press Inc., Totowa, NJ

epineurial situation may have an impact on nervi nervorum *(6)*, because pressure and local inflammation can induce nervi nervorum to signal pain. Although the same may well be true in most clinical cases of nerve injury, this dual patho-genetic mechanism makes it difficult to dissect effects of potential anti-hyperal-gesic drugs in animal experiments. In the case with our cytokine studies, the effect of a cytokine inhibitor in reducing pain-related behavior might have been via reduction of endoneurial cytokines, expressed in the course of Wallerian degeneration, or via reduction of epineurial cytokines, expressed by the inflam-matory cells attracted by the ligatures. Some authors even contend that epineur-ial inflammation is the main factor causing hyperalgesia in CCI *(7,8)*. The problem of a foreign body reaction around a ligature is also present in the model that was published by Seltzer et al. 1990 *(9)*. In this "partial sciatic nerve liga-tion" (PSNL) model, half of the diameter of the nerve is ligated with a suture, which remains *in situ* for the duration of the experiment.

We thus developed a modified PSNL model, where part of the sciatic nerve is transected proximal to the trifurcation, without a remaining foreign body. This model allowed us to relate animal behavior and drug effects to the endoneurial changes, undisturbed by major epineurial inflammation. We named this model "partial sciatic nerve transection" (PST). Indeed, a PST was first described by Ma and Bisby *(10,11)*, who studied the consequences of par-tial nerve lesion for neuropeptide expression in dorsal-root ganglion neurons and the gracile nucleus. However, the authors did not monitor their animals for the development of neuropathic pain. In a first step, we established the time-course of pain-related behavior in rats with PST *(12)*, later, we also adapted the model to mice *(13)*.

2. Materials

2.1. Animals

1. Female Sprague-Dawley rats (Charles River, Germany).
2. Female C57 BL/6 mice (Harlan Winkelmann, Germany).

2.2. Equipment and Materials

1. A surgical microscope (Leica, Germany) working at a magnification up to 10× equipped with a lightening system (WILD, Switzerland).
2. A no. 11 scalpel blade.
3. Fine watchmaker forceps.
4. A wound expander.
5. Fine iris scissors.
6. Prolene 7/0 ligature.
7. 4-0 silk suture.
8. Wound clamps.
9. Pentobarbital (Narcoren®).

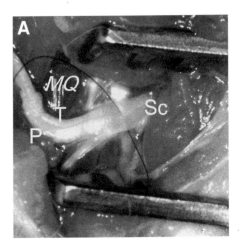 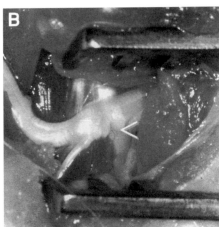

Fig. 1. Sciatic nerve in the rat before (**A**) and after (**B**) partial sciatic nerve transection. The gap between the two stumps is indicated by an arrow. P, peroneal; T, tibial fascicle; SC, sciatic nerve; MQ, quadratus femoris muscle; B, branch to the biceps femoris muscle.

3. Method

1. Anesthetize the animals with Pentobarbital (Narcoren) ip at a dose of 40 mg/kg body weight (0.25 mL) for rats and mice.
2. Dissect the skin and muscle using a no. 11 scalpel blade.
3. Expose the sciatic nerve at midthigh level with the aid of wound expander.
4. Mobilize the nerve gently using fine watchmaker forceps, then lift it and place a prolene 7/0 ligature through the midpoint of the nerve just cranial to the branch running to the musculus biceps femoris (*see* **Fig. 1A; Note 1**). This procedure is to prevent the transection of more than half of the diameter of the nerve (*see* **Note 2**).
5. When the prolene 7/0 ligature is in place, the inferior part of the nerve (which represents mostly the peroneal nerve) is transected until the ligature is free (*see* **Note 1**).
6. Then the ligature is removed such that no foreign material is left at the site. During the transection, a brief twitch of the hindlimb will be observed as described for CCI *(1)* (*see* **Note 3**). A gap of variable size may occur after partial transection of the sciatic nerve (**Fig. 1B**); (*see* **Note 2**).
7. The wound is closed in layers using silk sutures for the muscle and clamps for the skin.

4. Notes

1. The PST lesion site is chosen more proximal than that in CCI (10 mm in rats, 5 mm in mice). In our pilot experiments we used the same anatomical position as in CCI distal to the branch to the biceps femoris muscle. This leads to a complete lesion of the peroneal nerve in some animals, especially in animals with a high/proximal

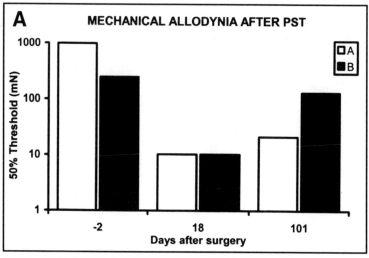

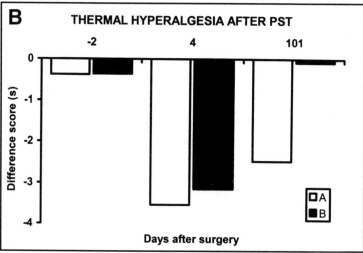

Fig. 2. Fifty percent withdrawal latencies in mN (**A**) and "difference score" in seconds (**B**) for thermal withdrawal latencies in two different female Sprague-Dawley rats with partial sciatic transection. Both animals developed thermal hyperalgesia with a maximum on d 4 after PST and mechanical allodynia with maximum on d 18 after PST. On d 101 after PST, animal B recovered, whereas thermal hyperalgesia and mechanical allodynia were still present in animal A. The same technique of PST was applied in both animals.

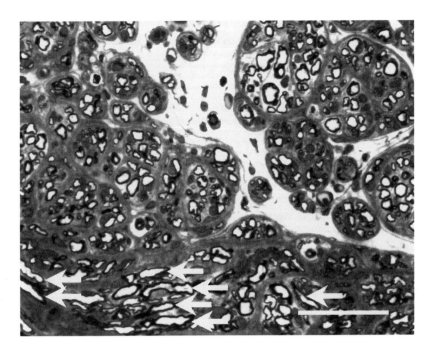

Fig. 3. Formation of a neuroma-in-continuity with aberrant fibers and epineurial minifascicles in a rat with signs of neuropathic pain on d 103 after PST. The aberrant fibers are indicated by arrows. Bar = 15 μm.

division of the sciatic nerve. This has the disadvantage that the animals cannot elevate their paw, which makes the observation of behavioral reactions to thermal and mechanical stimuli very difficult. Furthermore, some of these animals do not develop neuropathic pain. With the partial sciatic transection at the position described earlier, the peroneal portion of the sciatic nerve is mostly cut but not alone. Thus a proximal lesion is very important for the "success" of the model.

2. At 6 wk after PST, we observed that thermal hyperalgesia and mechanical allodynia still persisted in some, but not all, animals. As shown in **Fig. 2,** even 101 d after PST, animal A still had thermal hyperalgesia, whereas animal B had no signs of neuropathic pain. Persistence of neuropathic pain for this long duration is associated with the formation of a neuroma-in-continuity with aberrant fibers and epineurial minifascicles **(Fig. 3)**. Neuroma formation is likely to occur when the resulting gap after PST **(Fig. 1B)** is too big to allow sprouting of the proximal fibers into the distal part of the nerve. It is known from nerve transection studies that the size of the gap between nerve stumps determines the success of nerve regeneration *(14)*. A larger gap is thus likely to lead to neuroma formation in PST. This gap varies in size from animal to animal. The variability may be the result of slight differences in the size of the lesion, of variable elasticity of the epi- and perineurium,

and of a different amount of endoneurial prolaps owing to positioning of the nerve. We do not think that it is possible to overcome the problem of variable gap sizes entirely because we took great care to standardize the lesion (uniform handling, positioning of the animal, careful anatomical dissection) as much as possible. Because almost all animals with PST develop signs of neuropathic pain, "good regenerators" and "bad regenerators" will not be problematic for short-term experiments. This difference may even be considered an advantage in long-term experiments because animals with longstanding pain may be used to identify candidate molecules for the maintenance of neuropathic pain.

3. The model of PST is reliable because it causes signs of thermal hyperalgesia and mechanical allodynia in nearly all the animals (90–95%) comparable to CCI. We performed direct comparisons between PST and CCI in our laboratory. Animals with either CCI or PST were tested in the same session by an investigator blinded to the type of nerve lesion. In both rats and mice, no significant differences in the extent of thermal hyperalgesia and mechanical allodynia were found.

References

1. Bennett, G. J. and Xie, Y. K. (1988) A peripheral mononeuropathy in rat that produces disorders of pain sensation like those seen in man. *Pain* **33**, 87–107.
2. George, A., Schmidt, C., Weishaupt, A., et al. (1999) Serial determination of tumor necrosis factor-alpha content in rat sciatic nerve after chronic constriction injury. *Exp. Neurol.* **160**, 124–132.
3. Sommer, C., Marziniak, M., and Myers, R. R. (1998) The effect of thalidomide treatment on vascular pathology and hyperalgesia caused by chronic constriction injury of rat nerve. *Pain* **74**, 83–91.
4. Sommer, C. and Schäfers, M. (1998) Painful mononeuropathy in C57BL/Wld mice with delayed wallerian degeneration: differential effects of cytokine production and nerve regeneration on thermal and mechanical hypersensitivity. *Brain Res.* **784**, 154–162.
5. Vogel, C., Lindenlaub, T., Tiegs, G., et al. (2000) Pain related behavior in TNF-receptor deficient mice, in *Proceedings of the 9th World Congress on Pain, Progress in Pain Research and Management* (Devor, M., Rowbotham, M. C., and Wiesenfeld-Hallin, Z., eds.), IASP Press, Seattle, WA, pp. 249–257.
6. Bove, G. M. and Light, A. R. (1997) The nervi nervorum. Missing link for neuropathic pain? *Pain Forum* **6**, 181–190.
7. Clatworthy, A. L., Illich, P. A., Castro, G. A., and Walters, E. T. (1995) Role of periaxonal inflammation in the development of thermal hyperalgesia and guarding behavior in a rat model of neuropathic pain. *Neurosci. Lett. 184*, 5–8.
8. Maves, T. J., Pechman, P. S., Gebhart, G. F., and Meller, S. T. (1993) Possible chemical contribution from chromic gut sutures produces disorders of pain sensation like those seen in man. *Pain* **54**, 57–69.
9. Seltzer, Z., Dubner, R., and Shir, Y. (1990) A novel behavioral model of neuropathic pain disorders produced in rats by partial sciatic nerve injury. *Pain* **43**, 205–218.

10. Ma, W. and Bisby, M. A. (1998) Increase of calcitonin gene-related peptide immunoreactivity in the axonal fibers of the gracile nuclei of adult and aged rats after complete and partial sciatic nerve injuries. *Exp. Neurol.* **152,** 137–149.
11. Ma, W. and Bisby, M. A. (1998) Increase of preprotachykinin mRNA and substance P immunoreactivity in spared dorsal root ganglion neurons following partial sciatic nerve injury. *Eur. J. Neurosci.* **10,** 2388–2399.
12. Lindenlaub, T. and Sommer, C. (2000) Partial sciatic nerve transection as a model of neuropathic pain: a qualitative and quantitative neuropathological study. *Pain* **89,** 97–106.
13. Sommer, C., Lindenlaub, T., Teuteberg, P., et al. (2001) Anti-TNF-neutralizing antibodies reduce pain-related behavior in two different mouse models of painful mononeuropathy. *Brain Res.* **913,** 86–89.
14. Buti, M., Verdu, E., Labrador, R. O., et al. (1996) Influence of physical parameters of nerve chambers on peripheral nerve regeneration and reinnervation. *Exp. Neurol.* **137,** 26–33.

6

Modeling Diabetic Sensory Neuropathy in Rats

Nigel A. Calcutt

Summary

The procedures to induce insulin-deficient diabetes in rats using streptozotocin are described along with a number of insulin treatment regimes that can be used to maintain these animals at different degrees of glycemia for periods of weeks to months. Streptozotocin-diabetic rats develop tactile allodynia, hyperalgesia following paw formalin injection and abnormal responses to thermal stimulation and the detailed methods used to evaluate these behavioral indices of abnormal sensory function are provided.

Key Words: Diabetes; streptozotocin; neuropathy; tactile allodynia; formalin test; thermal hyperalgesia; nociception; neuropathic pain; rat.

1. Introduction

There are an estimated 150 million people suffering from diabetes mellitus in the world (1), of these approx 50% will develop some indication of peripheral nerve disorder during the course of their disease (2). Diabetic peripheral neuropathy is the most frequently encountered neuropathy in the developed world and has wide-ranging effects on the quality of life of diabetic patients. Although diabetic neuropathy encompasses a diverse range of presentations, the most common is a distal symmetrical polyneuropathy that is initially encountered in the hands and feet before progressing more proximally. Clinical indications of neuropathy include increased vibration and thermal perception thresholds that progress to sensory loss, occurring in conjunction with degeneration of all fiber types in the peripheral nerves. A proportion of neuropathic diabetics also describe abnormal sensations such as paresthesias, allodynia, hyperalgesia, and spontaneous pain that may co-exist with loss of normal sensory function.

Neuropathy occurs in both type 1 and type 2 diabetics, suggesting hyperglycemia as a primary pathogenic mechanism. However, the specific etiologic

From: *Methods in Molecular Medicine, Vol. 99: Pain Research: Methods and Protocols*
Edited by: Z. D. Luo © Humana Press Inc., Totowa, NJ

pathways that produce the various manifestations of diabetic neuropathy are largely unknown and investigations are constrained by the practical and ethical requirements that accompany clinical research. Diabetic animals develop indices of peripheral nerve dysfunction and have been widely studied as models of diabetic peripheral neuropathy to investigate etiologic mechanisms and screen potential therapeutic agents. Although no animal model unequivocally replicates the human condition of diabetic neuropathy, diabetic rats can provide useful models of certain aspects of hyperglycemia-induced peripheral neuropathy.

Short-term (weeks to months) diabetes induced by the pancreatic β-cell toxin streptozotocin (STZ) is the most widely studied animal model of diabetic neuropathy. STZ-diabetic rats exhibit a number of functional disorders of the nervous system that are similar to changes seen in diabetic patients, including nerve conduction velocity (NCV) slowing in large sensory and motor nerves *(3)*. Although the presence of spontaneous pain cannot be assessed directly in diabetic rats, they do exhibit altered behavioral responses to sensory stimuli applied to the hindpaws that indicate tactile allodynia *(4)*, mechanical and chemical hyperglycemia *(5)*, and a transient thermal hyperalgesia that can progress to thermal hypoalgesia *(6)*. These behavioral disorders develop within weeks of the onset of hyperalgesia and are corrected by insulin, which indicates that they are not a consequence of direct STZ-induced neurotoxicity. In contrast, structural abnormalities develop very slowly in STZ-diabetic rats and are restricted to a small reduction in myelinated fiber axonal caliber and subtle ultrastructural changes that may be precursors to more overt indications of neuropathy. In the absence of the progressive segmental demyelination and Wallerian degeneration that characterizes human diabetic neuropathy, STZ-diabetic rats are best considered as models of short-term hyperglycemia, with neurochemical and functional abnormalities that may reflect early and reversible stages in the pathogenesis of diabetic neuropathy. As such, they are being increasingly used to evaluate the therapeutic potential of agents targeted at preventing or alleviating the sensory loss and neuropathic pain states that are associated with diabetic neuropathy. In this Chapter, I will detail the approaches used in my laboratory to establish and maintain STZ-diabetic rats and the changes in behavioral responses to sensory stimuli that develop in these animals that can be used to model aspects of sensory neuropathy.

2. Materials

1. Adult (250–275 g bdy weight), female Sprague-Dawley rats (Harlan, San Diego, CA) (*see* **Note 1**).
2. Streptozotocin (Sigma, St. Louis, MO).
3. Ultralente insulin (Novo Nordisk) for injection.
4. Insulin slow-release capsules (Linshin, Canada) for implantation.
5. Strip operated reflectance meter (Ames Glucometer II, Elkhart, IN),

6. Thermal testing apparatus (UARD, San Diego, CA)
7. von Frey Filament series (Stoelting, Wood Dale, IL)
8. Custom-made perspex observation chambers to house rats individually.
9. Stock solution of 10% (v:v) buffered formaldehyde, pH 6.0–7.0–7.1, in water (Malinckrodt, KT), diluted in distilled water to provide 5.0%, 0.5%, and 0.2% formalin solutions, which are stored at room temperature.

3. Methods
3.1. Induction of Diabetes

1. Rats are allowed 1 wk to recover from transport to the vivarium, weighed, and then fasted from 4 PM until the following morning.
2. STZ is prepared in glass scintillation vials, each containing 100 mg.
3. Sterile 0.9% saline solution (2 mL) is added to a vial immediately prior to use, to give a 50 mg STZ/mL solution.
4. Each rat is injected intraperitoneally with a volume (in microliters) that is equivalent to its unfasted body weight (in grams), so that each animal receives 50 mg STZ/kg body weight (*see* **Note 2**).
5. One vial is sufficient for seven to eight animals and the solution should be used within 5 min of preparation to prevent loss of activity.
6. Food is restored 30 min after the final STZ injection.

3.2. Maintenance of Diabetic Rodents

1. Rats are maintained under a 12-h light–dark cycle with free access to food and water. They are observed daily and weighed weekly during the study period.
2. Because of the high volume of urine produced, diabetic rats are housed two per cage and the bedding changed daily. Bedding should be sawdust or paper but not wire grates, as these can induce pressure neuropathies in both normal and diabetic rats *(7)*.
3. Particular attention is paid to the animals during the initial 3 d after STZ treatment, as destruction of pancreatic β-cells by STZ leads to release of intracellular insulin that can produce a transient hypoglycemia. Any rats showing signs of lethargy during this time are treated by oral gavage with 1 mL of a saturated glucose and tap water solution to prevent hypoglycemic coma.
4. Four days after STZ injection, sugar concentration is measured in a sample of blood obtained from the tip of the tail by needle prick using a strip operated reflectance meter. Rats with a blood sugar level of 15 mmol/L or greater are accepted as diabetic and those below 10 mmol/L are rejected from the study.
5. Animals with a blood sugar of between 10 and 15 mmol/L are re-tested 3 d later and those that have crossed the 15 mmol/L threshold are included as diabetic. Approximately 90–95% of STZ-injected rats should become diabetic.
6. It is possible to provide a second STZ treatment to rats that did not develop hyperglycemia after the initial injection. This should be carried out, as described above, at least 1 wk after the first injection and with the STZ dose reduced to 45 mg/kg. Be particularly vigilant for hypoglycemia in these animals. Some deaths may be expected.

3.3. Insulin Treatment to Prevent Cachexia

1. In the absence of insulin treatment, a cohort of STZ-injected diabetic rats will survive for 10–16 wk before the number of deaths can become limiting. Weight loss, reflecting initial dehydration and subsequent muscle wasting, is variable between individual animals in the cohort, with some maintaining body weight near prediabetic values despite marked hyperglycemia. If rats show weight gain then regeneration of an incompletely destroyed β-cell population is to be suspected and blood sugar should be re-tested.

2. To prevent extreme muscle wasting and behavioral depression that could interfere with behavioral tests, rats that lose 20% of their initial body weight (approx 25–30 g) are treated twice weekly with 4 IU of ultralente insulin by subcutaneous (sc) injection into the scruff of the neck until weight is within 10% of the initial value. This dose of insulin does not produce protracted normoglycemia and this regime will allow most animals in a cohort to survive for 12–16 wk.

3. We have not noted any differences in the behavioral responses to sensory tests between untreated and insulin-treated animals within any cohort of diabetic rats, although we are careful to ensure that behavioral studies are not performed on the day that insulin is delivered.

4. Rats maintained in this manner will develop tactile allodynia and hyperalgesia in the formalin test within 4 wk of onset of diabetes *(4,8)*. They will also show a transient thermal hyperalgesia after 4 wk that progresses to hypoalgesia within 8 wk *(6)*. The hypoalgesia is not a consequence of simple behavioral depression owing to the catabolic excesses seen in this model as it is prevented by treatment with TX14(A), a neurotrophic peptide that does not alter weight loss, hyperglycemia, or other indices of systemic diabetes *(9)*.

3.4. Insulin Treatment to Maintain Body Weight With Persistent Hyperglycemia

1. This model was developed to produce diabetic rats that show near normal body weight and can survive for a year or more, despite marked hyperglycemia.

2. One week after the induction of STZ-induced diabetes as described earlier, rats are implanted with a 2.5-mm segment of an insulin capsule (cut down from the 7.5-mm length capsules as supplied by Linshin) placed sc at the scruff of the neck.

3. Blood sugar levels are tested 1 wk after implantation to ensure that the animal remains in the hyperglycemic range (15 mmol/L or above) and body weight is monitored weekly.

4. When body weight drops below 20% of starting weight, a new 2.5-mm segment of capsule is inserted.

5. Using this regime we have kept STZ-injected rats with blood sugar levels consistently above 27.7 mmol/L (the upper limit of our reflectance meter) at normal body weight for 13 mo. These animals exhibit NCV slowing, tactile allodynia, and hyperalgesia in the formalin test, emphasizing that these disorders are not associated with weight loss in STZ-diabetic rats (**Table 1**). Interestingly, these insulin-treated rats did not progress to the thermal hypoalgesia seen in the untreated STZ-diabetic rat model but remained hyperalgesic to thermal stimulation even after 13 mo of diabetes.

Table 1
Behavioral and Physiologic Responses of Control, Untreated STZ-Diabetic Rats and STZ-Diabetic Rats That Received 2 mm of an Insulin Slow-Release Implant

	Number of animals	Body weight (g)	Tactile 50% response threshold (g)	Sum 0.5% formalin flinches	Thermal response latency (s)	MNCV (m/s)	SNCV (m/s)
Control	10	271 ± 2^a	10.3 ± 1.5^a	37 ± 8^a	10.8 ± 0.7^a	61.6 ± 1.1^a	59.8 ± 1.4^a
8 wk untreated diabetic	10	189 ± 6^b	3.4 ± 0.5^b	86 ± 16^b	15.2 ± 0.9^b	46.6 ± 1.1^b	46.7 ± 1.7^b
8 wk insulin-treated diabetic	5	266 ± 16^a	3.1 ± 0.3^b	90 ± 10^b	11.1 ± 0.9^c	50.0 ± 1.3^c	48.9 ± 1.0^b
56 wk insulin-treated diabetic	5	286 ± 14^a	3.5 ± 0.6^b	–	5.1 ± 0.3^d	55.7 ± 0.5^d	49.4 ± 4.3^b
Statistical significance		a vs b $p < 0.001$	a vs b $p < 0.001$	a vs b $p < 0.05$	b vs a, c, d and d vs a, c: $p < 0.05$	a vs b, c, d and d vs b, c	a vs b $p < 0.05$

Mean ± SEM. Statistical comparisons by ANOVA with Student Newman Keuls post-hoc test.

3.5. Insulin Treatment to Maintain Normoglycemia

1. This model is used to confirm that any disorder identified in either of the two models of STZ-induced diabetes described earlier can be prevented by insulin treatment that restores normoglycemia and, thus that it is not caused by STZ-induced neurotoxocity but as a consequence of insulin deficiency or subsequent hyperglycemia.
2. One week after the induction of STZ-induced diabetes as described earlier, rats are implanted with a 7.5-mm insulin capsule (Linshin, Canada) placed sc at the scruff of the neck.
3. Blood sugar levels are tested 1 wk after implantation to ensure that the animal remains in the normoglycemic range (less than 15 mmol/L).
4. Blood sugar is monitored weekly and a new implant inserted when hyperglycemia reappears (usually after 4–8 wk).
5. We have previously shown that this regime prevents and reverses tactile allodynia and prevents hyperalgesia in the formalin test *(4)*.

3.6. Thermal Response Latency

1. Rats are placed in an observation chamber on top of the thermal testing apparatus and allowed to acclimate to the warmed glass surface (30°C) and surroundings for 30 min.
2. The mobile heat source is maneuvered to below the center of the right hindpaw and turned on, a process that activates a timer and locally warms the glass surface (*see* **Note 3**). When the rat withdraws the paw, movement sensors stop the timer and turn off the heat source. The rat should be watched during the test and the observer must be convinced that the paw movement was not a normal walking or grooming behavior.
3. At a current setting of 4.5 amps for the heat source, control rats usually respond after about 10 s and there is an automatic cut-off after 20 s to prevent tissue damage.
4. We make four measurements for each hindpaw, with a gap of 5 min between each measurement. The first of the four measurements is excluded from analysis and the median of measurements 2–4 is used as the thermal response latency for that paw. Both paws may be measured and the mean of the two scores used as a composite score for each rat.
5. Groups of animals are tested at monthly intervals. In my experience, weekly testing leads to acclimation and learning behaviors in the rats that can complicate interpretation of the effects of diabetes and treatment regimes on thermal responses.

3.7. Tactile Response Threshold

1. Rats are transferred to a testing cage with a wire mesh bottom and allowed to acclimate for 30 min.
2. Von Frey filaments (Stoelting, Wood Dale, IL) are used to determine the 50% mechanical threshold for foot withdrawal. A series of filaments, starting with one that possessed a buckling weight of 2 g, are applied in sequence to the plantar surface of the right hindpaw for 5 s with a pressure that causes the filament to buckle.

Lifting of the paw is recorded as a positive response and the next lighter filament is chosen for the next measurement. Absence of a response after 5 s prompts use of the next filament of increasing weight.

3. This paradigm is continued until four measurements have been made after an initial change in the behavior or until five consecutive negative (15 g) or four positive (0.25 g) responses have been obtained. The resulting sequence of positive and negative scores is used to interpolate the 50% response threshold using the formula: 50% threshold = (10 [Xf+kδ])/10,000 where Xf is the value (in log units) of the final filament used; k = tabular value for the sequence of positive and negative responses as listed by Chaplan and co-workers *(10)*; and δ = mean difference (in log units) between stimuli.

4. Animals can be tested repeatedly after a drug treatment to obtain a time:effect curve. However, I have found that multiple testing of rats over a number of days can lead to adaptive behaviors that can obscure the efficacy of drugs and erroneously suggests development of tolerance *(11)*.

3.8. Formalin-Evoked Flinching

1. Rats are restrained manually by wrapping in a towel and formalin (50 µL of 0.5% solution; *see* **Note 4**) is injected subdermally into the dorsum of the right hindpaw.
2. The rat is then placed in an observation chamber and flinching behavior is counted in 1-min blocks every 5 min for 1 h.
3. The sum of flinches counted during the hour (flinches during minutes 1–2, 5–6, 10–11, 15–16, 20–21, 25–26, 30–31, 35–36, 40–41, 45–46, 50–51, 55–56, and 60–61 postformalin injection) can be calculated to provide an overall score or the data can be subdivided to highlight specific phases of the test (phase 1 = sum of flinches during min 1–2 and 5–6; phase 2 = 10–11, 15–16, and 20–21; phase 3 = remaining scores).

4. Notes

1. We routinely use adult female Sprague-Dawley rats for studies of STZ-induced diabetic neuropathy. This is because insulin-deficient diabetes can have marked effects on the maturation of many tissues, including the peripheral nervous system (PNS), which can complicate data interpretation. For example, if diabetes is induced before peripheral NCV has stabilized at adult values, a few weeks of hyperglycemia will result in a difference between control and diabetic NCV values that can be attributed to the diabetic rats not continuing the normal maturational increase seen in control rats. In contrast, NCV values in rats made diabetic once they had attained maturity will show an absolute decrease from prediabetic levels **(Fig. 1)**.

   We use female Sprague-Dawley rats because they attain maximal body weight (250–280 g) and NCV values at an earlier age and smaller weight than male Sprague-Dawley rats or either sex of other strains such as Wistars. It should be noted that although serial weighing of rats can give an estimate of the approach to maturity, we find that NCV continues to increase by 1–2 m/s/wk for 3–4 wk after weight has stabilized. Although there could be concerns that hormonal status can contribute to a range of physiologic parameters, including sensory function and

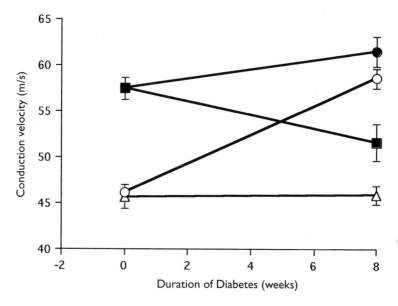

Fig. 1. Large-fiber sensory conduction velocity in the sciatic nerve of control (circles) and untreated STZ-diabetic (squares) female Sprague-Dawley rats. Values were measured before and after 8 wk of hyperglycemia in groups of juvenile (open symbols: starting weight = 185 ± 3 g) and adult (filled symbols: starting weight = 280 ± 5 g) rats. Data are mean ± SEM. n = 8–10/group (N. A. Calcutt, unpublished observations).

Table 2
Dose of STZ Necessary to Induce Hyperglycemia

Body Weight (g)	STZ Dose
175–200	60 mg/kg (10.5–12.0 mg/rat)
201–249	55 mg/kg (11.1–13.7 mg/rat)
250–299	50 mg/kg (12.5–15.0 mg/rat)
>300	45 mg/kg (13.6 mg/rat +)

pain perception, we have not noted sex-related differences between male and female rats on the effects of diabetes on behavioral responses *(4)*.

2. We usually use adult rats in the 250–275 g range and treat them with STZ at a dose of 50 mg/kg. However, if younger animals are to be used, the scale in **Table 2** is applied to calculate the dose of STZ necessary to induce hyperglycemia.

3. At the beginning, halfway through, and at the end of every testing session, we measure the upper surface temperature of the glass floor of the thermal stimulation device. This is done at 5-s intervals during a 20-s period when the heat source is

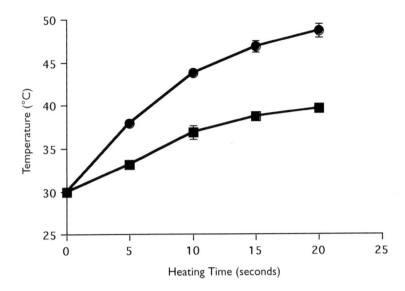

Fig. 2. Temperature change at the upper (filled squares) and lower (filled circles) surface of the glass floor of the thermal testing apparatus following activation of the directed heat source. Data points represent median ± SEM of 3 series of measurements made at different times during the course of 1 d testing (N. A. Calcutt and C. Morgan, unpublished observations).

turned on and allows construction of time vs temperature curves using the median of the three measurements at each time point (**Fig. 2**). Because we find day-to-day variations in these heating curves, studies that are performed over many days may be standardized by calculating the upper surface temperature that elicits a withdrawal response using the response latency of each rat and interpolating from the appropriate daily time vs temperature curves.

4. In control rats, the frequency of paw flinching following local injection of formalin is dependent on the concentration of formalin used, with no flinching seen using 0.2% formalin and maximal flinching seen at 1% and above *(12)*. In diabetic rats, different patterns of response are seen and these depend on the concentration of formalin. Diabetic rats treated with 5% formalin show increased flinching only during the quiescent interphase period *(8)*, presumably because flinching is already at a maximal rate during phases 1 and 2 in control rats. Using 0.5% formalin, which provokes submaximal bi-phasic flinching in control rats, reveals increased flinching in diabetic rats that is most consistently noted during the quiescent phase and phase 2 *(12)*. Although control rats do not respond to 0.2% formalin, diabetic rats show a response that differs from that seen using higher concentrations, because it is monophasic (**Fig. 3**). This can be viewed as allodynia (a response to a normally innocuous stimulus) rather than hyperalgesia (exaggerated responses to a normally painful stimulus).

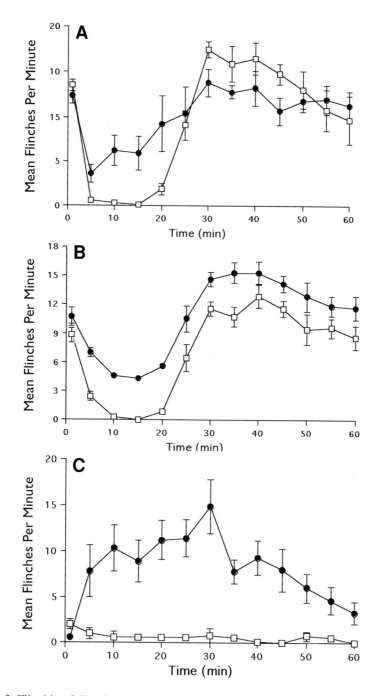

Fig. 3. Flinching following sc injection of 50 µL of 5% (**A**), 0.5% (**B**), and 0.2% (**C**) formalin into the hindpaw dorsum of control (open squares) and untreated STZ-diabetic (filled circles) rats. Data are mean ± SEM of n = 6–8 rats/group (N. A. Calcutt and J. D. Freshwater, unpublished observations).

References

1. Zimmet, P., Alberti, K. G. M. M., and Shaw, J. (2001) Global and societal implications of the diabetes epidemic. *Nature* **414,** 782–786.
2. Pirart, J. (1978) Diabetes mellitus and its degenerative complications: a prospective study of 4,400 patients observed between 1947 and 1973. *Diabetes Care* **1,** 168–188, 252–263.
3. Moore, S. A., Peterson, R. G., Felten, D. L., and O'Connor, B. L. (1981) A quantitative comparison of motor and sensory conduction velocities in short and long term streptozotocin and alloxan diabetic rats. *J. Neurol. Sci.* **48,** 133–152.
4. Calcutt, N. A., Jorge, M. C., Yaksh, T. L., and Chaplan, S. C. (1996) Tactile allodynia and formalin hyperalgesia in streptozotocin-diabetic rats: effects of insulin, aldose reductase inhibition and lidocaine. *Pain* **68,** 293–299.
5. Courteix, C., Eschalier, A., and Lavarenne J. (1993) Streptozotocin-induced diabetic rats: behavioral evidence for a model of chronic pain. *Pain* **53,** 81–88.
6. Kolta, M. G., Ngong, J. M., Rutledge, L. P., et al. (1996) Endogenous opioid peptide mediation of hypoalgesic response in long-term diabetic rats. *Neuropeptides* **30,** 335–344.
7. Mizisin, A. P., Kalichman, M. W., Garrett, R. S., and Dines, K. C. (1998) Tactile hyperesthesia, altered epidermal innervation and plantar nerve injury in the hindfeet of rats housed on wire grates. *Brain Res.* **788,** 13–19.
8. Calcutt, N. A., Malmberg, A. B., Yamamoto, T., and Yaksh, T. L. (1994) Tolrestat treatment prevents modification of the formalin test model of prolonged pain in diabetic rats. *Pain* **58,** 413–420.
9. Calcutt, N. A., Campana, W. M., Eskeland, N. L., et al. (1999) Prosaposin gene expression and the efficacy of a prosaposin-derived peptide in preventing structural and functional disorders of peripheral nerve in diabetic rats. *J. Neuropathol. Exp. Neurol.* **58,** 628–636.
10. Chaplan, S. C., Bach, F. W., Pogrel, J. W., et al. (1994) Quantitative assessment of tactile allodynia in the rat paw. *J. Neurosci. Methods* **53,** 55–63.
11. Calcutt, N. A., Freshwater, J. D., and O'Brien, J. S. (2000) Protection of sensory function and antihyperalgesic properties of a prosaposin-derived peptide in diabetic rats. *Anesthesiology* **93,** 1271–1278.
12. Calcutt, N. A., Li, L., Yaksh, N. A., and Malmberg, A. B. (1995) Different effects of two aldose reductase inhibitors on nociception and prostaglandin E. *Eur. J. Pharmacol.* **285,** 189–197.

7

Sciatic Inflammatory Neuropathy in the Rat

Surgical Procedures, Induction of Inflammation, and Behavioral Testing

Erin D. Milligan, Steven F. Maier, and Linda R. Watkins

Summary

Peripheral nerve damage involves inflammation, and is frequently causal to the development of neuropathic pain. However, inflammatory neuropathies often occur in the absence of trauma. We have recently developed an animal model of neuropathic pain where allodynia is induced by nerve inflammation rather than injury. This sciatic inflammatory neuropathy (SIN) model was developed to understand immunologic, neuropathic, and spinal mechanisms underlying allodynia in the territory of the sciatic nerve as well as in extraterritorial and contralateral ("mirror image") sites. A specially designed indwelling catheter system allows immune activators to be selectively injected around one healthy sciatic nerve in awake, behaving rats. Here, we provide detailed procedures on the construction and implantation of chronic indwelling perisciatic catheters used to create SIN. Detailed procedures for implantation of intrathecal catheters via a lumbar vertebra 5 and 6 approach in the same rat are also provided. Methods for testing allodynia and for data analysis are additionally described so to provide all the steps needed for behavioral experimentation.

Key Words: Allodynia; inflammation; perisciatic; von Frey hairs; intrathecal; zymosan; SIN; chronic catheterization; neuropathy; rat; neuropathic pain.

1. Introduction

Neuropathies associated with pathological pain are often a result of frank trauma to peripheral nerves, which always involves inflammation *(1)*. However, many other neuropathies, approximately half of clinical neuropathies, that involve inflammation and/or infection near peripheral nerves occur without significant physical nerve trauma *(2,3)*. Yet, the role of immune activation in pathological pain states is not clear. Until recently, animal models focused on understanding the mechanisms underlying neuropathic pain associated with nerve damage *(4–7)*.

From: *Methods in Molecular Medicine, Vol. 99: Pain Research: Methods and Protocols*
Edited by: Z. D. Luo © Humana Press Inc., Totowa, NJ

The sciatic inflammatory neuropathy (SIN) model was recently developed to examine how inflammatory pain is created without frank nerve trauma *(8–10)*.

The SIN model evolved from a prior procedure *(11)* with changes incorporated to allow examination of: (1) perisciatic immune activation not confounded by anesthetics, because these drugs can grossly alter immune responses *(12,13)*; (2) the earliest onset of immune activation-induced, low-threshold mechanical allodynia in awake, freely moving rats; (3) immune cell responses in and around the peripheral nerve that may underlie SIN-induced allodynia; (4) spinal-cord mediators of SIN-induced territorial, extraterritorial (saphenous), and mirror-image (contralateral) allodynias; and (5) the peripheral and spinal bases of persistent allodynia created by repeated immune challenges around the sciatic nerve for a period of weeks.

This chapter will describe chronic perisciatic catheterization and all of the steps needed for successful SIN experimentation. Additionally, surgery for both intrathecal (it) catheterization *(14)* and perisciatic catheterization in the same animal will be described, because there are slight changes required in each procedure to be successful. Testing for allodynia will also be described to address unexpected problems that have been observed by our team after these surgical procedures. Estimating a 50% threshold from the observed data using a computer software program will also be addressed.

2. Materials

2.1. Chronic Perisciatic Catheter Construction

1. Sterile gelfoam sheets (approx 2 × 6 cm; NDC no. 0009-0315-03; Upjohn, Kalamazoo, MI). Each sheet will produce four gelfoam pieces.
2. Silastic tubing (1.57-mm inner diameter, 2.41-mm outer diameter; Helix Medical Inc., Carpinteria, CA).
3. Sterile silk suture (4-0 and 3-0) with attached needle (cutting FS-2 and FS-1, respectively; Ethicon, Somerville, NJ).
4. Sterile polyethylene tubing (PE-50, Becton Dickinson, Sparks, MD).
5. Sterile 50-mL conical tube (Fisher Scientific, Houston, TX).
6. No. 11 scalpel blade.
7. Sterile metal metric ruler (15 cm).

2.2. Chronic Perisciatic Catheter Surgery

2.2.1. Equipment

1. Two micro-forceps.
2. Toothed forceps.
3. Blunt dissection scissors.
4. Suture hemostats with scissors.
5. No. 11 or no. 10 scalpel blades.

6. Scalpel handle.
7. Two small towel clips.
8. Four to eight glass Pasteur pipets with the tips previously melted into small hooks.
9. Ultra hot glass-bead sterilizer (World Precision Instruments, Sarasota, FL) to sterilize tools between use
10. Shaver.

2.2.2. Reagents

1. 70% alcohol.
2. Exidine-2 surgical scrub solution (undiluted, Baxter Healthcare, Deerfield, IL).
3. Sterile gauze (4 × 4 inches) to create a drape around the surgical site.
4. Sterile Q-tips to absorb blood.
5. Approximately 800 mL of both an antibacterial water mixture and water for cleansing hands between surgeries.
6. Sterile autoclave paper (12 × 12 cm) to provide a clean surface for placing sterilized tools.
7. One sleeve/rat that protects the exteriorized portion of the perisciatic catheter (cc-sleeve; described below).

2.2.3. Constructing the cc-Sleeve

1. 1-cc plastic syringe.
2. One-sided razor blade.
3. Manual metal tube-cutter with a cutting diameter range starting from 1/8 in.
4. Hand drill (Multipro Dremel Drill with variable speed; Dremel, Racine, WI) for creating 3-mm-sized holes with a drill bit (bit size code no. 150, 1/8 in; Dremel, Racine, WI).
5. Silastic 732 silicon sealant (Dow Corning, Midland, MI).

2.3. Chronic Intrathecal (it) Catheter Construction

2.3.1. Equipment

1. Polyethylene tubes (PE-10, Clay-Adams, Becton Dickinson, Sparks, MD) cut to 10 cm and stored in 70% alcohol in a previously autoclaved glass jar.
2. Two sterile 50-mL conical tubes.
3. Sterile gauze (4 × 4 inches).
4. Sterile, endotoxin-free isotonic saline (NDC# 0074-4888-10, Abbott Laboratories, North Chicago, IL).
5. 1-cc syringe.
6. Sterile 30-G 1/2-in. needle (Becton Dickinson, Franklin Lakes, NJ).
7. Black marker.
8. Sterile metal ruler.
9. One 7 cm (approx) metal rod (approx 1 mm diameter) that is placed in the glass-bead sterilizer and heated to heat-seal PE-10 tube (described in **Subheading 3.3.2, step 15**).
10. Ultra hot glass-bead sterilizer (to heat-seal PE-10 tube described below).

2.3.2. It Catheter Construction

1. Several days prior to surgery, the PE-10 catheters are air-dried in a sterile dry container (a 50-mL conical tube) with sterile gauze placed tightly over the top to allow alcohol evaporation.
2. The air-dried PE-10 catheters are flushed with sterile, endotoxin-free isotonic saline using a 1-cc syringe attached to a 30-G needle and heat-sealed with the heated metal rod.
3. The flushed catheters are marked between 7.7 and 7.8 cm (using a sterile metal ruler), from the open end of the catheter. These materials are stored in a sterile, dry container (50-mL conical tube with lid tightly secured) until the time of surgery.

2.4. Chronic it Catheter Surgery

1. Two micro-forceps.
2. Blunt dissection scissors.
3. Suture hemostats with scissors.
4. No. 11 or no. 10 scalpel.
5. Scalpel handle.
6. Sterile silk suture with attached needle (3-0 silk with cutting FS-1 needle, Ethicon, Somerville, NJ).
7. A sterile 18-G, 1 $\frac{1}{2}$-inch, hypodermic needle (Becton Dickinson, Franklin Lakes, NJ) with the plastic hub removed (referred to as a guide cannula for the PE-10 catheter in **Subheading 3.3.**). These are made in advance of surgery and stored in a sterile, dry container (a small, shallow autoclaved glass container with lid is recommended).
8. Spring-loaded diagonal cutting pliers (4 in.; Small Parts, Inc., Miami Lakes, FL).
9. The glass-bead sterilizer, shaver, and cc-sleeve used for the perisciatic surgery listed in **Subheading 2.2.** can also be used for this surgery.
10. Supplies needed for conducting it surgery are the same as those listed for the perisciatic surgery (containers for rinsing hands, sterile gauze, Q-tips, etc.) in **Subheading 2.2.**

2.5. Perisciatic Catheter Cleaners

1. Sterile 3-cc syringe.
2. One 23-G needle.
3. PE-50 tubing (Becton Dickinson, Sparks, MD).

2.6. Perisciatic Catheter Injectors

1. Sterile 23-G, 1-in. hypodermic needle (Becton Dickinson, Franklin Lakes, NJ).
2. PE-50 tubing (Becton Dickinson, Sparks, MD).
3. Autoclaved 100 µL Hamilton glass syringe (Fisher Scientific, Houston, TX).
4. Black permanent fine-tip marker.
5. Dental probe with a 45° angel (microprobe; Fisher Scientific).

2.7. Intrathecal Catheter Injectors

1. 30-G, $^1/_2$-in. hypodermic needles (Becton Dickinson, Franklin Lakes, NJ), with the plastic hub removed.
2. PE-10 tubing (Clay-Adams, Becton-Dickinson and Co., Sparks, MD).
3. Autoclaved 50 µL Hamilton glass syringe (Fisher Scientific).

2.8. Low Threshold Mechanical Probes

1. Rats are placed atop a mounted grid inside 4000 mL beakers (no. 02-591-15AA, Fisher Scientific) with the bottom sawed off.
2. Calibrated Semmes-Weinstein monofilaments (von Frey hairs; Stoelting, Wood Dale, IL). The hair stiffness ranges from 0.406 g through 15.136 g, in a logarithmic series of 10 monofilaments. Log stiffness of the hairs is defined as Log_{10} (g × 10,000). The 10 stimuli have the following log stiffness values: 3.61 (0.407 g), 3.84 (0.692 g), 4.08 (1.202 g), 4.17 (1.479 g), 4.31 (2.041 g), 4.56 (3.630 g), 4.74 (5.495 g), 4.93 (8.511 g), 5.07 (11.749 g), and 5.18 (15.136 g).

2.9. Estimation of 50% Threshold

The computer program, PsychoFit, used to estimate 50% threshold values is available for both Macintosh and PC computers and can be downloaded from L. O. Harvey's website (http://psych.colorado.edu/~lharvey).

3. Methods

The methods and procedures detailed here are for: (1) construction of supplies such as chronic perisciatic catheters, it catheters, microinjectors, perisciatic catheter cleaners, perisciatic catheter injectors, and protective cc-sleeves; (2) chronic perisciatic catheter and intrathecal surgeries; (3) cleaning and injecting drugs around the sciatic nerve, and it drug injections; (4) behavioral testing using a series of calibrated monofilaments (the von Frey test); and (5) applying the resultant psychometric data to estimate 50% threshold values using a simple computer software program. Importantly, all procedures described for constructing catheters are conducted in a sterile environment such as in an ultraviolet (UV) hood. The stainless-steel surface of the hood is wiped with 70% alcohol before making supplies. All instruments (forceps, scissors, and scalpels) used to handle or make the supplies are sterile. It is imperative that the catheters for these surgeries are endotoxin-free as well as sterile because: (1) endotoxin is not destroyed by autoclaving or gas sterilization and (2) endotoxin and bacterial contamination activates immune cells.

Extra steps are taken during the surgeries to minimize the introduction of endotoxin and other inflammatory agents. That is, all instruments are sterilized prior to conducting surgery on each animal using a glass bead mini-sterilizer.

A

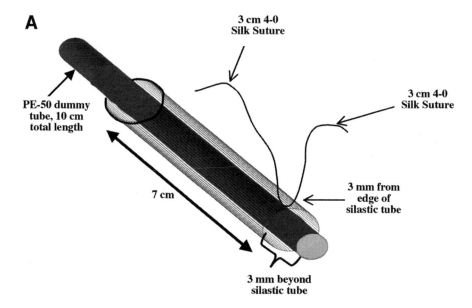

3 cm 4-0
Silk Suture

3 cm 4-0
Silk Suture

PE-50 dummy
tube, 10 cm
total length

7 cm

3 mm from
edge of
silastic tube

3 mm beyond
silastic tube

Fig. 1. **(A)** The silastic + Pe-50 gelfoam assembly. This is the assembly immediately prior to attaching it to the gelfoam. *(Figure continues)*

Hands are washed with antibacterial soap between animals. The skin surrounding the open wound is draped with sterilized gauze to prevent the suture material from contacting the fur when tying the catheter in place or closing the wound. This step further avoids bacterial and endotoxin contamination.

3.1. Chronic Perisciatic Catheter Construction

1. Sterile, 10-cm PE-50 tubing is inserted through and 3 mm (not cm) beyond a 7 cm sterile silastic tube. This 10-cm PE-50 tubing serves as a dummy catheter. That is, this dummy catheter is the same diameter as the PE-50 tubing that will later be used to inject drugs. The dummy catheter ensures that the silastic tube does not become blocked either by silk sutures used for making the silastic tube + gelfoam assembly or by the surgical anchoring step (described below).
2. A sterile, 6-cm length of 4-0 silk suture with attached needle is hooked through a small portion of the silastic tube at 3–4 mm from the tip where the PE-50 dummy catheter extends 3 mm beyond the silastic tube. It is critical that the 4-0 silk suture does not pierce the indwelling PE-50 tubing **(Fig. 1A)**. The approximate length of the silk-suture (6 cm) is needed to easily tie gelfoam (described below) to the silastic + PE-50 assembly as well as to tie the gelfoam ends together after enwrapping the sciatic nerve (described in **Subheading 3.2.**).
3. The silastic + PE-50 assemblies are stored in a sterile, dry 50-mL conical tube that is tightly capped until the prepared gelfoam is ready to be attached.

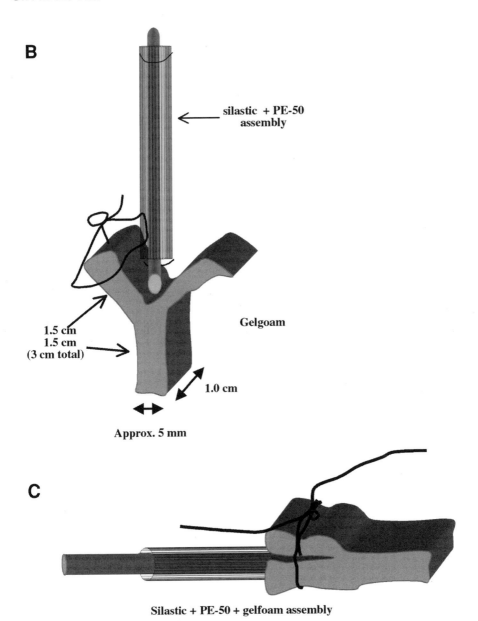

Fig. 1. *(continued)* (**B**) Attachment of the silastic + PE-50 gelfoam assembly to the gelfoam. Note that this is the size of the gelfoam after it has been cut from the gelfoam sheet. (**C**) The complete silastic + PE-50 + gelfaom assembly. Note that the gelfoam is securely tied around the silastic + PE-50 gelfoam assembly with 3-0 silk suture.

4. The perisciatic gelfoam is constructed from sterile gelfoam sheets (6 [L] × 1 [W] × 2 [H] cm) cut, using a sterile no. 11 scalpel blade on a sterile metal metric ruler, into 3 (L) × 1.0 (W) × 1 (H) cm strips.
5. One end of the gelfoam strip is bisected (0.5 cm W) to a depth of 1.5 cm (**Fig. 1B**).
6. The 4-0 silk suture end of the silastic + PE-50 assembly is inserted into the flap of the gelfoam to a depth of approx 1.5 cm and the 4-0 silk-suture is used to securely attach the assembly to the gelfoam. That is, both ends of the 4-0 silk suture are tightly tied and knotted around one side of the gelfoam flap and again around the opposing flap (**Fig. 1C**), closing the flaps tightly together around the silastic + PE-50 assembly.
7. The silastic + PE-50 + gelfoam assembly is stored in a sterile, dry 50-mL conical tube (which can store up to 6 silastic + PE-50 + gelfoam assemblies) until the time of surgery.

3.2. cc-Sleeve Construction and Chronic Perisciatic Catheter Surgery

3.2.1. cc-Sleeve Construction

1. Construction of the cc-sleeve is similar to that described previously *(14)*, with some minor changes. Briefly, cc-sleeves are constructed from sterile 1-cc plastic syringes, with the rubber plug removed from the internal plunger.
2. The rubber plug is cut in half with a one-sided razor blade, producing a rubber ring that is discarded, and a concave plug.
3. The concave plug serves as "stopper" for the silastic catheter, which is tucked inside the cc-sleeve (described below).
4. The concave plugs are stored in 70% alcohol until the time of surgery.
5. The barrel of the 1-cc syringe is cut to approx 8 mm from the flanged end, and an approx 3-mm hole is drilled through each flange.
6. As a final step, an aluminum sleeve, produced by cutting an aluminum tube (inner diameter of 8 mm) to approx 5–8 mm long, is sealed around the plastic barrel of the cc-sleeve with a small amount of Silastic 732 silicon sealant (Dow Corning, Midland, MI) dabbed on the inside of the aluminum tube. This aluminum tube protects the plastic cc-sleeve from being chewed by the rats.
7. The prepared cc-sleeve is placed in a clean area to air-dry for 1 d followed by storing in 70% alcohol until the time of surgery.

3.2.2. Chronic Perisciatic Catheter Surgery

1. Surgery is conducted under isoflurane anesthesia (Halocarbon Laboratories, River Edge, NJ), 2.5 vol% in oxygen, which is chosen because it has minimal effects on immune cell function compared to other commonly used anesthetics *(12,13)* (*see* **Note 1**).
2. The dorsal aspect of the rat faces up with the nose facing away from the surgeon, and the left and right hind legs are splayed laterally to the left and right of the surgeon. The fur is shaved from the left leg and lower back area.
3. The exposed skin is cleaned with 70% alcohol-soaked gauze.

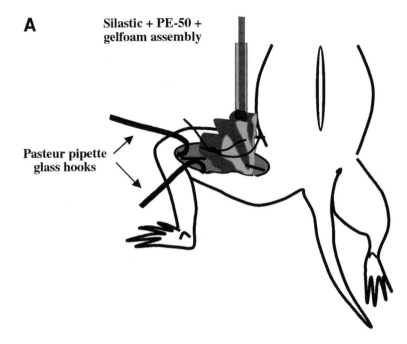

A **Silastic + PE-50 + gelfoam assembly**

Pasteur pipette glass hooks

Fig. 2. **(A)** The process of enwrapping the gelfoam portion of silastic + PE-50 + gelfoam assembly around the sciatic nerve. *(Figure continues)*

4. A small amount of concentrated Exidine-2 surgical scrub solution applied to fresh gauze is then used to further clean the surgical area. The two steps in cleaning are done to remove cage-bedding flakes and dander as well as kill bacteria.
5. A midline incision at the lower back area is then made with either a no. 10 or no. 11 surgical scalpel blade and the skin around the cut is separated from its underlying loose connective tissue using blunt dissection scissors. This is done to provide space for subcutaneous implantation of the cc-sleeve (described below).
6. To prepare for the perisciatic implant, a second incision is made along the lateral aspect of the left thigh.
7. Separation of the skin from underlying connective tissue extends beyond the incision site to the midline incision where the exterior portion of the catheter will be encased by the cc-sleeve.
8. The shaved and cleaned skin surrounding the wound is lightly retracted using small-toothed towel clips followed by draping with sterile gauze.
9. Exposure of the sciatic nerve is achieved by blunt dissection, and connective tissue is gently removed using glass Pasteur pipet hooks sterilized in the glass-bead mini-sterilizer before each use.
10. At approximately mid-thigh level, a portion of the sciatic nerve is gently and minimally lifted using a sterile glass Pasteur pipet hook.

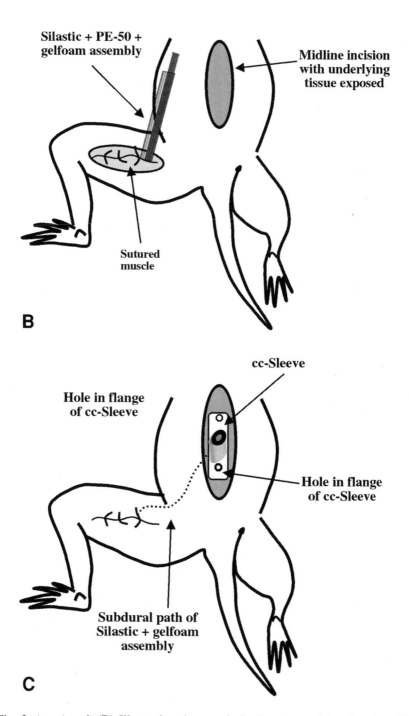

Fig. 2. *(continued)* **(B)** Illustrating the exteriorized portion of the silastic + PE-50 catheter after the gelfoam has been implanted and muscle walls have been closed with sutures. **(C)** cc-Sleeve attachment to the lower back area after the silastic + PE-50 + gelfoam assembly has been implanted.

11. A few drops of sterile isotonic, endotoxin-free saline are added to keep the nerve moist.
12. The gelfoam of the silastic + PE-50 + gelfoam assembly is then gently threaded around the sciatic nerve (**Fig. 2A**) starting from the quadriceps side of the sciatic nerve in order to avoid obscuring the surgeon's view of the implant site.
13. The 4-0 silk-suture that is part of the silastic + PE-50 + gelfoam assembly (*see* **Subheading 3.1.**) is used to tie together the proximal and distal ends of the gelfoam once it forms a U-shape around the sciatic nerve (**Fig. 2A**).
14. The surrounding muscle walls are then closed around the gelfoam-enwrapped sciatic nerve, leaving the silastic + PE-50 portion exteriorized.
15. The silastic tube is anchored to the muscle by threading a sterile 4-0 silk suture with attached suture needle through the muscle at the most proximal portion of the dissection site, followed by threading the suture through the silastic tube, but avoiding the internal PE-50 dummy tube, and then through the opposing muscle.
16. The remaining overlying muscle is closed with one or two more sutures through the muscle (**Fig. 2B**).
17. The exposed portion of the silastic catheter is tunneled sc to exit through the lower back incision (**Fig. 2C**).
18. The skin overlaying the sutured muscle is closed with wound clips.
19. The PE-50 dummy catheter is carefully removed while holding the silastic catheter in place to ensure that the gelfoam does not become torn or displaced.
20. The exposed portion of the silastic catheter is threaded through the cc-sleeve.
21. The cc-sleeve is then anchored to the muscle overlaying the lumbosacral area by threading one or two 3-0 silk sutures with attached suture needle through each flange (**Fig. 2C**).
22. The skin is then closed with 3-0 silk sutures.
23. The remaining exteriorized portion of the silastic tube is folded into the cc-sleeve and an air-dried concave plug is inserted inside the tip of the sleeve.
24. As a final step, a small amount of silastic silicon sealant is coated over the end of the plug and cc-sleeve with a moistened Q-tip.
25. The wound area around the hind leg and lower back are lightly cleaned with 0.9% saline. Total surgical time is typically 15–20 min.

3.2.3. Postsurgical Care for Chronic Perisciatic Catheterization

1. Beginning 4–5 d following surgery when catheters are used to induce chronic allodynia for extended periods of time (as long as 3 wk), the wound areas of the hind leg and lower back are cleaned with 0.9% saline every 2 d. This decreases the amount of inflammation, such as redness, slight bleeding, and scabbing of the skin around the surgical sites (*see* **Notes 2** and **3**).
2. The cc-sleeve and the indwelling perisciatic silastic catheter are also cleaned with separate single-use perisciatic catheter cleaners (*see* **Note 4**).
3. The cc-sleeves are discarded *after use* in the chronic SIN model. However, for uses less than 7 d, the cc-sleeve can be reused after thoroughly cleaning in 10% bleach and alconox, followed by water rinses.

3.3. 18-G Guide Cannula Construction and Chronic Intrathecal Catheter Surgery Combined With Perisciatic Catheter Surgery

3.3.1. 18-G Guide Cannula Construction

1. The plastic hub of the 18-G, 1 $^1/_2$ inch needle is removed by deforming the plastic off of the embedded needle using spring loaded 4-in. diagonal pliers. Pinch into the plastic hub, starting at a point midway along the needle hub where the embedded portion of the 18-G needle ends. This embedded portion of the needle has a white coating and can be easily identified through the plastic hub. Do not cut through or crimp the 18-G needle itself.

2. This step is repeated approximately four additional times, making one quarter turns at each pinch and moving toward the beveled tip at 1–2 mm increments.

3. At the fifth pinch, grasp between the pliers the white coating that is now exposed, and pull the 18-G needle away from the plastic hub.

4. The 18-G needle is now fully exposed, with a total length of 2 $^3/_{16}$ inches (4.5 cm), and is placed directly into a sterile container with the beveled tip facing away from the container opening. This is referred to as the 18-G guide cannula during surgical procedures.

3.3.2. Chronic Intrathecal Catheter Surgery Combined With Perisciatic Catheter Surgery

1. If both surgeries are being conducted in the same animal, the intrathecal catheterization procedure should be conducted first, followed by the chronic perisciatic surgery. The order is important because the perisciatic catheter placement is more sensitive to perturbations than the firmly anchored intrathecal catheter. All procedures for chronic intrathecal catheter surgery are similar to those described previously *(14,15)*.

2. Briefly, under isoflurane anesthesia (2.5 vol% in oxygen), the animal is shaved and cleaned as described in **Subheading 3.1.**

3. A 2–3 cm dorsal mid-line incision is then made at the lower pelvic area followed by forming a subcutaneous pocket underneath the incision to create room for the cc-sleeve.

4. At this point in the surgery, a mark is made with a black permanent marker on the white-coated portion of the 18-G guide cannula on the same plane as its beveled side.

5. From here, the lumbar vertebral gap between lumbar vertebra 5 (L5) and lumbar vertebra 6 (L6) is manually located with the forefinger. The L5/L6 vertebral gap is located at the rostral edge of the pelvis. Sacral vertebra 1 (S1) is then identified with the forefinger by feeling and counting one dorsal vertebral process caudal to the L6 dorsal vertebral process.

6. Parallel to the small gap between S1 and L6, and at a point approx 5 mm lateral to midline, the 18-G guide cannula is inserted at a 30° angle from the muscle surface with the beveled side facing up and with the hips flat.

7. The tip of the 18-G guide cannula is then "walked" rostrally along the L6 vertebra, over the L6 spineous processes *(16)*, and slipped down into the L5–L6 vertebral

gap at a 45° angle, aiming medially. Typically, a tail flick and cerebrospinal spinal fluid (CSF) efflux are observed from the 18-G needle hub end. The 18-G guide cannula should not be inserted between L5 and L6 too tightly, because this can compress and damage the exiting nerves. Moreover, if blood efflux from the 18-G guide cannula results during placement, start again with a new, sterile 18-G guide cannula. This avoids blood contamination of the spinal canal, which can increase inflammation at the entry site.

8. The sealed PE-10 catheter is slowly inserted into the 18-G guide cannula until the 7.7 cm mark on the PE-10 tubing aligns with the blunt exterior end of the 18-G cannula. Hind limb and tail twitching are commonly observed during this step. Although a tail flick and CSF efflux are good indications that the needle tip is subdural, both are not always required for successful catheter placement. Often, while threading the PE-10 catheter, a slight tail-twitch along with hind leg twitching are strong indications of subdural catheter placement. In addition, it is critical that the 18-G guide cannula be maintained at a 45° angle while threading the PE-10 catheter. Threading the PE-10 catheter at a more shallow angle can lead to supradural catheter placement. This is especially critical when the experimental protocol involves drugs that do not readily cross the dura into the CSF space.

9. After the it catheter is in place, the sealed end of the PE-10 catheter is cut to allow the 18-G guide cannula to pass.

10. The guide cannula is then carefully removed and discarded.

11. A mark is made with fine point permanent marker where the juncture of the PE-10 catheter and the muscle surface meet.

12. A loose loop-knot is then carefully created in the PE-10 catheter at the site of the mark. Attention to the mark is made to detect displacement of the PE-10 catheter (typical displacement is up to 5 mm away from the muscle surface, either into or out of the rat). Displacement of the mark from the muscle surface is immediately corrected by sliding the catheter back into place where the mark meets the muscle surface.

13. The loop-knot is then securely anchored to the muscle with three 3-0 silk sutures through the loop-knot (*see* **Note 5**).

14. A 10–15 µL sterile saline flush is done to verify that the catheter remained patent and free of leaks.

15. The catheter is re-sealed by pinching the cut end of the PE-10 catheter between the tips of forceps heated in the glass-bead sterilizer.

16. After implantation of the perisciatic silastic catheter, the exteriorized silastic tube is tunneled sc to exit through the lower back incision.

17. Here, both catheters are threaded through the protective cc-sleeve that is then anchored to the underlying muscle, and the surrounding skin is closed with 3-0 silk sutures.

18. Both catheters are folded into the cc-sleeve, the concave plug inserted, and silicon sealant added over the plug and sleeve. Total time for both surgeries is 25–30 min.

3.4. Perisciatic Catheter Cleaners and Injectors and Injection Procedures

3.4.1. Perisciatic Catheter Cleaners

1. The cleaners are used to suction out fluid accumulation within the indwelling silastic catheter starting 4–5 d after surgery and prior to drug injections. The catheter cleaners are made from the same supplies as the injectors, except the Hamilton 100 µL micro-syringe is replaced with a sterile 3-cc syringe.
2. Additionally, the cleaners are constructed in the same way as the injectors (described above) except that the 3-cc syringe is attached to the 23-G needle. Prepared perisciatic catheter cleaners are stored in a sterile, dry place (typically, an autoclavable box) until the time of injections.

3.4.2. Perisciatic Catheter Injectors

1. The beveled end of a sterile 23-G, 1-in. hypodermic needle is inserted into one end of a 35 cm PE-50 tube.
2. A mark is made 7.3 cm from the opposite end, using a black permanent fine-tip marker. The mark must line up with the exterior end of perisciatic silastic catheter upon PE-50 tubing insertion. This alignment assures that the interior end of the PE-50 tubing is within the gelfoam.
3. Prepared perisciatic catheter injectors are stored in a sterile, dry place (typically, an autoclavable box) until the time of injections.
4. The 23-G needle is attached to a sterile Hamilton 100 µL micro-syringe at the time of injection.

3.4.3. Perisciatic Catheter Injections

1. The sterile glass Hamilton micro-syringe and the perisciatic catheter injector are flushed with sterile, endotoxin-free water and tightly connected making the syringe and injector air tight.
2. An air bubble is then created in the 30 cm PE-50 tubing of the perisciatic catheter injector by drawing up 1–2 µL of air followed by drug. Always double-check that the air-bubble is identifiable between the water and drug. Thus, during the injection, drug enters the gelfoam immediately because the internal portion of the PE-50 injection tubing is directly touching the gelfoam. Thus, there is no internal catheter volume that must be voided prior to drug entry into gelfoam.
3. Keep in mind, the length of the injection catheter will vary depending on the volume of drug injection. A 1.0 µL volume occupies approx 0.41 cm of PE-50 tubing.
4. Animals are gently placed in crumpled soft cotton towels and allowed to move freely underneath the towels (*see* **Note 6**).
5. The cc-sleeve area is exposed, the indwelling concave rubber plug is removed with a dental probe, and the folded portion of the silastic catheter is exteriorized.
6. Fluid that had accumulated in the indwelling silastic catheter is suctioned off with the perisciatic catheter cleaner and discarded.

7. This is followed by drug injection using the prepared PE-50 injectors (described above). The 7.3 cm mark on the PE-50 tubing of the perisciatic catheter injector is flush with the edge of the silastic catheter to ensure that the tip of the PE-50 tubing is 2–3 mm inside the gelfoam and near (but not touching) the sciatic nerve. All drug injections are followed by a 20 μL saline flush (*see* **Note 7**).

8. Chronic allodynia is maintained for more than 2 wk by repeated injections every 2 d that are conducted in steps identical to that described in **steps 1–7.**

9. In chronic allodynia, an additional step of cleaning the inside of the cc-sleeve with a separate perisciatic catheter cleaner is done to decrease bacterial build-up. Perisciatic catheter and cc-sleeve cleaning followed by drug injections are done every 2 d to maintain chronic allodynia. Using this paradigm, unilateral and bilateral allodynia remain stable during the entire testing period in terms of both pattern (i.e., unilateral does not change to bilateral nor the reverse) and magnitude.

3.5. Intrathecal Catheter Injectors and Injections

3.5.1. Intrathecal Catheter Injectors

1. The blunt end of a sterile 30-G, $^1/_2$-inch hypodermic needle, with the plastic hub removed (using the same method used for removing the plastic hub from the 18-G needle, as described in **Subheading 3.3.1.**), is inserted into a 30 cm length PE-10 tube.

2. Additionally, an intact sterile 30-G, $^1/_2$-inch hypodermic needle is inserted into the open end of the PE-10 tube.

3. Prepared catheter injectors are stored in a sterile, dry place until the time of injections.

3.5.2. Intrathecal Catheter Injections

1. A 50 μL autoclaved Hamilton glass syringe and a PE-10 it catheter injector are flushed with sterile, endotoxin-free water and are connected to each other, and made air-tight, as described in **Subheading 3.4.3.**

2. Additionally, air bubbles are then created in the PE-10 tubing of the it catheter injector between the sterile water, 8 μL saline and drug as described in **Subheading 3.4.3.**

3. Animals are placed in crumpled soft cotton towels, the cc-sleeve area is exposed, the indwelling concave rubber plug is removed with a dental probe, and the it catheter is exteriorized.

4. These injections are completed over a 2–3 min period for careful drug delivery. The two air bubbles are watched carefully for compression or fast decompression indicating problems with drug delivery within the spinal canal that may lead to alterations in behavioral testing independent of drug effects (*see* **Note 8**).

5. The tip of the it catheter is re-sealed using heated forceps and folded back into the cc-sleeve after the injection.

6. All drug injections are followed by an 8 μL saline flush for complete drug delivery.

3.6. Low-Threshold Mechanical Allodynia

1. The von Frey test measures stimulus response thresholds to a series of calibrated light-pressure monofilaments to the ventral aspect of the rat hind paws. All animals are habituated and tested as previously described *(17)*. Briefly, rats are placed in testing chambers in a dimly lit, quiet room for 4 d, 1 h/d prior to surgery (*see* **Note 9**).
2. The testing chambers are clear Plexiglas cylinders (24 cm [H] × 16.5 cm [D]) made from 4000 mL beakers with the bottom sawed off and placed atop an elevated plastic coated grill (bars spaced approx 2.2 cm).
3. Weighted cardboard squares are placed on top of the cylinders to deter the rats from exploring/jumping out of the containers.
4. Four to five d after surgery, any animal that showed detectable hind paw retraction is excluded. We have observed less than 1% of the total animals implanted with perisciatic catheters display hind paw retraction.
5. Animals are placed in the testing chamber and allowed to adjust to the experimental context for 20–30 min. Baseline (BL) responses to the monofilaments are then assessed, consisting of two to three trials spaced approx 15 min apart. The left and right hind paws are probed randomly with the monofilaments according to specific procedures, as describe previously *(17)*.
6. Here briefly described, the monofilament at about the mid-range of the logarithmic series, labeled 2.041 g, is applied for 8 s twice at 10-s intervals (at minimum) to the left and right hind paws.
7. In the event of a paw withdrawal to the 2.041 g monofilament for two consecutive trials to the same hind paw, the 0.407 g monofilament (the lightest monofilament of the logarithmic series) is then presented. This is done to assess the 100% threshold (responses for two out of two trials) to the *lightest* stimulus presentation in the logarithmic series.
8. Thus, in the absence of a response to the 0.407 g monofilament, presentation of monofilaments continues in ascending order (0.692 g, 1.202, and so on), until a clear response for two consecutive trials (indicated 100% threshold to that stimulus) is elicited and no further probing is conducted. All single responses (one out of two trials) are recorded and entered into the "PsychoFit" software program to assess 50% threshold values (described below).
9. If the 2.041 g monofilament fails to elicit a response for two consecutive trials, the next higher monofilament is used (3.630 g). Again, presentation of monofilaments continues in ascending order and stops when a monofilament elicits clear responses for two consecutive trials. All single responses are recorded and used to assess 50% threshold values. Testing the stability of the 100% response threshold either repeatedly for 2 h (at 20-min intervals) or for several weeks (two trials per day), consistently yields responses between 4.74 (5.495 g) and 5.18 (15.136 g).
10. Data collected from left and right hind paws can be averaged prior to analysis or analyzed separately depending on the experimental paradigm. For example, we have previously shown that bilateral allodynia is produced by spinal inflammation

compared to controls *(17,18)*. No reliable left and right hind paw differences were observed, therefore data from both hind paws were averaged. Alternatively, we have also shown that data from left and right hind paws, analyzed separately, revealed unilateral and bilateral allodynia after induction of left sciatic inflammatory neuropathy *(8–10)*.

3.7. Testing for Low-Threshold Mechanical Allodynia After it and Perisciatic Catheterization

1. Procedures used prior to surgery for habituation to the testing context are the same as described in **Subheading 3.6.** However, several steps are added when both catheterization procedures are conducted.
2. Rats are weighed to roughly assess recovery from it and perisciatic catheterization. These rats typically lose 5% of body weight by 5 d after surgery. Animals that lose more than 10% of their presurgery body weights (<2% of animals) are excluded.
3. At the time body weights are recorded, the it catheter is removed from the hub of the cc-sleeve and is visually inspected for blood inside the catheter. Rats with it catheters containing blood (<1%) are also excluded. We have observed hind paw retraction in approx 2% of all rats implanted with only the it catheter. However, after both the perisciatic and it catheterization procedures are conducted, we have observed (at postoperative d 5) up to 5% of animals display hind paw retraction that must be excluded. The reason for this difference is unknown.

3.8. Interpolation of 50% Threshold

The behavioral data are a collection of psychometric responses that are best described by 50% response thresholds; that is, absolute threshold. Thus, the log stiffness that would have resulted in a 50% paw withdrawal rate is computed by fitting a Gaussian integral psychometric function to the observed withdrawal rates for each of the tested monofilaments at each time point using a maximum-likelihood fitting method *(19,20)*. The slope of the psychometric function is set at 3.32 and corresponds to a standard deviation of 3.01 of the underlying Gaussian probability distribution. The range of the response probability is from 0.0 to a maximum of 1.0. Previous reports that have fit psychometric data to a Gaussian integral function estimate 50% thresholds using a different methodology that yields the same results *(21,22)*. However, with the ease of computer software, the method described here is advantageous in that: (1) all patterns of responses are reflected in the estimated 50% thresholds, and (2) it is flexible in the number of trials desired for testing (i.e., four trials presented/stimulus intensity) requiring trivial adjustments in the software program. The estimated thresholds derived from a Gaussian integral function are part of a continuous data set and yield a mathematical continuum that are appropriate for parametric statistical analysis *(8,17,18,20)*.

The "PsychoFit(fat)" software program for: (1) fitting psychometric data to a Gaussian integral function, and (2) computing estimated 50% thresholds using the maximum-likelihood fitting method, is available for both Macintosh and PC computers. The program is written in Microsoft Word and saved as a "text only" file.

3.8.1. PsychoFit (fat) Software Program: Setting Alpha and Beta Values in Initial Four Lines of Program

After downloading the program and information from L. O. Harvey's website (http://psych.colorado.edu/~lharvey), open the "example" file and set the terms as follows (*see* **Fig. 3**):

1. The minimum alpha to 0.0,
2. The maximum alpha to 10.0,
3. Minimum beta to 0.001 and
4. Maximum beta to 11.0. These terms are specified once and take up the first three lines of the program.

3.8.2. PsychoFit (fat) Software Program: Setting Parameters Within Each Trial

Additionally, change labels and parameters within each trial as follows (*see* **Fig. 3**).

1. Change "Title" to the appropriate rat identification and trial number.
2. In the next line, change "1 1 1 0 0 Do Logistic, Weibull, Gaussian but not Poisson and Step" to "0 0 1 0 0 Fit Gaussian Integral."
3. Change the Alpha and Beta flags from "1 1" to "1 0."
4. Set the Alpha (starting value) to 3.610000.
5. Set the Beta (starting value) to 10.00000.
6. Set the Gamma (fixed value) to 0.000000.
7. Set the Delta (fixed value) to 0.000100.
8. Set the Percent Confidence Interval to 95.00000.
9. Change the "31 Log Contrast, Number Correct, Number Incorrect" to "10 Log Force, Number Withdrawals, Number Nonwithdrawals," which range from 0 to 2 (or to however many stimulus presentations are used; the experimenter can as many as desired.
10. Change each log force according to the stimulus intensity of the von Frey hair used (numbers 1–10 in the far left column; *see* **Fig. 3**). The range of log force stimulus intensities given in **Fig. 3** are based on previously published methods (*17,22*). The settings for the first trial serve as a template for all trials that follow. For example, if three baselines are assessed for the left leg of one rat, then parameters for three trials (each trial consisting of 10 log force stimulus presentations, repeated three times) are created, only changing the pattern of withdrawals vs nonwithdrawals.

```
    00.0          minimum alpha
    10.0          maximum alpha
    00.001        minimum beta
    11.0          maximum beta
Rat1Baseline-1Left
    0 0 1 0 0 Fit Gaussian Integral
    1 0           Alpha and Beta flags
    3.610000      Alpha (starting value)
    10.00000      Beta  (starting value)
    0.000000      Gamma (fixed value)
    0.000100      Delta (fixed value)
    95.00000      Percent Confidence Interval
    10      Log Force, Number Withdrawals, Number Nonwithdrawals
    1       3.61              0                          2
    2       3.84              0                          2
    3       4.08              0                          2
    4       4.17              0                          2
    5       4.31              0                          2
    6       4.56              1                          1
    7       4.74              1                          1
    8       4.93              2                          0
    9       5.07              0                          0
    10      5.18              0                          0
Rat1Trial-1-1Left
    0 0 1 0 0 Fit Gaussian Integral
    1 0           Alpha and Beta flags
    3.610000      Alpha (starting value)
    10.00000      Beta  (starting value)
    0.000000      Gamma (fixed value)
    0.000100      Delta (fixed value)
    95.00000      Percent Confidence Interval
    10      Log Force,   Number Withdrawals, Number Nonwithdrawals
    1       3.61              1                          1
    2       3.84              1                          1
    3       4.08              2                          0
    4       4.17              0                          0
    5       4.31              0                          2
    6       4.56              0                          0
    7       4.74              0                          0
    8       4.93              0                          0
    9       5.07              0                          0
    10      5.18              0                          0
```

Fig. 3. A portion of a data file showing the terms needed to run the "PsychoFit(fat)" program. The data also illustrate two trials for the left hindpaw only. The first trial shows data from a nonallodynic normal rat responding to stimulus intensities at baseline levels. The second trial shows the response patterns to stimulus intensities when that rat became allodynic.

3.8.3. Generating Interpolated 50% Threshold Values

After completion of data entry, be sure to do the following.

1. Do not leave blank spaces or lines between trials.
2. Save the response data as a text only file.
3. Open the "PsychoFit(fat)" program and enter the file name of the response data set. Once the PsychoFit(fat) program recognizes the file, four questions will appear (below). Respond to each as indicated to the right:

Output each iteration from pfit() (y or n)?	n
Print parameter confidence limits (y or n)?	n
Write data to file "PsychoFit.alt" (y or n)?	y
Use bootstrap (enter number of trials or 0)?	0

4. After running the program, the output file is automatically labeled "PsychoFit.alt" (*see* **Note 10**).
5. Import the file into Microsoft Excel and rename it appropriately.
6. Delete all columns except "label", "Function," and "Log Alpha." The data in the "Log Alpha" are the interpolated 50% threshold values.

4. Notes

1. Although the procedure for chronic perisciatic catheter surgery is successful in rats that weigh 250 g, we have found greater ease of enwrapping the sciatic nerve in rats 350 g and heavier. This is likely related to the area the surgeon must work within because manipulating the gelfoam around the sciatic nerve must be done while minimizing nerve stretching.
2. The chronic perisciatic catheter placement can last at least 3.5 wk (we have not tested this procedure for longer periods of time). The cc-sleeve must be sutured to the underlying muscle with two to three 3-0 silk sutures through each flange because the integrity of the silastic catheter is dependent on a long-lasting and regularly cleaned cc-sleeve. We have found that only touching the indwelling perisciatic catheter and all catheter injectors with 70% alcohol-swiped forceps greatly decreases bacterial build-up within the perisciatic silastic catheter and around the cc-sleeve. These areas remain clean throughout the 2-wk period.
3. Placement of the chronic perisciatic catheter can be verified by injecting Evans blue dye (25 µL; 50 mg/mL in 0.9% saline), using a PE-50 microinjector (described above) to verify drug delivery around the sciatic nerve within the gelfoam. It is critical that the dye is found in direct contact with the sciatic nerve. Dye not found to be in direct contact with the nerve is perfectly correlated with failure of zymosan injection to produce allodynia. Indeed, we have previously reported that injection of zymosan into adjoining muscle fails to produce allodynia *(8)*.
4. The cc-sleeve must be kept as clean as possible before and during surgical placement. This is critical to ensure the least amount of inflammation of the muscle and overlaying skin during postsurgical recovery.

5. The it catheter must be anchored securely in place with three 3-0 silk sutures through the PE-10 loop knot and the tough white dense connective tissue that covers the lumbosacral vertebrae. During the 10–15 µL saline injection, it is imperative that the bubble is followed through the PE-10 catheter until it passes into the muscle to ensure a fully patent and leak-proof catheter.

6. Animals placed for several minutes underneath soft cotton towels will typically explore less, and thus injections are easier to conduct. Moreover, injecting unrestrained animals is advantageous because behavioral testing can be reliably assessed within 15 min of injection. Less stressful handling such as this leads to a lower tendency for freezing behavior.

7. Often times, the PE-50 injector will not be able to easily pass beyond the 4-0 silk sutures that are threaded through the silastic tubing (as described in several steps in **Subheadings 3.2.2.** and **3.4.3.**). To troubleshoot this, gently straighten the silastic tube between the thumb and forefinger, and hold the PE-50 tubing of the perisciatic injector between the thumb and forefinger of the other hand at a point past the 7.3 cm marking (i.e., 7.5 cm to avoid bacterial contamination from fingers). Gently twist the PE-50 tubing while inserting it through the silastic catheter. This movement will allow the PE-50 tubing to slip past the 4-0 silk suture.

8. Allowing at least 3 min to conduct the it injection typically results in an overall better injection because the animal shows little to no discomfort after the injection. Some signs of discomfort are typically biting, licking, or scratching of the left hind paw or hind leg area that can last for several minutes after the injection. Better injections are also accomplished in freely moving animals under crumpled cotton towels. However, exploratory movements may become too frequent for ease of injections. Reorienting the animal under the towels usually stops exploration for a short while.

9. Allow 4–5 d for surgical recovery. Often, rats will display weakness in one hindpaw a day or two after surgery and by the third day postsurgery, no abnormal motor movements are observed. Freezing behavior in response to von Frey hair probing is typical in a rat that is not completely habituated. Finally, close temperature regulation (79°F ± 2°), quiet and a dimly lit room enhances habituation to the experimental context and reliability of testing results. Stability of behavioral testing chambers is also essential because vibrations and wiggles cause rats to show elevated paw withdrawal response thresholds to von Frey hairs.

10. The "PsychoFit" program will successfully run only if no blank lines or spaces occur anywhere in the entire data set. Label animal identification and time point without blank spaces. Additionally, when naming the "PsychoFit" data file, do not use special characters or blank spaces. The PsychFit(fat) program will only recognize data files within the same folder where the PsychFit(fat) program occurs. The "PsychoFit" data file is tab delimited to allow the converted data set to be easily imported into Microsoft Excel and to a statistics program such as Statview. Further information about this software program can be found at L. O. Harvey's website (http://psych.colorado.edu/~lharvey).

Acknowledgments

The authors would like to thank Marucia Chacur and Charles B. Armstrong for their outstanding technical assistance. This work was supported by NIMH grants 45045, MH01558, MH50479; NIH grant NS38020; the University of Colorado Undergraduate Research Opportunities Program; and the Hughes Initiative for Undergraduate Research.

References

1. Frisen, J., Risling, M., and Fried, K. (1993) Distribution and axonal relations of macrophages in a neuroma. *Neuroscience* **55,** 1003–1013.
2. Said, G. and Hontebeyrie-Joskowicsz, M. (1992) Nerve lesions induced by macrophage activation. *Res. Immunol.* **143,** 589–599.
3. Bourque, C. N., Anderson, B. A., Martin del Campo, C., and Sima, A. A. (1985) Sensorimotor perineuritis: an autoimmune disease? *Can. J. Neurol. Sci.* **12,** 129–133.
4. Bennett, G. J. and Xie, Y. K. (1988) A peripheral mononeuropathy in rat that produces disorders of pain sensation like those seen in man. *Pain* **33,** 87–107.
5. DeLeo, J. A., Coombs, D. W., Willenbring, S., et al. (1994) Characterization of a neuropathic pain model: sciatic cryoneurolysis in the rat. *Pain* **56,** 9–16.
6. Kim, S. H. and Chung, J. M. (1992) An experimental model for peripheral neuropathy produced by segmental spinal nerve ligation in the rat. *Pain* **50,** 355–363.
7. Seltzer, Z., Dubner, G., and Shir, Y. (1990) A novel behavioral model of neuropathic pain disorders produced in rats by partial sciatic nerve injury. *Pain* **43,** 205–218.
8. Chacur, M., Milligan, E. D., Gazda, L. S., et al. (2001) A new model od sciatic inflammatory neuritis (SIN): induction of unilateral and bilateral mechanical allodynia following acute unilateral peri-sciatic immune activation in rats. *Pain* **94,** 231–244.
9. Gazda, L. S., Milligan, E. D., Hansen, M. K., et al. (2001) Sciatic inflammatory neuritis (SIN): behavioral allodynia is paralleled by peri-sciatic proinflammatory cytokine and superoxide production. *J. Periph. Nerv. Syst.* **6,** 111–129.
10. Milligan, E. M., Twining, C. M., Chacur, M., et al. (2003) Spinal glia and proinflammatory cytokines mediate mirror-image neuropathic pain. *J. Neuroscience* **23,** 1026–1040.
11. Eliav, E., Herzberg, U., Ruda, M. A., and Bennett, G. (1999) Neuropathic pain from an experimental neuritis of the rat sciatic nerve. *Pain* **83,** 169–182.
12. Lockwood, L. L., Silbert, L. H., Laudenslager, M. L., et al. (1993) Anesthesia-induced modulation of in vivo antibody levels. *Anesthesia Analgesia* **77,** 769–775.
13. Sato, W., Enzan, K., Masaki, Y., et al. (1995) The effect of isoflurane on the secreation of TNF-alpha and IL-1 beta from LPS-stimulated human peripheral blood monocytes. *Masui* **44,** 971–975.
14. Milligan, E. D., Hinde, J. L., Mehmert, K. K., et al. (1999) A method for increasing the viability of the external portion of lumbar catheters placed in the spinal subarachnoid space of rats. *J. Neurosci. Methods* **90,** 81–86.

15. Storkson, R. V., Kjorsvik, A., Tjolsen, A., and Hole, K. (1996) Lumbar catheterization of the spinal subarachnoid space in the rat. *J. Neurosci. Methods* **65,** 167–172.
16. Greene, E. C. (1935) Nervous system, in *Anatomy of the Rat,* vol. 27. The American Philosophical Society, Philadelphia.
17. Milligan, E. D., Mehmert, K. K., Hinde, J. L., et al. (2000) Thermal hyperalgesia and mechanical allodynia produced by intrathecal administration of the human immunodefiency virus-1 (HIV-1) envelope glycoprotein, gp120. *Brain Res.* **861,** 105–116.
18. Milligan, E. D., O'Connor, K. A., Nguyer, K.T., Armstrong, C. A., et al. (2001) Intrathecal HIV-1 envelope glycoprotein gp120 induces enhanced pain states mediated by spinal cord proinflammatory cytokines. *J. Neurosci.* **21,** 2808–2819.
19. Harvey Jr, L. O. (1986) Efficient estimation of sensory thresholds. *Behav. Res. Methods Intrum. Comput.* **18,** 623–632.
20. Treutwein, B. and Strasburger, H. (1999) Fitting the psychometric function. *Perception Psychophys.* **61,** 87–106.
21. Dixon, W. (1980) Efficient analysis of experimental observations. *Annu. Rev. Pharmacol. Toxicol.* **20,** 441–462.
22. Chaplan, S., Bach, F., Pogrel, J., et al. (1994) Quantitative assessment of tactile allodynia in the rat paw. *J. Neurosci. Methods* **53,** 55–63.

8

A Rat Pain Model of Vincristine-Induced Neuropathy

Emiliano S. Higuera and Z. David Luo

Summary

Vincristine belongs to the family of vinca alkaloids used for treatment of malignant tumors. Clinical application of these agents is often associated with dose-dependent painful neuropathy due to damages to the peripheral axons. A rat model of vincristine-induced hyperalgesia was developed through intravenous injection of vincristine by Aley et al. (1996) and was later modified by Nozaki-Taguchi et al. (2001) using continuous intravenous infusion of vincristine. This model provides consistent and long-lasting neuropathic pain states mimicking vincristine-induced pain conditions in human patients. Therefore, this model is a valuable means of studying the mechanisms and pharmacology of vincristine-induced neuropathic pain. In this chapter we describe in detail steps the generation of vincristine-induced neuropathy in rats through continuous intravenous infusion of vincristine.

Key Words: Rats; vincristine; neuropathic pain; chemotherapy; continuous infusion; Alzet mini-pumps; intravenous catheterization; tactile allodynia; allodynia testing.

1. Introduction

Neuropathic pain is a common clinical syndrome caused by nerve injuries. In addition to physical nerve injuries, other common etiologies include metabolic disorders (such as diabetic neuropathy) and viral infections (such as shingles, and HIV-induced neuropathies). Neurotoxic agent-induced neuropathy is also a common cause of neuropathic pain among patients receiving chemotherapy and antiviral treatments. Experimental data have indicated that neurotoxic-agent induced neuropathic pain has distinct pharmacology and biochemical changes in the spinal cord and dorsal-root ganglia compared with other neuropathies, even though the behavioral manifestations are similar among different pain-inducing pathologies (1). This suggests that similar neuropathic pain states may have distinct underlying mechanisms depending on the pathology

From: *Methods in Molecular Medicine, Vol. 99: Pain Research: Methods and Protocols*
Edited by: Z. D. Luo © Humana Press Inc., Totowa, NJ

of the disorder. Thus, appropriate models mimicking pain-inducing conditions in human patients are critical in studying mechanisms of nociception.

In this chapter, we describe in detail the generation of a rat pain model derived from vincristine-induced neuropathy. Vincristine belongs to the family of vinca alkaloids that are used for treatment of malignant tumors. It is believed that these agents exert their anti-tumor efficacy by inhibiting mitosis through binding to tubulin in mitotically active cells, disrupting microtubule formation in the mitotic spindle *(2,3)*. Thus, clinical application of these agents is often associated with dose-dependent painful neuropathy owing to damages to the peripheral axons *(4)*. To mimic vincristine-induced pain conditions in human patients, a rat model of vincristine-induced hyperalgesia was first developed by Aley et al. in 1996 by daily intravenous (iv) injection of vincristine for 2 wk *(5)*. This model was later modified later by Nozaki-Taguchi et al. in 1999 by continuous iv infusion of vincristine for the same duration *(6)*. We found that the latter approach can provide consistent and long-lasting neuropathic pain states without the need for daily injections, thereby limiting the stress to the animal and investigator alike. Therefore, this model is a valuable means of studying the mechanisms and pharmacology of vincristine-induced neuropathic pain.

2. Materials

1. Male Sprague-Dawley rats (300–400 g; Harlan Industries).
2. Vincristine Sulfate Salt (Sigma Cat. no. V8879).
3. Alzet mini-osmotic pumps (Durect Corporation Cat. no. 2002).
4. PE-50 tubing (BD Cat. no. 427411).
5. PE-60 tubing (BD Cat. no. 427416).
6. 28-G and 20-G stainless-steel wire.
7. 20 G Luer stub adaptors (blunt-tip needles) (BD Cat. no. 427546). In place of the 20-G stainless steel wire, a 20-G Luer stub adaptor can be removed from the plastic fitting and plugged with clay, to be used as a plug for the PE-60 tubing.
8. 16-G needle 1 $1/2$ inches or similar gauge Trocar.
9. Sterile water and sterile heparanized saline.
10. 1 mL syringes with 20-G Luer stub needles attached. One filled with vincristine and one filled with heparanized saline.
11. Surgical scrub.
12. Isopropanol.
13. Scalpel handle and blades.
14. Blunt tipped scissors.
15. Micro-forceps.
16. Vessel dilator (not necessary, but nice).
17. Curved forceps (small, 10 cm long).
18. Toothed forceps or suture tying forceps.
19. Needle holders.

20. A nonabsorbable, sterile, surgical, monofilament suture Ethilon or the like (Ethilon by Ethicon Cat. no. G698G).
21. 3-0 silk suture.
22. Touch Test Sensory Evaluator Kit/von Frey filaments (Stoelting Company no. 58011).

3. Methods

The methods described below include catheter fabrication **(Subheading 3.1.)**, drug preparation **(Subheading 3.2.)**, jugular vein catheterization **(Subheading 3.3.)** and allodynia testing **(Subheading 3.4.)**.

3.1. Catheter Fabrication

A source of hot air, from a hot air gun or the like, is necessary for the fabrication of the catheter. The fabrication will be the easiest if the stream of air is both slow and narrow (e.g., metal tubing similar to the size of an 18-G needle).

1. Take a piece of PE-50 tubing (about 20 cm), feed a guide wire (28-G, 15 cm) through one end of the tubing.
2. On the side with the wire, slowly heat the tubing about 6–7 cm from the end, rolling gently to melt the tubing evenly. As the tubing begins to melt, push the tubing together to form a bubble. Quickly remove from the air and roll the tubing between your thumb and forefinger, until it is completely cooled.
3. Remove the guide wire and check for patency by flushing the catheter with sterile water (20-G needles fit well into PE-50). If no leaks are present, feed the guide wire about 3–5 cm into the opposite end of the tubing. Place a piece of PE-60 tubing (about 5 cm long) on the exposed piece of guide wire pushing the PE-50 and -60 together. As mentioned in **step 2,** place the two pieces of tubing in the hot air to melt both ends, and push them together to form a bubble. Again, quickly remove the tubing and roll between your thumb and forefinger (*see* **Note 1**).
4. Remove the guide wire when it is completely cooled, flush with sterile water, and check for leaks by blocking the opposite end of the catheter.
5. Before surgery you can soak your catheters in 70% isopropanol, followed by a rinse with sterile water. Just prior to surgery, connect the PE-60 end of your catheter to a 1-mL syringe filled with sterile heparanized saline and fill all dead space of the catheter.

3.2. Drug Preparation

Vincristine should be purchased as close to the usage date as possible. The intravenous dose is 30 µg/kg/d in physiological saline. Because the flow rate of the Alzet mini-pump is 12 µL/d, the vincristine working solution should be about 0.75 µg/µL for a 300 g rat. It is necessary to double the solution needed to fill all pumps. Fill the pumps according to the manufacture's instructions. It is important to prime the pumps, usually overnight, for iv placement. This should also be done following manufacture's instructions.

3.3. Intravenous Catheterization and Pump Placement

It is important to start with 300–400 g rats as they will lose body weight as much as 10–20% owing to the vincristine treatment. Please follow your IAACUC's protocol on weight loss and euthanization.

1. Induce rat anesthesia with 3–5% isoflurane and maintain it with 2–3% isoflurane in clean dry air and O_2.
2. Shave the throat and neck/upper back, scrub with surgical wash (Betadine, Povidine, or similar scrub) and rinse with 70% isopropanol.
3. Position the rat in supine (face up) position, head toward the investigator and tail away from the investigator. Looking down on the rat, identify the left or right clavicle. Just rostral to the clavicle there should be a pulsating mass. This is the external jugular, which travels under the clavicle and connects to the subclavian vein to form the cranial vena cava.
4. Make a 2 cm long skin incision lateral and cephalad (toward the head) of the pulsating mass. Using a pair of blunt-tipped scissors, blunt dissect through the fascia and adipose layers of the throat until the jugular vein is readily visible. Be careful to dissect gently so as not to tear the jugular vein or any of the smaller vessels feeding into it (*see* **Note 2**).
5. Expose the jugular vein about 2 cm in length, and dissect a 1 cm portion free of the surrounding connective tissue. Pass two pieces of 3–0 silk suture (about 7 cm long) under the jugular vein. Place one suture as rostral as possible and the other as caudal as possible. Ligate the rostral suture tightly without tearing the vein or the suture. Use a square knot so that the ligation will not come loose. Make a single loose knot through the suture at the caudal end of the jugular vein so that it will not impede the insertion of the catheter. Place the curved forceps under the vein and open them gently so that they provide traction and gently elevate the vein. Once the forceps are properly placed they do not need to be held. Use micro-forceps to grasp the outer wall of the vessel, and use micro-spring scissors to make an incision in the jugular vein (about one-fourth of the total diameter).
6. With the curved forceps still in place, use the vessel dilator or micro-forceps to open the jugular vein. Insert your catheter, still connected to the 1-mL syringe, as far as possible. Gently remove the vessel dilator and the curved forceps while holding the catheter in place with your free hand. Use forceps to apply gently traction on the rostral silk suture (previously ligated), and advance the catheter, following the natural bend of the vessel, until the "anchoring" bubble is flush against the opening of the jugular vein. While holding the catheter in place, very gently release back traction, readjust the catheter as necessary, and use the curved forceps to readjust the caudal suture so that it is just distal to the bubble. After making sure that the catheter is secure, gently tie the suture around the vessel and the implanted catheter with a pair of toothed forceps or suture tying forceps. It is important to make sure that the suture is as tight as possible, so that there is no possibility of vessel leakage (*see* **Note 3**). Likewise, tie the proximal ligation around the catheter, to help anchoring it. At this point you should be able to draw blood into the catheter freely.

Inject a small amount (0.2–0.4 mL) of heparinized saline slowly and look for vessel damage and/or leakage of the injected saline.

7. Turn the rat over and place it in the prone position (face down). Make sure that the catheter stays in a natural orientation and lay the syringe down next to the rat. Make a 2-cm midline incision starting at the base of the neck and continuing in between the shoulder blades (scapulae). Burrow subcutaneously (sc) (above adipose and muscle layers) toward the jugular vein using a 16-G needle or trocar, turning the rat on its side when necessary. Once the needle is externalized through both incisions, use a 20-G stainless-steel wire to plug the catheter, crimping the catheter while removing the syringe to prevent backflow from the jugular vein. Feed the plugged catheter through the trocar and externalize the catheter on the back (*see* **Note 4**). Remove the trocar, turn rat over, and inspect the catheter. If it is necessary, add more sutures to hold the catheter in a natural position.

8. Remove the stainless-steel wire plug and connect the catheter with the syringe filled with heparanized saline, again crimping to prevent backflow. Flush the catheter with a small amount of saline (0.2–0.4 mL) to ensure that the catheter is patent and there is no extra vascular pooling. Suture the skin on the throat using sterile, 5-0, monofilament nylon suture (Ethilon or the like).

9. Using needle holders or hemostatic forceps, bluntly dissect a compartment between the scapulae large enough to hold the mini-pump. Place the pump into the pocket and exchange the saline-filled syringe for the vincristine-filled syringe. Inject 0.25 mL of the vincristine to fill the catheter (*see* **Note 5**). Note the length of the metal stub on the mini-pump. Remove the syringe and trim the PE-60 portion of the catheter to the length of the metal stub while crimping the catheter (PE-50 side) (*see* **Note 6**). Connect the pump to the catheter. It maybe necessary to force the pump further down into the pocket, so that the entire pump is below the incision (including the metal stub). This will ensure that the pump will not be encapsulated in scar tissue and thus will work properly. Close the skin with sterile, 5-0, monofilament, nylon suture (Ethilon or the like).

3.4. Testing for Tactile Allodynia

A presurgery test is important to determine presurgery threshold. It is also critical to allow a recovery of 2–3 d postsurgery before testing rats. Typically rats should begin to develop allodynia 7–10 d postsurgery and the allodynia state lasts at least 30 d *(6)*. Respiratory distress may develop in the later stage of vincristine treatment and is the most common reason that rats need to be euthanized on or around postoperative d 30. These results have not been quantified or reported in the literature.

The behavioral testing methods described by Chaplan et al. (1994) *(7)* measure the 50% withdrawal threshold of the hind paw to von Frey filament stimulation in awake, unrestrained rats. Briefly, rats are placed in an acrylic-testing chamber with a wire mesh floor so as to permit access to the bottom of the rat's paw. The rats are allowed to acclimate to the testing surroundings until there is little or no exploratory behavior observed (*see* **Note 7**).

Once rats are calm, a series of von Frey filaments with roughly exponential incremental target force (0.4, 1.0, 1.4, 2.0, 4.0, 6.0, 8.0, and 15.0 g) are applied to the bottom of the rat paw, behind the front pads and lateral to the medial pads of the rat. The filament is presented perpendicular to the rat paw and applied with enough force to cause a slight bend. It is held steadily against the paw for a period of 5 s. A response is positive if, within the 5-s period, the rat withdraws from the stimulus or briskly withdraws immediately after the filament is removed. A negative response is one in which the rat does not withdraw within the given time. Testing is usually initiated using the middle filament (2.0 g). A negative response requires the use of next filament with greater bending force. A positive response requires the use of next filament with less bending force. A total of six determinations, starting from the value before the first positive change, are required for the 50% withdrawal threshold calculation described later in this chapter. If a rat does not respond to the 15.0 g filament, the threshold is recorded as 15 g (a maximum value). If a rat respond to the 0.4 g filament, this is typically recorded (a somewhat random designation) as 0.25 g. For vincristine-treated rats, both paws are tested and the average of the two is recorded. By convention, for a rat to be considered allodynic, neither paw can have a threshold of greater than 6 g and the average must be below five grams (*see* **Note 8**). As shown in **Table 1,** we use "X" as a marker of a withdrawal response and "O" as a marker of no response. The 50% response threshold is interpolated using the following formula *(7):*

$$50\% \text{ g threshold} = (10^{[X_f + k\delta]})/10{,}000$$

where X_f = value (in log units) of the final von Frey filament used; k = tabular value found in Chaplan et al. *(7)* and δ = mean difference (in log units) between stimuli. This formula can be plugged into an Excel spreadsheet to calculate the 50% withdrawal threshold in grams. **Table 1** depicts a series of tests to illustrate the testing method.

4. Notes

1. There maybe another way of making the catheter, but we have found the "bubble" method useful as an anchoring source when placing the catheter in the jugular vein. Also, it may seem convenient to make the PE-60 longer and the PE-50 shorter so that you only have to make one anchoring bubble. This is a mistake, because PE-60 is quite stiff and will make running the catheter to the back of rats difficult and may cause shifting of the catheter, discomfort to the animal, and possible vessel leakage.
2. Do not dissect too caudally; stop before the jugular vein enters the pectoral muscle and clavicle. If the dissection is too caudal, nerve damage may occur, leading to partial paralysis of the front ipsilateral paw.
3. Vincristine is extremely toxic and can cause severe tissue damage; therefore, it is very important that there is no leakage around the catheter when vincristine is being infused. Leakage may necessitate euthanizing the animal.

Table 1
Examples of Six Individual von Frey Filament-Testing Results in Rats

Filament	Chart 1	Chart 2	Chart 3	Chart 4	Chart 5	Chart 6
3.61	X	O O O				
4.08	X	X X				
4.17	X	X	O O O			
4.31	X	X	O O	X	O	O
4.56			X X X	X X	O	
4.74				O	O	
4.93				O	O	O
5.18				O	X X X	O

O, Negative response; X, positive response.
Numbers in the left column of each chart (from top to bottom) represent the size of each filament corresponding to the target force in gram of each filament indicated in **Subheading 3.4.**

97

4. It is important to make sure that the catheter is oriented naturally, so that there is no undue pressure on the vein and the catheter is lying straight with no kinks. This will help to minimize any discomfort to the rat and hopefully prevent any irritation owing to the catheter.

5. It is important to ensure that the pump actually pumps vincristine systemically and not just fills the volume of the catheter, because its pumping volume is only about 168 μL. Likewise, the volume necessary to fill the catheter will depend on the total length of the catheter. Therefore, it maybe necessary to check the volume needed to fill, but not overflow the catheter. The volume of 0.25 mL to fill the catheter is just an approximation.

6. It is exceedingly important not to allow any backflow at this step, because the catheter is already primed with vincristine and cannot be flushed again if blood flows into it.

7. For the sanity of the person testing, it is a good idea to test in a quiet environment. Likewise, to maximize objectivity in determining a positive (painful) response, the rats should not be walking/ exploring their testing chamber.

8. This will ensure that experimental rats show consistent and reliable allodynia.

References

1. Luo, Z. D., Calcutt, N. A., Higuera, E. S., et al. (2002) Injury type-specific calcium channel alpha 2 delta-1 subunit up-regulation in rat neuropathic pain models correlates with antiallodynic effects of gabapentin. *J. Pharmacol. Exp. Ther.* **303,** 1199–1205.

2. Himes, R. H., Kersey, R. N., Heller, B. I., and Samson, F. E. (1976) Action of the vinca alkaloids vincristine, vinblastine, and desacetyl vinblastine amide on microtubules in vitro. *Cancer Res.* **36,** 3798–3802.

3. Dumontet, C. and Sikic, B. I. (1999) Mechanisms of action of and resistance to antitubulin agents: microtubule dynamics, drug transport, and cell death. *J. Clin. Oncol.* **17,** 1061–1070.

4. Kaplan, R. S. and Wiernik, P. H. (1982) Neurotoxicity of antineoplastic drugs. *Semin. Oncol.* **9,** 103–130.

5. Aley, K. O., Reichling, D. B., and Levine, J. D. (1996) Vincristine hyperalgesia in the rat: a model of painful vincristine neuropathy in humans. *Neuroscience* **73,** 259–265.

6. Nozaki-Taguchi, N., Chaplan, S. R., Higuera, E. S., et al. (2001) Vincristine-induced allodynia in the rat. *Pain* **93,** 69–76.

7. Chaplan, S. R., Bach, F. W., Pogrel, J. W., et al. (1994) Quantitative assessment of tactile allodynia in the rat paw. *J. Neurosci. Methods* **53,** 55–63.

9

Loop Dialysis Catheter

A Technology for Chronic Spinal Dialysis in a Freely Moving Rat

Martin Marsala

Summary

To permit long-term measurement of time-dependent changes in levels of dialyzable drugs and transmitters in the spinal intrathecal (IT) space of the unanesthetized rat, we developed a dialysis catheter for chronic placement. This was accomplished by constructing a loop-flexible probe 9 cm in length from PE-5 polyethylene tubing and 4 cm dialysis membrane. This loop catheter was inserted through an incision in the cisternal membrane and passed to the lumbar enlargement. The ends of the catheter were then externalized on the top of the head. For dialysis, an external end of the loop catheter was connected to a syringe pump and perfused with artificial cerebrospinal fluid (CSF) and the out flow collected. Using this system we demonstrate: a) a significant increase in spinal CSF concentrations of amino acids after spinal traumatic injury, b) the permeability of a drug (methylprednisolone) through the blood–brain barrier into the spinal extracellular space after systemic delivery, c) effect of IT injection of *N*-methyl-D-aspartate on secondary amino acid release, and c) clearance of sufentanyl after IT delivery and corresponding development of thermal nociception. The loop dialysis catheter provides a robust experimental tool for studying time-dependent changes in the concentration of diffusible substances in spinal CSF over an extended postimplantation interval and allows comparison of these changes with concurrently assessed behavioral indices.

Key Words: Spinal Cord; intrathecal microdialysis; rat; neurotransmitter release.

1. Introduction

An important experimental method for assessing the role of specific neurotransmitter systems is to determine the extravascular-extracellular levels of the agent in the vicinity of the terminals from which the neurotransmitter is released. Ex vivo methods, such as minces or slices, have advantages because they permit exposure of specific brain or spinal-cord sites. On the other hand, such methods typically remove the connectivity that is essential for the inter-

From: *Methods in Molecular Medicine, Vol. 99: Pain Research: Methods and Protocols*
Edited by: Z. D. Luo © Humana Press Inc., Totowa, NJ

pretation of mechanism. The use of in vivo models, although inherently more complex, has found favor because they permit assessment of the physiology of an intact system. Several approaches for measuring the extracellular levels of neurotransmitters and/or peptides have been developed. The use of voltametric electrodes may be an advantage, but they are limited to the nature of the product they can measure and they retain problems of selectivity. Accordingly, sampling from the extracellular space followed by assays of the spinal perfusate has been the method of choice. In brain, local perfusion techniques, such as the push–pull cannula *(1)*, or superfusion of portions of the cerebrospinal *(2)* or spinal *(3)* axis have been employed. Such superfusion techniques are limited in that they involve unpredictable perfusion pathways and depend on unobstructed patency to avoid tissue injury. Therefore, the application of dialysis membrane devices has attracted increasing attention. Such probes, typically concentric in nature, have been described and widely employed in brain research *(4)*.

In the past 15 yr, there has been an increasing interest in the transmitter pharmacology of the spinal cord. Dialysis systems have been developed in which a concentric cannula is inserted into the tissue *(5)* or a single fiber is inserted transversally through the parenchyma *(6,7)*. These models, although sampling the parenchyma, are typically unstable and difficult to maintain for extended periods in the unanesthetized animal and require an extensive exposure after removing portions of the paravertebral musculature and a partial laminectomy. In recent work, we have developed an alternative model, the loop dialysis catheter, which limits surgical exposure and permits extended dialysis sampling of the lumbar intrathecal space in the unanesthetized and relatively unrestrained rat for intervals in excess of 10 d *(8)*, (**Fig. 1A**). In this chapter, we describe the construction of the catheter and representative experiments emphasizing the utility of this experimental preparation.

2. Materials

1. Microdialysis hollow fibers (300 µm OD; 11 kDa cut-off; Filtral, AN 69-HF).
2. Nichrome-Formvar wire (OD-0.0026 ″; A-M Systems, Inc.).
3. Polyethylene (PE)-10 tubing (Marsil Scientific, San Diego, CA; Spectranetics, Colorado Springs, CO).
4. Double lumen PE-5 tubing (Marsil Scientific; Spectranetics).
5. Polycarbonate tubing (OD-194 µm, ID-102 µm; Polymicro Technologies Inc., Phoenix, AZ).
6. Cyanoacrylate: Super glue.
7. Stereotaxic headholder (Marsil Scientific).
8. Artificial cerebrospinal fluid (ACSF; in mM): 2.5 mM Na$_2$HPO$_4$, 2.6 mM KCl; 1.3 mM CaCl$_2$, 3.9 mM dextrose; 125 mM NaCl, 21 mM NaHCO$_3$, 0.9 mM MgCl$_2$.

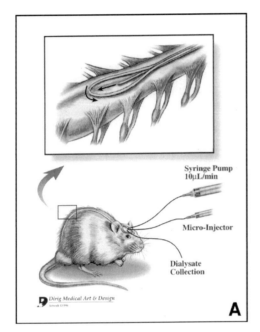
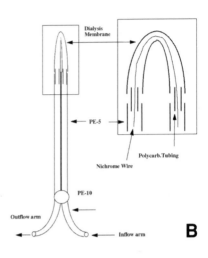

Fig. 1. **(A)** Schematic drawing of the triple loop-style intrathecal dialysis catheter implanted into the lumbar intrathecal space. **(B)** Details of the dialysis loop catheter (see text for details).

3. Methods

The methods outlined here describe: (1) construction of the dialysis catheter, (2) in vivo implantation of the loop catheter, (3) preparation of animals for dialysis sample collection, and (4) a sample of representative experiments outlining the experimental utility of this system.

3.1. Construction of the Dialysis Catheter

Intrathecal loop dialysis catheters are constructed from dialysis hollow fibers attached to a double lumen PE-5 catheter **(Fig. 1B)**. The whole procedure of catheter construction can be divided into several sequential steps:

1. Two pieces of PE-10 tubing (4.5 cm in length) are heat-connected to a double lumen PE- 5 catheter (9 cm length).
2. Patency of the PE-10/PE-5 connection is then tested by perfusing both arms of the catheter by saline followed by air flush to dry the PE tubing (*see* **Note 1**).
3. Two pieces of polycarbonate tubings (1 cm length each) are inserted (0.5 cm deep) into the distal ends of the double lumen of the PE-5 catheter.
4. A 4 cm long piece of dialysis tubing is then cut and Nichrome-Formvar wire (8 cm length) is then passed through the dialysis fiber (*see* **Note 2**).

5. Both ends of the Nichrome-Formvar wire are then inserted into two pieces of poly-carbonate tubing previously inserted into PE-5 double lumen catheter.
6. The wire is gently pushed into the polycarbonate tubing to the point where both ends of microdialysis membranes are in contact with both ends of the double lumen PE-5 catheter.
7. Two small drops of Superglue are then applied at the junction of both ends of the microdialysis fiber using a 30-G needle tip. Any excess Superglue is wiped of.
8. After 20–30 min, the catheter is flushed with hexane followed by air. If any leakage is observed at the microdialysis vs PE-5 tubing joint, Superglue is applied again and the catheter retested with hexane.
9. A microdialysis loop is then bent at the tip forming a U-shape catheter tip.
10. Completed catheters are stored in self-seal pouches (V. Mueller; Cat. no. 92308) and sterilized using ethylene oxide (*see* **Notes 3** and **4**).

3.2. Implantation of the Loop Dialysis Catheter in Rat

1. The rat is anesthetized with 2.5% halothane in a room air and oxygen mixture (1:1), and the back of the head and neck are shaved. Anesthesia is maintained with 1.5% halothane delivered by mask throughout the entire surgical procedure.
2. After induction the animal is placed in a stereotaxic headholder with the head flexed forward (*see* **Chapter 9**).
3. The back of the head is prepared with Betadine solution.
4. A midline incision is made on the back of the neck, the muscle is freed at the attachment to the skull and retracted with a flat elevator, exposing the cisternal membrane.
5. The membrane is opened with a 22-G needle and retracted with a small dural hook.
6. The loop portion of the catheter is then inserted through the cisternal opening and passed caudally 9 cm into the intrathecal space. This places the active dialysis loop section of the catheter at the T11-L5 spinal segment (*see* **Notes 5** and **6**).
7. After implantation animals are allowed to recover for a minimum of 2–3 d prior to experimentation. Rats showing motor weakness or paresis upon recovery from anesthesia are euthanized (*see* **Note 7**).

3.3. Catheter Perfusion, Dialysis Sample Collection, and Analysis

1. On the day of dialysis, one of the externalized PE-10 arms (**Fig. 1B**, Inflow arm) is attached to 30 cm of PE-10 tubing and the other arm to 25 cm of PE-10 (**Fig. 1B**, Outflow arm) (*see* **Notes 8** and **9**).
2. A syringe pump is connected and the dialysis tubing perfused with ACSF at a rate of 2–10 µL/min.
3. All experimental manipulations are preceded by a 30-min washout period and collection of two control samples (10 min each); dialysate samples are collected on ice and frozen at −20°C until analysis for amino acids and/or PGE$_2$; where both are assayed, samples were split prior to freezing.
4. Dialysis samples are routinely analyzed for a variety of amino acids; analysis is accomplished by the use of the PITC (phenyl isothiocyanate) derivatization proce-

dure using a Waters high-performance liquid chromatography (HPLC) with a reverse-phase C18 column (3.9 × 300 mm, 4 μm particle) and ultraviolet (UV) detector; amino acid content is measured from single 25 μL aliquots; methionine sulphone is added to each amino acid sample and used as an internal standard (sensitivity is 5–10 pmol/injection); amino acid peak heights are initially normalized to the methionine sulphone peak and then quantified based on a linear relationship between peak height and amounts of corresponding standards; external standards are run daily.

5. Dialysate concentration of PGE_2 is determined using a commercially available assay (Advanced Magnetics Inc., Cambridge, MA); the antibody is selective for PGE_2 with less than 1.0% cross-reactivity to PGF_{1a}, 6-keto PGF_{1a}, PGD_2, or PGs of the A, B, or D series, but cross-reacts with PGE_1. Assay sensitivity is 2.8 fmol/sample.

3.4. Experimental Studies

3.4.1. Traumatic Spinal-Cord Injury

To induce spinal compression in halothane anesthetized animals with previously implanted dialysis catheters, a 2F-Fogarty catheter was placed at the L1–L2 level in the spinal epidural space, through a partial laminectomy of the L5 vertebra. The balloon was inflated with saline for 60 s. After compression, animals recovered and survived for an additional 4 h, during which time dialysate samples were collected and analyzed for aspartate, glutamate, and prostaglandin E_2 (PGE_2). During the postcompression period, motor and sensory functions were evaluated by assessing flaccidity/spasticity and the response to hindpaw pinch. The placement of the epidural catheter had no effect on baseline concentrations of amino acids and PGE_2. Spinal-cord compression evoked significant increases in the concentration of aspartate (1242%; $p < 0.01$) and glutamate (1036%; $p < 0.01$) detected during the initial 10 min after compression, followed by a gradual decrease over the 4-h postcompression period. However, both amino acids showed significant increases at the end of 4 hr ($p < 0.05$) (**Fig. 2**). Similarly, PGE_2 levels increased immediately after compression (325%; $p < 0.05$) with gradual normalization in 1–2 h after trauma. Between 2 and 4 h postcompression, a secondary increase occurred and the concentrations reached even higher levels than those seen immediately after the compression. Neurologically, all animals displayed complete flaccid paralysis with loss of sensory function. This state remained unchanged for 4 h.

3.4.2. Systemic Drug Delivery and Spinal Cerebrospinal Fluid Concentration

To study the permeability of a drug through the blood–brain barrier into the spinal extracellular space after systemic delivery, methylprednisolone (MP) (20 mg/kg) was injected intravenously (iv) (left jugular vein) during a 30-s

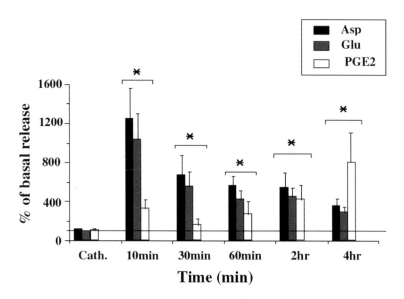

Fig. 2. The effect of spinal-cord compression on the spinal CSF glutamate, aspartate, and PGE_2 levels for the period of 4 h after injury. Note a biphasic PGE_2 release with the second peak seen at 4 h (*$p < 0.05$).

interval in halothane-anesthetized rats ($n = 3$). After injection, spinal dialysate samples were collected in 10-min intervals for 2 h. The concentration of MP in dialysate was determined by FID-gas chromatography (GC) using dexamethasone as an internal standard. After injection the concentrations of MP in the spinal cerebrospinal fluid (CSF) were as follows: (μmol/ml): 10 min < 0.01; 20 min = 0.08 ± 0.02; 30 min = 0.4 ± 0.1; 40 min = 2.3 ± 1.3; 50 min = 3.2 ± 2.4; 60 min = 4 ± 1.9; 70 min = 3.8 ± 2.2; 80 min 4.1 ± 2.5; 90 min = 3.9 ± 2.8; 100 min = 3.2 ± 1.7; 110 min = 2 ± 1.8; 120 min = 1.8 ± 1.6.

3.4.3. Intrathecal NMDA Injection and Spinal Amino Acid Release

To demonstrate the spinal CSF levels of amino acids after intrathecal (it) injection of N-methyl-D-aspartate acid (NMDA), rats were implanted with intrathecal dialysis catheters and an additional it catheter for spinal drug delivery. Two days after implantation, the animals were anesthetized with 2% halothane and maintained with 0.5–0.7% halothane. After baseline samples were collected, NMDA (1 μg) dissolved in saline was injected intrathecally. Five sequential dialysate samples were collected at 8-min intervals. Injection of NMDA evoked a significant release of glutamate and taurine with the peak seen 8 min after injection (**Fig. 3**).

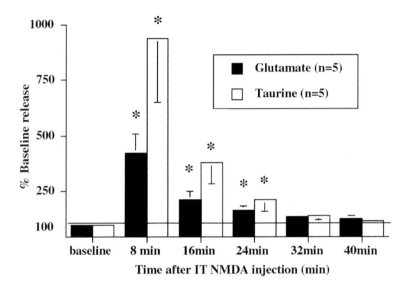

Fig. 3. The effect of it injection of NMDA (5 μg) on spinal CSF glutamate and taurine concentrations. Significant increase in the concentration of both neurotransmitters during the initial 24 min after injection was seen ($*p < 0.05$).

3.4.4. Clearance of Sufentanyl from Intrathecal Space and Corresponding Development of Thermal Nociception

Animals previously implanted with triple dialysis catheters were injected with 3H-sufentanil (1 μg; Janssen, Belgium). Before and after injection, the baseline thermal nociceptive response was measured at 5-min intervals using a hot plate. During the same period, dialysate samples were collected in 60-s intervals and the activity of the drug in the it space was determined using a γ-scintillation counter. Immediately after injection, all animals showed a significant increase in thermal withdrawal latencies and this behavioral effect corresponded with a peak concentration of the injected drug **(Fig. 4A,B)**. Thermal withdrawal latencies returned back to baseline at 50 min after injection. At the same time, an approximate sixfold decrease in the it sufentanyl activity, as compared to immediate postinjection activity, was observed.

4. Notes

1. The patency and a possible leakage of each catheter have to be checked by perfusing the catheter with hexane only. Perfusion with saline or any other "water"-based solution will cause the dialysis membrane to shrink and bend once the perfusion fluid is vaporizing.

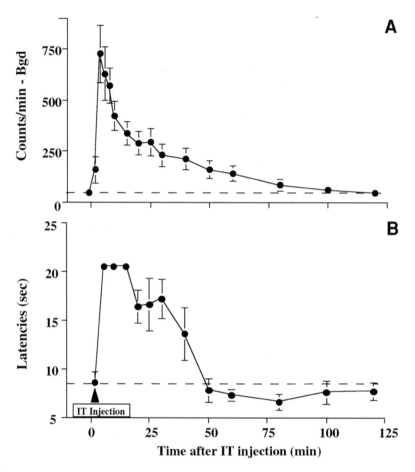

Fig. 4. Spinal CSF levels of sufentanil and corresponding changes in thermal nociceptive threshold after it injection of sufentanil (10 μg). Note the peak of it drug concentration **(A)** and corresponding loss of thermal sensitivity **(B)** immediately after it
sufentanil injection.

2. The length of the dialysis membrane can vary. We typically use membrane lengths
   between 1.8 and 4 cm, which corresponds to a recovery rate between 15 and 30%
   for glucose and glutamate at a perfusion rate between 2 and 10 μL/min.
3. Completed and hexane-tested catheters can be stored in sterilization pouches for
   several months once the catheters are sterilized.
4. If it is desired to inject an agent it in addition to a microdialysis sample collection,
   a triple lumen PE-5 catheter is used **(Fig. 1A)**. The procedure to construct the triple
   dialysis catheter is identical to the procedure described above. The middle lumen of
   the triple catheter is used for it drug injection.

5. The initial attempts to implant dialysis catheters can be quite challenging, particularly when no previous experience or supervision of an experienced experimentator is available. It is suggested to initiate the training by using a simple it catheter (PE-10 or PE-5; 8.5 cm length; *see* Chapter 9). The optimal weight of animals used for implantation is between 300 and 400 g.

6. Particular attention should be paid to the occurrence of it bleeding resulting from the rupture of posterior spinal arteries. It is typically caused by a forced insertion of the catheter. Should this happen, it is suggested to sacrifice the animal, because the presence of a blood clot at the vicinity of the dialysis membrane can significantly affect the profile of measured amino acids/prostaglandin concentration.

7. Placement of the catheter in the hands of a trained operator takes approx 20 min. In a prospective series of more then 500 rats, 35 rats were sacrificed owing to motor dysfunction, whereas 22 rats were sacrificed because of occlusion of the dialysis catheter. The median study time in the prospective groups was 7 d.

8. Sterility of the catheter and it implantation procedure represents one of the key factors in determining a reliable and consistent baseline amino acid and PGE_2 release, particularly if a long-term (up to 10 d) dialysis sample collection is planned. In our experience, the presence of bacterial infection in the vicinity of the catheter loop is associated with a significant increase in glutamate and PGE_2 levels. Although not systematically assessed, we believe that these changes can result from local inflammatory changes.

9. As a routine procedure, it is suggested to dissect each implanted catheter after animal sacrifice and to verify the position of the catheter loop as well as the development of any inflammatory changes. Under optimal conditions, the loop portion of the catheter should be localized on the surface of the dorsal portion of the lumbar spinal cord. The presence of inflammatory changes typically is expressed as a presence of yellow fibrotic masses in the vicinity of the dialysis loop.

Acknowledgments

This research was supported by grants NS32794, NS 40386 (M.M). Illustration in **Fig. 1** provided by Dirig Medical Art & Design.

References

1. Yaksh, T. L. and Yamamura, H. I. (1974) Factors affecting performance of the push-pull cannula in brain. *J. Appl. Physiol.* **37,** 428–434.

2. Feldberg, W. and Sherwood, S. (1954) Injections of drugs into the lateral ventricles of cats. *J. Physiol. Lond.* **123,** 148–167.

3. Yaksh, T. L. and Noueihed, R. (1985) The physiology and pharmacology of spinal opiates. *Annu. Rev. Pharmacol. Toxicol.* **25,** 433–462.

4. Benveniste, H., Drejer, J., Schousboe, A., and Diemer, N. H. (1984) Elevation of the extracellular concentrations of glutamate and aspartate in rat hippocampus during transient cerebral ischemia monitored by intracerebral microdialysis. *J. Neurochem.* **43,** 1369–1374.

5. Brodin, E., Linderoth, B., Gazelius, B., and Ungerstedt, U. (1987) In vivo release of substance P in cat dorsal horn studied with microdialysis. *Neurosci. Lett.* **76,** 357–362.
6. Skilling, S. R., Smullin, D. H., Beitz, A. J., and Larson, A. A. (1988) Extracellular amino acid concentrations in the dorsal spinal cord of freely moving rats following veratridine and nociceptive stimulation. *J. Neurochem.* **51,** 127–132.
7. Sorkin, L. S., Steinman, J. L., Hughes, M. G., Willis, W. D., and McAdoo, D. J. (1988) Microdialysis recovery of serotonin released in spinal cord dorsal horn. *J. Neurosci. Methods* **23,** 131–138.
8. Marsala, M., Malmberg, A. B., and Yaksh, T. L. (1995) The spinal loop dialysis catheter: characterization of use in the unanesthetized rat. *J. Neurosci. Methods* **62,** 43–53.

10

Intrathecal Catheterization and Drug Delivery in the Rat

Shelle A. Malkmus and Tony L. Yaksh

Summary

The spinal cord represents a complex system that serves in the encoding of sensory information and organization of autonomic and somatomotor outflow. As such, it has become a target of investigation for subjects ranging from pain to hypertension to motor spasticity. A primary method in such investigations is the specific delivery of drugs into the spinal intrathecal space to assess such agents with the actions limited to the spinal cord. The rat has served as a primary model in these investigations. It provides for the ability to deliver such agents both acutely and chronically in the absence of anesthesia or restraint. These goals can be accomplished by the placement of intrathecal catheters in the spinal space. This model, first demonstrating the feasibility of routinely catheterizing the lumbar intrathecal space in 1976, led directly to enabling a large number of studies focusing on spinal drug actions. As a test model, it has provided for the acquisition of an exceptional amount of information on the pharmacological and physiological mechanisms of spinal function, drug screening, drug efficacy and safety studies, and pharmacokinteics of spinally delivered drugs. The modified surgical method of intrathecal catheter placement, microinjection drug delivery, and behavioral parameters are described in detail.

Key Words: Rat; intrathecal; catheter; spinal cord; clinical observations; behavior; spinal pharmacology; animal model.

1. Introduction

The spinal cord represents a complex system that serves in the encoding of sensory information and organization of autonomic and somatomotor outflow. As such, it has become a target of investigation for subjects ranging from pain to hypertension to motor spasticity. A primary method in such investigations is the specific delivery of drugs into the spinal intrathecal (it) space to assess such agents with the actions limited to the spinal cord. The rat has served as a primary

From: *Methods in Molecular Medicine, Vol. 99: Pain Research: Methods and Protocols*
Edited by: Z. D. Luo © Humana Press Inc., Totowa, NJ

model in these investigations. It provides for the ability to deliver such agents both acutely and chronically in the absence of anesthesia or restraint. These goals can be accomplished by the placement of it catheters in the spinal space. This model, first demonstrating the feasibility of routinely catheterizing the lumbar it space in 1976 *(1)*, led directly to enabling a large number of studies focusing on spinal drug actions. As a test model, it has provided for the acquisition of an exceptional amount of information on the pharmacological and physiological mechanisms of spinal function, drug screening, drug efficacy and safety studies *(2)*, and pharmacokinetics of spinally delivered drugs *(3)*. In the following chapter, the modified surgical method of it catheter placement, microinjection drug delivery, and behavioral parameters are described in detail.

2. Materials

2.1. Animals

A large body of data on the effects of spinally delivered drugs exists for the Sprague-Dawley or Holtzman Rat strains (Harlan Industries, Indianapolis, IN), male, with a body weight of approx 250–350 g *(4,5)*. Although the same surgical procedure would be followed for other strains and body weights, their use is not as well-characterized.

2.2. Catheter

1. Polyethylene tubing (PE-5, no. E100-0620, PE-10, no. E100-0621, Spectranetics, Colorado Springs, CO).
2. Orthodontic resin (Dentsply, no. 651006).
3. Orthodontic pink liquid (Dentsply, no. 651002).
4. Ethylene oxide gas (ETO) or electron-beam (e-beam) sterilization source.

2.3. Surgical Supplies

1. Modified stereotaxic head holder with retractor (www.marsilsci.com).
2. Autoclave, glass-bead, or cold sterilization solution (Cetylcide-G, Pennsauken, NJ).
3. No. 15 scalpel blade and handle.
4. Periosteal elevator.
5. Retractor.
6. Serrated micro-dissection forceps.
7. Rat tooth (1 × 2) micro-dissecting forceps.
8. Needle holders.
9. Skin suture and suture needle.
10. 22-G $^3/_4''$ injection needle.
11. 19-G 1–1/2″ injection needle.
12. 30-G 1/2-in. injection needle.
13. Cotton-tipped applicator.
14. 28-G stainless-steel wire.

2.4. Micro-Injection Supplies

A variety of micro-injector systems may be employed.

1. Motor-driven systems (e.g., Harvard Apparatus, pump 22) to a simple hand-held syringe capable of delivering several 10-µL aliquots.
2. A simple device may be constructed from a microinjector syringe mounted on a plastic block delivering through a three-way stopcock.
3. Hamilton Microinjector with Threaded Plunger (500 µL), mounted.
4. Polyethylene tubing (PE90), (Intramedic PE90, Cat. no. 427421).
5. Three-way stopcock.
6. Reservoir syringe (5 mL).
7. 20-G to 30-G tubing connector.

3. Methods

3.1. Surgical Considerations

Instruments should be sterilized by a standard method (autoclave, glass-bead, or cold sterilization) prior to use. Surgical technique employs the use of gloves and a mask. The surgery area should be clean and neatly laid out. Clean surgical technique should be followed, as the it catheter is an externalized indwelling device.

3.2. Catheter Fabrication

1. To prepare a standard it catheter, a loose overhand knot that does not occlude the tubing is tied in a 10 cm length of PE-10, leaving 3 cm (external end) and 7 cm (indwelling end) on either side (*see* **Note 1**). Several catheters are prepared at a time.
2. To secure the catheter knot, a small amount (1 mL) of dental acrylic is prepared, the knot is dipped in the acrylic so that it is completely covered, and the acrylic is allowed dry. The final size of the knot is about 3 mm, rounded and smooth.
3. To soften and to decrease the size of the indwelling catheter tubing, the tubing is stretched. To do this, the indwelling end of the catheter is grasped with a hemostat in one hand, and the knot is secured to a surface with downward pressure using the other hand. The hemostat is pulled parallel to the surface away from the knot, ensuring an even stretch throughout the length of the catheter, to approx 60–90%. This amount varies with each roll of tubing. A good rule of thumb is to pull the tubing until a slight give can be felt, then pull until the give is exhausted. Stop pulling, and slowly release the tubing from the stretch. Care is taken not to flatten the catheter with compression, or stretch the catheter unevenly. Do not stretch or alter the external end of the tubing. Catheters should be left overnight to allow for any shrink back of the tubing before cutting them to length (*see* **Note 2**).
4. The indwelling catheter end is measured to 8.5 cm, and cut to length, ensuring the tip is smooth and square. The external end will be sized after implantation in the rat. The external end of the catheter is plugged with a short length of 28-G stainless steel, and packaged for sterilization.

5. Catheters are packaged individually or in units of several catheters, then sterilized by ethylene oxide gas or e-beam radiation.

3.3. Presurgical Evaluation

1. Rats are housed in micro-isolator filter cages, given ad libitum access to water and food, and allowed a minimum of 2 d to acclimate after receipt prior to any surgically related procedures.
2. A presurgical body weight is obtained and baseline clinical observations (*see* **Subheading 3.11.**) are recorded.

3.4. Anesthetic Protocol

Many anesthetic protocols are followed in rodent research. For this procedure, induction and maintenance of anesthesia is accomplished using a volatile gas, such as halothane or isoflurane, delivered in a mix of oxygen (50%) and air (50%). This allows rapid induction and recovery, and the ability to easily control the depth of anesthesia. Maintenance concentrations will vary among vaporizers; monitoring is done by close observation of respiratory rate and plantar paw surface color, which should remain pink. Anesthesia in rats is box-induced, indicated by loss of responsiveness and spontaneous movement, and then the rat is prepped for catheter placement.

3.5. Surgical Preparation

The hair of the dorsal head and neck is clipped using a no. 40 surgical clipper blade. The rat is then placed in a modified stereotaxic unit (*see* **Fig. 1**). Proper placement in the stereotaxic unit is checked by ensuring that: (1) the head is symmetrical in the device; (2) the pinnas are in a normal, relaxed position; (3) there is no exopthalmus; and (4) the head moves freely up and down, but does not move laterally. A petroleum ophthalmic lubricant is placed in the eye, and the surgical area is prepped with alcohol and Nolvasan solution. The catheter can now be flushed with sterile saline and is ready for placement.

3.6. Surgical Procedure

3.6.1. Skin Incision

With the animal placed in the stereotaxic unit, find the groove in the nuchal-crest (the dorsal, midline of the skull) using the dull side of the scalpel blade; this is the first reference to midline (*see* **Fig. 2**). To make a midline skin incision, push the skin evenly toward the nose, seat the sharp side of the blade in the groove with enough pressure to cut the skin, then pull the skin in a caudal direction through the blade a length of 1 cm. This method of skin incision prevents cutting the muscle on midline (*see* **Note 3**).

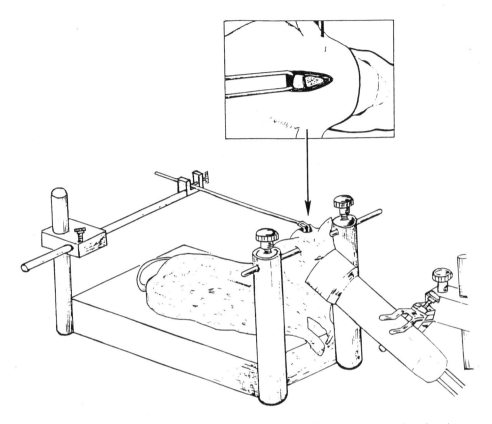

Fig. 1. Rat positioned in modified stereotaxic unit with retractor exposing the cisternal membrane. Reprinted with permission from ref. *(4)*.

3.6.2. Muscle Incision

Find the point on the dorsal head where the bone ends and the muscle begins. To do this, with the surgical blade at an angle, gently grate the blade over the skull in a caudal direction. You will feel bone (firm), then muscle (soft). You can also see that the bony area is white in color, becoming pink where the muscle begins. On the levator auris muscle, you will see the linea alba (white line); this is now your reference to midline. Cut the muscle where it attaches to the occipital crest about 3 mm lateral on both sides of the muscle midline, without leaving fragments attached to the crest. Care is taken not to split the muscle on midline.

3.6.3. Exposing the Cisternal Membrane (Dura)

Using the narrow end of a periosteal elevator the muscles (interscutularis) are scraped from the occipital crest, using the retractors to help peel the muscle

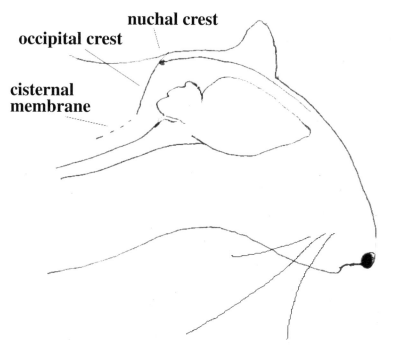

nuchal crest

occipital crest

cisternal membrane

Fig. 2. Schematic of the anatomical landmarks used in catheter placement.

from the bone and dura, to expose the cisternal membrane at the base of the skull. The fascia and tissue are removed from the membrane by scraping it with the elevator until approx 3–4 mm² of the cisternal membrane is exposed. Care is taken not to press too hard on the dura or the membrane may be ruptured with damage to the underlying brainstem. Once there is good exposure, the retractor is secured in the stereotaxic unit.

3.6.4. Dural Incision

Bend the bevel end of a 22-G needle to a 75° angle for use as a scalpel to incise the dura. To make a 1–2 mm lateral incision in the cisternal membrane, gently pierce the membrane using the bevel edge of the needle. Do not force the needle downward, or it will poke through the membrane and onto the brain stem. Cerebrospinal fluid (CSF) will appear when the membrane has been incised. A cotton-tipped applicator is used to absorb excess CSF, but as little as possible is swabbed to retain CSF volume in the it space.

3.6.5. Inserting the Catheter

Prior to inserting the catheter, it is flushed with sterile saline to ensure free flow of fluid through the catheter with no leakage. The catheter is held 2 cm from its tip in the right hand. The caudal edge of the incision is lifted using the dura hook. The objective is to create the maximum space available between the cisternal membrane and the spinal cord so that the catheter can be inserted without piercing the spinal cord. One to two mm of the tip of the catheter is inserted into the incision, then the catheter is repositioned parallel to the spinal column and cord. The catheter is guided toward the skull base, so that it loops and feeds into the spinal space in a dorso-caudal direction. This prevents the tip from being fed downward into the spinal cord. The external end is held and supported when repositioning your hand to advance the catheter in order to avoid unwanted twisting of the catheter. The catheter is slowly advanced, observing the trunk for muscle twitching. After about 30% of the catheter is indwelling, it can be advanced directly into the it space, and passed caudal to the lumbar level, until the knot lies just behind the nuchal crest.

3.6.6. Resistance and Twitching

As the catheter is advanced in the it space, resistance or mild twitching of the musculature may be noted. If twitching is seen, spinal nerves are being stimulated and may be damaged if the catheter is further advanced (twitch vs twang). In this case, the catheter may be retracted approx 1 cm, rotated away from the area being stimulated, and slowly advanced until the resistance has passed and no twitching is observed. The tail may be pulled gently (at its base) to align the spinal cord.

3.6.7. Catheter Externalization and Wound Closure

The catheter exit site is on the top of the skull approx 1 cm cranial to the incision, between the ears. A 19-G needle is inserted from this site subcutaneously (sc) out through the incision, the external end of the catheter is placed into the needle, and the catheter is tunneled forward when the needle is removed. The length of the external catheter will be trimmed to about 2 cm, or enough to grasp the end for injection or infusion. Once in place, 20–30 µL of sterile saline is injected through the catheter to clear the tip of any possible blood or tissue and a small length of 28-G stainless-steel wire is used to plug the catheter. The incision is sutured with silk or Vetafil (3-0), ensuring the catheter knot is secured under the muscle, behind the occipital crest (*see* **Note 4**).

3.7. Postsurgical Care and Recovery

The rat is given 5 mL of Lactated Ringers Solution or Saline SQ, or IP, postoperative analgesics as per protocol, and the tail is marked with an ID. Animals are placed in a warm Plexiglas box and monitored during anesthetic recovery. Following recovery behavioral, motor coordination and muscle-tone parameters are evaluated to ensure that no nerve damage occurred during catheter placement (*see* **Subheading 3.11.**). Food pellets are offered on the cage bottom

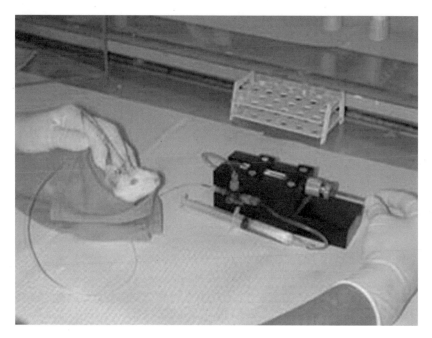

Fig. 3. Micro-injector system.

for 3 d following surgery so that the animals have easy access to food during initial recovery (*see* **Note 5**).

3.8. Maintenance of Catheterized Animals

Animals are housed separately and checked daily for body weight and clinical observations. A minimum of 5 d surgical recovery is recommended prior to any study-related procedures. Catheters should be flushed with 10 µL of sterile saline on a weekly basis to maintain patency if no drugs are administered.

3.9. Criteria for Entering Animals into a Study

Following the clinical observations, animals will be assessed for health and recovery 5 d postsurgery before they are considered for a study. General health criteria to be met also include the recovery of body weight, weight gain equal to the normal growth curve, normal appearance, and grooming activity.

3.10. Micro-Injection Technique

3.10.1. Micro-Injector

A micro-injector is comprised of a Hamilton glass micro-injection syringe with a threaded plunger, mounted on a platform to enable delivery of small amounts of drug at a slow rate, using only one hand (*see* **Fig. 3**). The Hamilton syringe is attached to an extension line, which is attached to a three-way stopcock. A reservoir syringe for flushing the system and the injection line are also attached to the three-way stopcock.

3.10.2. Injection Line

To make the injection line, one 25 cm length of PE-90 tubing is marked at 10 µL increments (marks are approx 1.9 cm apart), and calibrated by using a 100 µL Hamilton syringe. The injection line attaches to the stopcock via a 20-G luer stub adapter. The entire system is filled with distilled water. There should be scrupulous attention to being certain that there are no air bubbles in the tubing, the valve, or the syringe.

3.10.3. Connector

A connector is prepared to attach the PE-90 injector line to the PE-10 catheter. This can be accomplished by soldering a 1 cm length of 30-G stainless steel tubing inside a 0.5 cm length of 20-G stainless-steel tubing (injection needles with the sharp ends removed can be used as the tubing).

3.10.4. Preparing for Injection

To prepare the injection line for drug delivery, a small 2-mm air bubble is aspirated into the line, then saline is aspirated until the air bubble reaches the first mark on the tubing. Another 10 µL of saline is aspirated to the next mark, this saline will be used to flush the catheter after drug delivery. Transfer the injector tip into the drug solution and aspirate 10 µL of drug, using the position of the bubble as a guide. No air should be aspirated, and care is taken not to inject saline into the drug solution. You now have 10 µL of drug and 10 µL of saline flush ready to be delivered to the rat.

3.10.5. Injecting

To deliver drug, the rat is restrained in a cloth towel, or similar restraint. The external portion of the catheter is wiped with alcohol, and the wire plug is removed using forceps. The injector tip is connected to the catheter. The injector drive is turned slowly, while the injector/catheter junction is observed for leakage. Injection is immediately stopped if fluid is seen. The position of the bubble is moved two marks, corresponding to the delivery of 10 µL of drug solution and 10 µL of saline flush. This injection takes approx 15 s. If there is resistance, and the bubble does not move, the catheter may be clogged. The catheter is always unclogged with saline, not with the drug being injected. Following injection, the catheter tip is pinched to prevent leakage of the drug while the injector line is disconnected and the wire plug is replaced. This is considered time 0 for testing paradigms.

Table 1
Suggested Scoring System for Clinical Observations

0	Absence of deficit, normal behavior (baseline)
1	Slight deficit, noticeable change in parameter being evaluated, 5–25% change from baseline (occasional episode)
2	Moderate deficit, significant difference apparent upon first observations, 26–50% change from baseline (frequent episodes)
3	Marked or severe deficit, debilitating, >50% change from baseline (constant occurrence)

3.11. Clinical Observations

3.11.1. Evaluation

Many of the clinical observations being evaluated are subjective and may vary among observers. Therefore, extensive experience in evaluating these behaviors is essential in describing the clinical symptoms and drug side effects. The behaviors examined may include some or all of the following parameters. Each behavior is given a score based on the change in the baseline clinically observed, determined by the guidelines, and may be further defined by stating the distribution and degree of that clinical observation (*see* **Table 1**) A positive (+) or negative (–) sign can be used to indicate an increase or decrease in parameter, where appropriate.

3.11.2. Daily Observations/General Health Parameters

1. Appearance. Note general appearance of animal, eyes, haircoat, posture, and activity level. Also note behavior and responses when approached (sleep, quiet, active, or excited). Animal should appear bright, alert, and responsive (BAR).
2. Body weight. Increase or decrease. Normal weight gain expected for. growth curve (Harlan Sprague-Dawley 4–7 g/d). This is a measurable observation and should be monitored daily.
3. Respiratory rate. Normal rate, observe effort of breaths, note dyspnea, and so forth.
4. Appetite. Check for normal consumption of food and water.
5. Stool and urine production. Normal consistency, color, and volume.
6. Environmental changes. Note any changes or problems with cage, bedding, or housing environment.

3.11.3. Behavioral Status/Arousal

1. Startle response. Normal response to a handclap, finger snap, or other stimulating noise.
2. Agitation. Response to handler when approached, e.g., jumpiness, fear, escape behavior.

3. Allodynia. Squeaking or agitation in response to light touch or stroking of the spine with a pencil.

3.11.4. Motor Coordination and Function

1. Placing and stepping. Ability to replace limbs to normal position without stumble or lag. With rat on all four feet, lift the tail at its base raising hind feet slightly off of surface, then let go of the tail. Watch for extension of hind limbs when lifted and normal return of hind paws to surface when released.
2. Righting reflex. Roll or place rat on dorsal aspect; watch for a normal, immediate return to sternal recumbency.
3. Spinal symmetry, posture. Axis of spine is straight when viewed from above (dorsal), normal curvature when viewed from the side (lateral). May be asymmetric, curved, or exaggerated along either axis.
4. Symmetric ambulation. Normal placing of all four limbs. Does not walk with a wobble or favor any limb (limp).
5. Leaning/circling, head tilt. Animal shows head tilt, leaning, or circling to one side when ambulating indicating vestibular involvement; differentiate from limb favoring or limp.
6. Hunched back. Animal stands or walks with a hunched back, appears stiff, indicating reluctance to ambulate or pain in spinal area.

3.11.5. Muscle Tone

1. Truncal rigidity. Palpation of the chest gives sensation of a rigid, barrel-like structure; animal retains rigidity upon change of directional aspects, indicates catalepsy or guarding behavior (pain).
2. Flaccidity. Flaccid, without tone, animal will drape over arm when held.
3. Catalepsy. Animal will remain fixed in a placed position (greater than 6 s).
4. Tremor. High-frequency shaking; may resemble shivering but more intense.
5. Seizures. Involuntary rhythmic contraction of trunk or limb musculature, chattering of the jaw.

3.11.6. Other Parameters and General Observations

1. Vocalization. Excessive vocalizing, spontaneous or provoked, indicates fear, pain.
2. Pinna reflex. Evoked twitching of the ear or shaking the head when the ear canal opening is stimulated with a length of flexible PE tubing.
3. Blink (corneal) reflex. Blinking of the eye when the rim of the eye is lightly touched with a small length of flexible tubing.
4. Optic abnormalities. Bulging eyes, sunken eyes, corneal ulcers, pupil abnormalities.
5. Guarding behavior. Animal displays behaviors to avoid normal motor coordination, such as hunched back, cornering in cage, favoring a limb, and so forth. Usually indicates pain.
6. Urine-stained belly. Yellow staining of inguinal area, owing to incontinence.

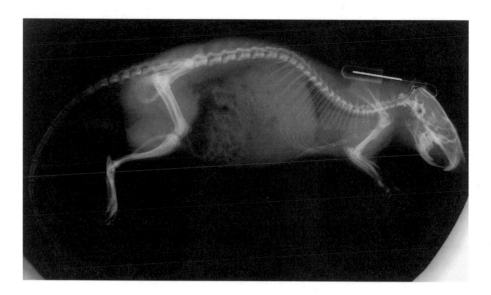

Fig. 4. Radiograph showing placement of the intrathecal catheter connected to a sc Alzet mini-osmotic pump (a stylette wire was used to demonstrate placement).

7. Chromodacryorhea. ("bloody tears") Black crusty residue resembling blood around the margins of the eyes, nose, or mouth. These porphyrins from the hardarian gland usually indicate stress or pain.
8. Salivation. Wetness around the mouth or chin, visible appearance of saliva, also seen on forepaws if animal is grooming. Usually a drug effect.
9. Piloerection. Erection of the hair, usually on the neck and back area, may indicate pain.
10. Straub tail. Stiff, cataleptic tail.
11. Flushed ears. Redness and flushing of the ears, usually a drug effect.
12. Alopecia. Loss of hair, balding.
13. Pruritus. Scratching.

4. Notes

1. Catheters can be configured with various modifications to allow for continuous delivery of drug, multiple lumen delivery, microdialysis (6), or toxicology studies. Single, double, or triple lumen polyethylene tubing in micro sizes is available for use as catheter material (Spectranetics).
2. Catheter materials have been described, including those constructed of small-gauge polyurethane and polyimide (7). The important variable in all cases is to achieve a small diameter profile.
3. The placement of an it catheter as described in this chapter is that of a cisternal approach. Other investigators have reported on the use of a dissection that permits

placement through the L5/6 inter space *(8)*. The relative merits of the two approaches likely depends on the facility with which either technique is accomplished.

4. Continuous infusion. A mini-osmotic pump (Alzet, Durect Corp., Cupertino, CA) is easily connected to the it catheter to allow for continuous infusion of test articles in a closed system. These pumps are available in various volumes, rates, and durations. The it catheter is prepared as described, with the external end measuring 3 cm. Hot air is used to heat-crimp a 1 cm length of polyethylene 60 (PE-60) tubing to the external it catheter for connection to the osmotic pump. The pump is connected and placed in the dorsal sc space between the shoulders, so that it does not impede normal movement and activity of the rat. The catheter tubing is buried sc and the incision is closed **(Fig. 4)**.

5. On average, a single trained individual, using gaseous anesthetic induction, should be able to accomplish four to five rat preparations per hour or about 18–20 rats d. This number is usually dictated by the postoperative testing schedule. In a prospective analysis of 100 rats each, three skilled technicians failed to obtain a satisfactory outcome (e.g., no sensory or motor dysfunction) in less than 2% of the 300 rats implanted. It should be stressed that no change from un-implanted controls in the measured end points and moderate, reversible weight loss are important criteria for defining the successful acquisition of the technique.

References

1. Yaksh, T. L. and Rudy T. A. (1976) Chronic catheterization of the subarachnoid space. *Physiol. Behav.* **17,** 1031–1036.
2. Malkmus, S. A., Myers, R. R., and Yaksh, T. L. (1997) Rat chronic spinal intrathecal infusion model for drug safety evaluation. *Fundam. Appl. Toxicol.* **36S,** 276.
3. Kohn, F. R., Malkmus, S. A., Brownson, E. A., et al. (1998) Fate of the predominant phospholipid component of DepoFoam drug delivery matrix after intrathecal administration of sustained-release encapsulated cytarabine in rats. *Drug Delivery* **5,** 143–151.
4. Yaksh, T. L. and Malkmus, S. A. (1999) Animal models of intrathecal and epidural drug delivery, in *Spinal Drug Delivery* (Yaksh, T. L., ed.), Elsevier Press, Amsterdam, Netherlands, pp. 317–344.
5. Fletcher, T. F. and Malkmus, S. A. (1999) Spinal anatomy of experimental animals, in *Spinal Drug Delivery* (Yaksh, T. L., ed.), Elsevier Press, Amsterdam, Netherlands, pp. 71–96.
6. Marsala, M., Malmberg, A. B., and Yaksh, T. L. (1995) The spinal loop dialysis catheter: characterization of use in the unanesthetized rat. *J. Neurosc. Methods* **62,** 43–53.
7. Sakura, S., Hashimoto, K., Bollen, A. W., Ciriales, R., and Drasner, K. (1996) Intrathecal catheterization in the rat. Improved technique for morphologic analysis of drug-induced injury. *Anesthesiology* **85,** 1184–1189.
8. Storkson, R. V., Kjorsvik, A., Tjolsen, A., and Hole, K. (1996) Lumbar catheterization of the spinal subarachnoid space in the rat. *J. Neurosci. Methods* **65,** 167–172.

11

Trigeminal Neuronal Recording in Animal Models of Orofacial Pain

Koichi Iwata, Yuji Masuda, and Ke Ren

Summary

The electrical signal associated with nerve cells, mainly as a result of changes in the membrane potential during functional activity, can be recorded extracellularly to study central mechanisms underlying sensory processing. The secondary neurons in the spinal trigeminal complex receive inputs from peripheral neurons that innervate the orofacial region and forward information to the higher levels of the nervous system. Analyzing activity patterns of trigeminal neurons related to pain perception has proven to be an efficient method in studying orofacial pain mechanisms. Here we describe some basic techniques and tips for extracellular single neuron recording from the subnucleus caudalis of the trigeminal spinal nucleus in rats with orofacial injury. Two different rat models with temporomandibular joint inflammation and inferior alveolar nerve transection are described.

Key Words: Electrophysiology; extracellular recording; single-unit; rat; orofacial pain; subnucleus caudalis; medullary dorsal horn; nociceptive neurons; temporomandibular joint (TMJ); inferior alveolar nerve; inflammation; complete Freund's adjuvant; nerve injury; tungsten microelectrodes; receptive field; action potential.

1. Introduction

The neural network in the central nervous system (CNS) contributes to a variety of physiological functions such as sensation and movements. A central neuron receives either excitatory or inhibitory input, or both. The neuronal circuits constructed from excitatory and inhibitory neurons process information and output the result to other parts of the nervous system. The electrical signal associated with nerve cells, mainly resulting from changes in the membrane potential during functional activity, can be recorded extracellularly to study central mechanisms underlying sensory processing.

The secondary neurons in the spinal trigeminal complex receive inputs from peripheral neurons that innervate the orofacial region and forward information

From: *Methods in Molecular Medicine, Vol. 99: Pain Research: Methods and Protocols*
Edited by: Z. D. Luo © Humana Press Inc., Totowa, NJ

to the higher levels of the nervous system. Analyzing activity patterns of trigeminal neurons related to pain perception has proven to be an efficient method in studying orofacial pain mechanisms *(1–7)*. Here we describe some basic techniques and tips for extracellular single neuron recording from the subnucleus caudalis of the trigeminal spinal nucleus in rats with orofacial injury. Two different rat models with temporomandibular joint (TMJ) inflammation and inferior alveolar nerve (IAN) transection will be described.

2. Materials

1. Standard equipment for extracelullar recordings (*see* **Note 1**). A Hum-Bug noise eliminator (Quest Scientific) is useful for reducing 50–60 Hz noise. A regular commercial Stereo Receiver can be used for audio monitoring.
2. Microelectrodes. Two types of microelectrodes, metal and glass microelectrodes, can be used for extracellular recordings (*see* **Note 2**). The thin-walled borosilicate glass capillaries (Glass, Standard, 0.75 mm × 0.4 mm, 6 in., A-M SYSTEMS, Carlsburg, WA) can be used to pull glass microelectrodes with higher impedance (3–20 MΩ). Metal electrodes usually have lower impedance (1–10 MΩ). The commercially available tungsten wire electrodes are well-designed and can be purchased from many sources (approx $10/per electrode). To reduce the cost of the experiment and customize the tip of the electrode to our needs, we have used enamel- or glass-coated tungsten microelectrodes for extracellular recordings from the trigeminal spinal nucleus. The methods for making such electrodes are described here.

    a. Enamel-Coated Tungsten Microelectrodes

    Ten-centimeter tungsten wires (0.2–0.3 mm in diameter, FHC) are polished electrically. The electrode tip (1 cm in length from the tip of the wire) is put into a polishing solution and DC current (1–2 A, 3–6 V) is passed through the solution for polishing and sharpening. The polishing solution is made of distilled water saturated with $NaNO_3$ (or KNO_3 dissolved to the saturated concentration). The tip of the electrode is examined under a microscope as illustrated in **Fig. 1.** After polishing, the electrodes are coated with enamel (FHC). Enamel should be diluted to a solvent (approx 50%). The tungsten wire is coated with enamel more than three times. Between the coatings, the electrodes are baked (150–180°C) in an oven for 30 min. After the coating, the impedance of the electrodes is measured (1000 Hz) (*see* **Note 3**).

    b. Glass-Coated Tungsten Wire Electrode

    Prepare a 5-cm tungsten wire (0.2 mm in diameter) and thin-walled glass pipet (0.75 mm in diameter). The tungsten wire is first polished electrically using the polishing solution as described earlier. Only the tip of the tungsten wire should be polished. The tungsten wire is then placed into the glass pipet with polished tip upward. The bottom of the glass pipet is closed with clay to prevent the tungsten wire from slipping off from the pipet. The glass pipet with polished tungsten wire is set in a longitudinal puller as illustrated in **Fig. 2** and pulled slowly using a high-intensity current (~25 A). Check the tip of the electrode under the microscope after pulling (*see* **Note 4**).

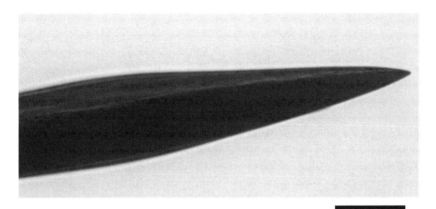

100 μm

Fig. 1. The photomicrograph of the tip of the tungsten wire after polishing. The tip of the electrode looks slightly blunt. Do not make the tip too sharp.

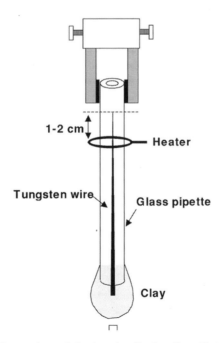

Fig. 2. A schematic illustration of the longitudinal puller. The tip of the electrode should be set at 1–2 cm above the heater. The amount of the clay should be adjusted according to the power of the heater. The size of the clay is usually about 1 cm in diameter.

3. Animal models. Sprague-Dawley rats are used.
4. Complete Freund's adjuvant (CFA, Sigma, Cat. no. F5881) can be used as an inflammatory agent for the inflammation model. Dilute CFA with the same amount of saline (1:1) to make an oil/saline emulsion (*see* **Note 5**). Incomplete Freund's adjuvant (Sigma, Cat. no. F5506) can be used as a control. Prepare a 1-cc syringe with a 27-G needle. The rats are anesthetized with pentobarbital Na (50 mg/kg, ip) and placed on a stereotaxic frame. CFA (0.05 ml, 1:1 oil/saline) is injected into the TMJ capsule (*see* **Note 6**).
5. The IAN transection was developed as trigeminal nerve injury model *(7)*. Previous studies have shown that chronic constriction injury of the IAN induced hypersensitivity of the subnucleus caudalis neurons to mechanical and thermal stimulation of the face *(7)*. Compared with nerve injury models at the spinal level (*see* Chapters 4–6), one advantage of the IAN injury is that it only affects sensory afferents (*see* **Note 7**). Rats are initially anesthetized with pentobarbital sodium (50 mg/kg, ip). For the IAN transection, rats are placed on a warm mat and a small incision is made on the surface of the facial skin over the masseteric muscle and to the alveolar bone through the masseteric muscle. The surface of the alveolar bone is exposed and the bone surface covering the IAN is removed to expose the IAN. The IAN is tightly ligated at two points: immediately above the angle of the mandible and 1 mm proximal from the angle of the mandibular bone. For sham-operated rats, the facial skin and the masseter muscle are cut and the surface of the alveolar bone is removed. Penicillin G potassium (20,000 U, im) is injected after the surgery to prevent infection.

3. Methods
3.1. Animal Preparation

Rats are initially anesthetized with pentobarbital sodium (50 mg/kg, ip) and the trachea and left jugular veins are cannulated to allow artificial respiration and intravenous (iv) administration of drugs. Anesthesia is maintained with halothane (2–3%) mixed with oxygen (95%) during surgery. The rats are mounted in a stereotaxic frame, the medulla is exposed, and a mineral oil pool is made with the skin flaps surrounding the laminectomy. A head holder is rigidly secured to the skull by stainless-steel screws and dental acrylic resin, and the ear bars and nose holder are removed as illustrated in **Fig. 3**. This setup allowed convenient access to orofacial receptive fields (RFs) during recordings.

After surgery, anesthesia is maintained by continuous inhalation of halothane (2–3%) mixed with oxygen (*see* **Note 8**). During recording sessions, the rats are immobilized with pancuronium bromide ($\leq$1 mg/kg/h, iv; *see* **Note 9**) and ventilated artificially. The expired CO_2 concentration is monitored and maintained between 3 and 4% (*see* **Note 10**). Rectal temperature is maintained at 37–38°C by a thermostatically controlled heating pad (*see* **Note 11**) and the electrocardiogram is monitored. Blood pressure is measured

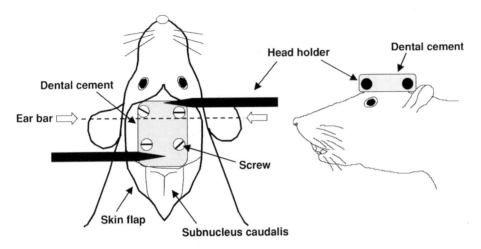

Fig. 3. A schematic illustration of the head holder for fixing rat's head without ear bars and nose holder. Four screws are implanted in the skull and head holder and screws are rigidly secured with dental acrylic cement. The tip of the head holder is completely embedded with the dental acrylic cement. Avoid putting acrylic on the brain surface.

every 30 min indirectly from the tail (*see* **Note 12**) and kept at 90–120 mmHg during the experiments.

3.2. Extracellular Recording

3.2.1. Isolation of Single Unit

The microelectrode is advanced into the subnucleus caudalis region at about 2–6 mm caudal to the obex, 2–3 mm lateral to the midline, and 0.5–2.5 mm ventral to the surface of the medulla. As illustrated in **Fig. 3,** the rat's head is fixed rigidly to the head holder with dental acrylic cement before removing the ear bars. Thus, the stereotaxic coordinates are maintained without the ear bars. After opening the dura matter, the photograph of the brain surface is taken using a Polaroid camera as illustrated in **Fig. 4.** While paying attention to background firing of neurons, the caudalis neurons are searched for by applying mechanical stimuli (pressure or brush) to the orofacial skin. The electrode should be advanced in 1 μm steps and the penetration stopped whenever clear action potentials are encountered. Carefully advance or withdraw the electrode to achieve clear recording from one unit (*see* **Note 13**). When a single neuron is isolated, the responses to mechanical stimulation of the facial skin are carefully examined and the RFs are mapped. The RFs are drawn to scale on standard diagrams of a rat head as shown in **Fig. 5.**

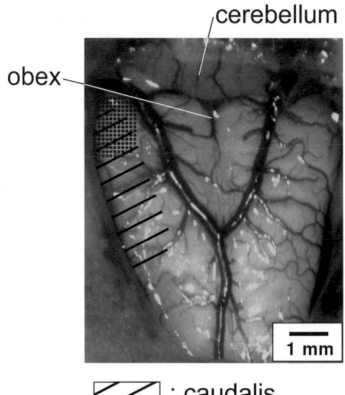

Fig. 4. A photograph of the brain surface. This picture can be used to guide the electrode penetration.

3.2.2. Classification of Medullary Sensory Neurons

Each neuron is classified as either: (1) a low-threshold mechano-receptive (LTM) neuron that has only transient firing at the onset and termination of the mechanical stimulus or has tonic responses during mechanical stimulation of the RFs but decreases its firing frequency after noxious mechanical stimulation; (2) a wide-dynamic-range (WDR) neuron that responds to both non-noxious and noxious mechanical stimuli and increases its firing frequency as stimulus intensity increases (*see* **Note 14**); or (3) a nociceptive specific (NS) neuron that responds exclusively to noxious mechanical stimulation of the RFs (*see* **Note 15**).

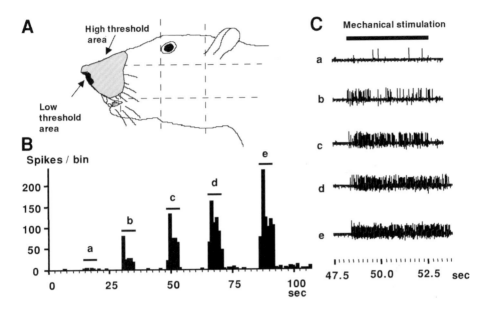

Fig. 5. An example of a WDR neuron. (**A**) The orofacial receptive field (gray and solid areas indicated by arrows). (**B**) PST histograms following graded mechanical stimulation of the low-threshold area of the receptive field. (**C**) The original recordings of activities of this WDR neuron. The intensities of stimulus are indicated: a, 1.2 g; b, 5.5 g; c, 15.1 g; d, 28.8 g; e, 75.9 g.

After characterization of neurons with mechanical stimuli, thermal stimuli (heating and cooling) are applied to the most sensitive area of the cutaneous mechanical RFs of nociceptive neurons, including WDR and NS neurons. When LTM neurons are identified, a cold stimulus is applied to the most sensitive areas of the mechanical RFs. The tip of the thermal probe is 5 mm in diameter and the rate of temperature change is set at 10°C/s. Before application of the thermal stimulus to the RF, the surface temperature is adapted to 38°C for 180 s. Skin heating ranges from 42–55°C and lasts for 10 s. Cold stimuli consist of cooling of the skin to 10–30°C. It is important that the thermal stimuli are applied to the RFs at 190-s intervals (adaptation time: 180 s; stimulus time: 10 s) to avoid sensitization of nociceptors.

3.2.3. Identification of Projection Neurons

Standard antidromic activation techniques are used to verify projection neurons (*5,8–10*). A monopolar or bipolar metal electrode for antidromic stimulation can be placed in one of the rostral projection sites, such as the parabrachial nucleus (*see* **Note 16**). Refer to a rat brain atlas for coordinates *(11)*. After isolation and characterization of a neuron, electrical pulses (0.1–0.2 ms pulse width, 0.3–0.5 mA and 1 Hz) are applied to the antidromic activation site. The following criteria should be satisfied to qualify for a projection neuron: (1) Constant latency and threshold to stimulation. Neurons projecting to the parabrachial nucleus should respond with a constant latency of 1–2 ms. (2) Ability to follow high-frequency antidromic stimulation (>200 Hz). Applying a pair of pulses (separated by 3–5 ms interval) is sufficient. (3) Collision of antidromic action potential with orthodromic action potential generated by background firing, mechanical stimulation of the RFs, or stimulating the peripheral nerve. Electric pulses should be applied first to the peripheral nerve and then the antidromic activation site with stimulus intervals ranged from 5 to 30 ms. If the antidromic spike is blocked by an orthodromic spike occurred before the onset of an antidromic stimululs, the neuron is defined as a projection neuron.

3.2.4. Verification of the Recording Site (see **Note 17**)

At the conclusion of the experiment, 20-μA anodal DC current is applied through the tip of the electrode for 10 s to make electrolytic lesions at the site of recording or antidromic stimulation. The rats are overdosed with sodium pentobarbital (100 mg/kg) and perfused transcardially with 50 mL 0.01 *M* phosphate-buffered saline (PBS), pH 7.4, followed by 10% formaline in 0.1 *M* PB. The brain is removed and placed in cold fixative for a few days, and transferred to cold phosphate-buffered 30% sucrose for 48 h. Serial sections (50 μm-thick) are cut along the path of the electrode penetration. The sections are counterstained with thionin or cresyl violet. The recording site can be identified under a microscope as illustrated in **Fig. 6** and images digitized for documentation.

3.3. Data Analysis

3.3.1. Data Analysis using Spike2 Software (CED, Cambridge, UK)

The neuronal activity is digitized and saved as Spike2 files. The sampling rate of extracellular recording data should be more than 10 Hz to help identify spike shape (*see* below). Pay attention to the timing of neuronal firing. The analysis of mean firing frequency and the construction of peristimulus time histograms (PSTH) require the timing of neuronal firing data. Two ways can be used to determine the timing of the spikes from the original recorded data. One way is to use the spike amplitude. If all spikes from the isolated neuron have similar amplitude, the timing of the spikes can be derived from a certain point of an action potential, either during the rising or falling phase. The other way is

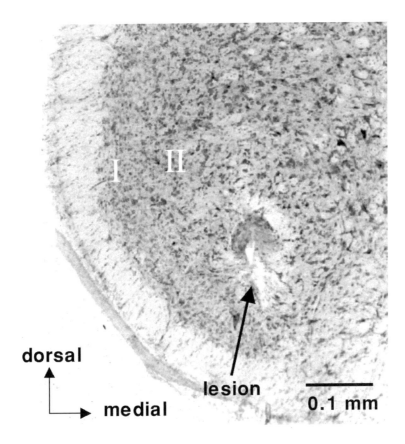

Fig. 6. Histological verification of the recording site. The electrical lesion is located in the ventral part of the trigeminal subnucleus caudalis (Vc) indicated by the arrow. Roman numerals indicate the laminae of the subnucleus caudalis.

to refer to the waveform of the spikes. To establish a specific waveform of a neuron, several parameters, including the spike amplitude, duration, and rising time, should be considered. The template of the spikes from a particular cell can be conveniently generated using Spike2 and used to match spikes. With the help of the Spike2 software, more than one unit with different spike waveforms can be analyzed simultaneously. **Figure 7** shows an example of such recordings from two subnucleus caudalis neurons that have large and small action potentials (**Fig. 7A**), respectively. The two neurons, 01 and 02, are separated using the Spike2 software (**Fig. 7B**).

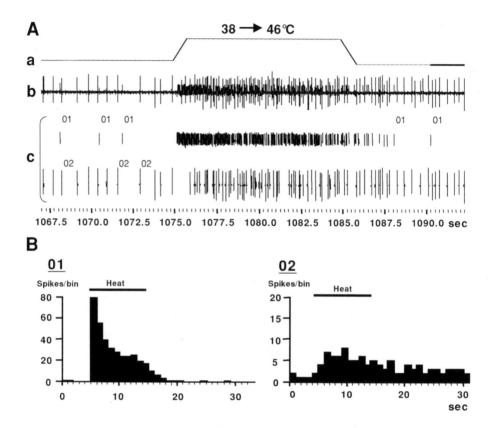

Fig. 7. An example of spike sorting from two WDR neurons responding to heating of the face. Two neurons with different amplitudes of action potentials are recorded. (**A**) a, Trace of the temperature change. b, the original recording of neuronal activities. c, Spikes from the two neurons are isolated as 01 and 02. (**B**) Peristimulus time histograms from neurons 01 and 02.

The derived timing of the spikes is expressed numerically in s or min. An array variable may be set for these numerical data. When calculating the mean firing frequency during a certain period, the items in the array variable for the period are counted and then divided by the elapsed time. The firing rate can be seen visually from a histogram. As shown in **Fig. 7B,** both 01 and 02 units increased their firing frequency in response to heat stimulation of the face. The bin width of the PSTH can be set between 0.001 to 1 s depending on the purpose of the analysis. In the PSTH, the timing of peripheral stimulus (e.g., electrical stimulus) is determined and items in the array variable (spike firing point) are transported to the point relative to each stimulus.

3.3.2. Multiple Parameter Analysis

Multiple parameters can be analyzed depending on the purpose of experiments:

1. Background activity (Hz): there may be an increase in firing rate after injury.
2. Receptive fields: there may be an expansion of the RFs or appearance of novel RFs after orofacial injury.
3. Response threshold: there may be a reduction in thermal and mechanical response thresholds after injury.
4. Evoked responses: Post- or peristimulus time histogram of neuronal discharges can be constructed using Spike2. The number of action potentials during a specified time period can be quantified. The level of background firing should be estimated from a period prior to stimulation and subtracted from the responses. An increase or decrease in responses can be detected by the total number of spikes in a certain period or response frequency. A linear correlation between the stimulus intensity and firing frequency suggests an involvement in encoding stimulus intensity. The after-discharges following a stimulus suggest the level of sensitization and descending modulation. Long-lasting, high-frequency afterdischarges recorded after the secession of the stimulus suggest central sensitization or deficit in descending inhibition.
5. The interspike interval histogram can be constructed to analyze the firing pattern of neurons. A lack of interspike intervals within the range of the refractory period of the action potential (0.5–1 ms) confirms recording from single neuron.

4. Notes

1. Although it is essential to have a stable table for the recording, it is not necessary to pursue a vibration-isolated table for these experiments. A heavy marble table is sufficient to host good extracellular recordings.
2. The impedance of the electrodes (1–10 MΩ) is similar to that used for patch-clamp recordings, but relatively low when compared to that used in intracellular recordings (80–120 MΩ). Different type of electrodes should be used according to the goal of experiments. It is easier to isolate clear single neuronal activity by using glass-pipet microelectrodes with higher impedance (3–10 MΩ). Glass-pipet microelectrodes are better for recording from neurons that are located in the superficial laminae of the subnucleus caudalis and have high background activity. When using glass-pipet microelectrodes, one should be aware that tissues may stick to the tip of the electrode, and thus preventing repeated use.
3. If the impedance is too high (>20 MΩ), the electrode can be put into saline solution and DC current (10 μA) can be applied for 10 s or less to reduce the impedance to about 10 MΩ.
4. The tip of the tungsten wire is often covered by some melted glass after pulling. The small amount of glass should be taken away from the tip of the electrode. To do this, prepare a small glass ball (about 1 mm in diameter) with a glass pipet. Place the glass ball on the microscope stage to the left side and loosely fix the electrode to a glass plate with a small amount of clay opposite to the glass ball. The glass ball and the tip of the electrode can be seen under the microscope. Move the tip of the

electrode toward the surface of the glass ball until touching its surface. This procedure can take away the tiny amount of glass mass from the tip of the electrode. Further details on making this type of electrode can be found elsewhere *(12)*.

5. The CFA solution is light-sensitive. The bottle containing diluted CFA solution should be wrapped with aluminum foil and refrigerated.

6. To inject CFA into the TMJ, the skin above the joint is reflected and the zygomatic arc exposed to see the bottom of the arc. The TMJ capsule is located immediately beneath the bottom of the zygomatic arc. Pull down the lower jaw slightly and insert the needle into the capsule. After injection of CFA, use a cotton pellet to wipe off CFA flowing back from the capsule. The reflected skin flap is closed with skin sutures. Antibiotics (e.g., Penicillin G potassium, 20,000 U, im) are injected intraperitoneally (ip) to prevent infection after the procedure. (Also *see* **refs.** *13,14* for this procedure). The injection of CFA into the TMJ induces localized inflammation, behavioral hyperalgesia, and hyperexcitability of trigeminal neurons *(15)*.

7. To produce animal models of neuropathic pain, most studies have targeted the sciatic nerve, which includes sensory as well as motor fibers. Thus, the effect of sciatic nerve lesion on nociception may be confounded by motor-nerve damage. One unique feature of the trigeminal nerve is that most trigeminal nerve branches, such as IAN, are purely sensory without a motor component. The injury of such trigeminal nerve branches is ideal for dissecting the effect of sensory nerve lesion on nociception. The other advantage of trigeminal nerve lesion is that the innervation territories of three trigeminal nerve divisions are well-demarcated. The study of reorganization of primary afferent terminals in the trigeminal nuclei after injury is facilitated.

8. We primarily use pentobarbital Na (50 mg/kg, ip) as initial anesthetic followed by continuous inhalation of halothane (2–3% mixture with O_2) during experiments. Gas anesthetic is very convenient to use and can maintain a stable level of anestheia for a relatively long period of time.

   α-Chloralose (40–60 mg/kg, iv) can be used as an alternative anesthetic to maintain anesthesia during recordings. Mix 0.3 g α-chloralose with 0.37 g sodium borate in 10 mL saline, heat and stir for 5 min until it is dissolved, and adjust pH to 7.8 with 1 *N* HCl. The chloralose solution should be freshly prepared for each experiment.

9. Pancuronium bromide (1 mg/kg/h, iv) immobilizes animals with little effect on the heart. However, it has a slight effect on blood pressure. Arterial blood pressure is gradually increased when pancuronium is used repeatedly. If posssible, use pancuronium at a lower dose than we normally use.

10. The expired CO_2 concentration should be monitored and kept at 3–4%. Low expired CO_2 concentration indicates bad ventilation, which may lead to the death of animal. Try sucking out mucus accumulated in the tracheal cannula to allow better aeration.

11. The immobilized animals tend to lose body temperature during recordings, resulting in suppression of neuronal activity. The body temperature should be carefully monitored and kept at 37–38°C. In addition to a heating pad, a heating lamp may be necessary to help to maintain the body temperature. The heating lamp is particu-

larly useful during brainstem neuronal recordings because the exposed brain surface is easily cooled down during recordings.

12. The arterial blood pressure is a very useful index for monitoring animals' conditions during the recording. Usually, the blood pressure responds more quickly than the expired CO_2 concentration. We monitor the blood pressure from the rats' tail every 30 min through a noninvasive approach. The blood pressure may be monitored continuously through the femoral artery line or other monitoring systems (IITC, Woodland Hills, CA).

13. The amplitude of an action potential should be in the range of 50–100 microvolts. Do not be ambitious to obtain action potential with very large amplitude, which suggests that the electrode is very close to the cell body. An unusually large action potential often quickly leads to so-called "death firing" of a neuron: high-frequency discharges with rapidly diminishing amplitude. Thus, it is often wise to withdraw electrode slightly to reduce the amplitude of action potentials when signal-to-noise ratio can be maintained at a reasonable level.

    A very large action potential may also be owing to recording from a nerve fiber. Different from the cell body, action potentials from nerve fibers usually exhibit more than two phases with first phase positive and with narrower spike width. The nerve fiber spikes make a high-pitched sound through the audio monitor as compared with the sound of action potentials from cell bodies.

    During recordings, the rat's brain is always vibrating as a result of blood flow and ventilation, which may result in change in the shape of spike. If the height of spike is gradually decreased, the electrode needs to be advanced or withdrawn to maintain the waveform and recoding from the same neuron. To ensure recording from the same neuron, monitor the waveform configuration during continuous recordings.

14. Graded mechanical stimuli are applied to the most sensitive area of the RFs. The mechanical stimuli consist of brushing with a camel hairbrush, pressure produced by a large arterial clip, and pinch produced by a small arterial clip. Noxious mechanical stimuli are applied only to small areas of the RFs to avoid sensitization owing to repeated stimulation. If the non-noxious RFs of first and secondly encountered nociceptive neurons overlap each other, the second neuron should not be included in the analysis. A set of Semmes-Weinstein monofilaments (von Frey filaments, Stoelting) can be used to assess mechanical response threshold.

15. A proprioceptive neuron only responds to stretch of the muscle and not to cutaneous stimuli. Thus, some proprioceptive neurons act like NS neurons because they respond to a forced pinch that may activate muscle spindle receptors and appear to respond exclusively to noxious stimuli. Carefully applying noxious mechanical stimulus to the cutaneous and not involving deep tissues will validate the neuronal type.

    To avoid sensitization of the RFs, do not attempt exhausted and repeated noxious stimuli to search for NS neurons. If a neuron shows weak responses to a pressure stimulus and not to brushing, noxious pinch can be applied to verify if it is an NS neuron.

16. The electrode can be placed either ipsilateral or contralateral to the side of recording depending on the known anatomical pathways. To aid the placement of

the stimulating electrode, try to evoke and audibly monitor multiple unit activity of the target site by tactile stimulation of the orofacial skin. Multiple electrodes or systematic tracking method can be used to increase the efficiency of antidromic activation.

17. It is helpful to take a photograph of the surface of the medulla before the start of recording using a Polaroid camera. The picture is very useful for further histological identification of the location of the recording sites **(Fig. 4)**.

Acknowledgments

The authors thank Dr. R. Dubner for his comments on the manuscript. The authors' work is supported by USPHS grant DE11964 (K.R.) and Grants-in-Aid for Scientific Research (7457442, 9671907, and 9771551) from the Japanese Ministry of Education, Science and Culture, and the Ministry of Health and Welfare (H11-Choju-006).

References

1. Price, D. D., Dubner, R., and Hu, J. W. (1976) Trigeminal neurons in nucleus caudalis responsive to tactile, thermal, and nociceptive stimulation of monkey's face. *J. Neurophysiol.* **39**, 936–953.

2. Broton, J. G., Hu, J. W., and Sessle, B. J. (1988) Effects of temporomandibular joint stimulation on nociceptive and non-nociceptive neurons of the cat's trigeminal subnucleus caudalis (medullary dorsal horn). *J. Neurophysiol.* **59**, 1575–1589.

3. Hu, J. W. (1990) Response properties of nociceptive and non-nociceptive neurons in the rat's trigeminal subnucleus caudalis (medullary dorsal horn) related to cutaneous and deep craniofacial afferent stimulation and modulation by diffuse noxious inhibitory controls. *Pain* **41**, 331–345.

4. Chiang, C. Y., Hu, J. W., and Sessle, B. J. (1994) Parabrachial area and nucleus raphe magnus-induced modulation of nociceptive and non-nociceptive trigeminal subnucleus caudalis neurons activated by cutaneous or deep inputs. *J. Neurophysiol.* **71**, 2430–2445.

5. Meng, I. D., Hu, J. W., Benetti, A. P., and Bereiter, D. A. (1997) Encoding of corneal input in two distinct regions of the spinal trigeminal nucleus in the rat: cutaneous receptive field properties, responses to thermal and chemical stimulation, modulation by diffuse noxious inhibitory controls, and projections to the parabrachial area. *J. Neurophysiol.* **77**, 43–56.

6. Iwata, K., Tashiro, A., Tsuboi, Y., et al. (1999) Enhancement and depression of medullary dorsal horn neuronal activity after noxious and non-noxious stimulation of the face in rats with persistent temporomandibular joint and cutaneous inflammation. *J. Neurophysiol.* **82**, 1244–1253.

7. Iwata, K., Imai, T., Tsuboi, Y., et al. (2001) Alteration of medullary dorsal horn neuronal activity following inferior alveolar nerve transection in rats. *J. Neurophysiol.* **86**, 2868–2877.

8. Lipski, J. (1981) Antidromic activation of neurones as an analytic tool in the study of the central nervous system. *J. Neurosci. Meth.* **4**, 1–32.

9. Ren, K., Randich, A., and Gebhart, G. F. (1991) Effects of electrical stimulation of vagal afferents on spinothalamic tract cells in the rat. *Pain* **44,** 311–319.

10. Malick, A., Strassman, A. M., and Burstein, R. (2000) Trigeminohypothalamic and reticulohypothalamic tract neurons in the upper cervical spinal cord and caudal medulla of the rat. *J. Neurophysiol.* **84,** 2078–2112.

11. Paxinos, G. and Watson, C. (1998) *The Rat Brain in Stereotaxic Coordinates,* 4th ed. Academic Press, San Diego, CA.

12. Sugiyama, K., Dong, W. K., and Chudler, E. H. (1994) A simplified method for manufacturing glass-insulated metal microelectrodes. *J. Neurosci. Methods* **53,** 73–80

13. Haas, D. A., Nakanishi, O., MacMillan, R. E., et al. (1992) Development of an orofacial model of acute inflammation in the rat. *Arch. Oral Biol.* **37,** 417–422.

14. Zhou, Q-Q., Imbe, H., Dubner, R., and Ren, K. (1999) Persistent trigeminal fos protein expression after orofacial deep or cutaneous tissue inflammation in rats: implications for persistent orofacial pain. *J. Comp. Neurol.* **412,** 276–291.

15. Imbe, H., Iwata, K., Zhou, Q-Q., et al. (2001) Orofacial deep and cutaneous tissue inflammation and trigeminal neuronal activation: implications for persistent temporomandibular pain. *Cells Tissues Organs* **169,** 238–247.

12

In Vivo Electrophysiology of Dorsal-Horn Neurons

Louise C. Stanfa and Anthony H. Dickenson

Summary

The dorsal horn of the spinal cord is a key relay in the transmission of sensory information to the brain. Furthermore, this circuitry of spinal-cord neurons, and hence the spinal processing of sensory information, is subject to a great deal of plasticity, both pharmacological and physiological, in persistent pain states. This chapter describes in detail the procedure by which the activity and pharmacological modulation of these dorsal-horn neurons can be recorded in vivo in anesthetized rats, allowing a comprehensive study of spinal sensory processing in an intact and integrated system. The chapter covers the surgical preparation of the animal for electrophysiological recording; isolating and recording the activity of a single dorsal-horn neuron; and identifying the type of dorsal-horn neuron recorded by characterizing the neuronal response to a variety of peripheral stimuli. The study of these neuronal responses in a variety of persistent pain states, such as carrageenan-induced inflammation and neuropathy induced by L5/L6 spinal nerve ligation, together with the study of their pharmacological modulation by locally or systemically administered drugs, is also described.

Key Words: In vivo electrophysiology, dorsal-horn neuron, halothane anesthetized rat, laminectomy, noxious/innocuous mechanical and thermal stimuli, transcutaneous electrical stimulation, C-fiber evoked activity, wind-up.

1. Introduction

Pain transmission is not a hard-wired system. The dorsal horn of the spinal cord is a key relay in the transmission of sensory information to the brain. Here, sensory information from the periphery is integrated, modulated, and relayed to the higher brain centers. Located within the dorsal horn is a complex network of interneurons. This is a dynamic circuitry, capable of a great deal of plasticity either as a result of pharmacological intervention or pathophysiological changes resulting from insult or trauma to the peripheral nervous system (PNS), the net result of which is to alter the relationship between the sensory input arriving at the spinal cord and the sensory output relayed from the spinal cord to the brain.

From: *Methods in Molecular Medicine, Vol. 99: Pain Research: Methods and Protocols*
Edited by: Z. D. Luo © Humana Press Inc., Totowa, NJ

This can arise from changes in channels, e.g., the increased role of N-type Ca^{2+} channels seen after nerve injury *(1)*, transmitters or their receptors, e.g., the enhanced potency of spinal opioids following peripheral inflammation *(2)* or even anatomical changes such as the Aβ-fiber sprouting proposed after nerve injury *(3)*. Using the techniques described in this chapter, the physiology and pharmacology of the spinal processing of sensory information can be investigated both in naïve animals and, by studying the activity of dorsal-horn neurons in various animal models of nociception, e.g., carrageenan-induced inflammation, neuropathy induced by L5/L6 spinal nerve ligation, can give us an insight into how the processing and pharmacological modulation of nociceptive (and innocuous) sensory information is altered in persistent pain states.

This chapter describes the procedure for recording the evoked activity of dorsal-horn neurons in vivo in anesthetised rats. The chapter will cover the surgical preparation of the animal for electrophysiological recording, isolating and recording the activity of a single dorsal-horn neuron, and identifying the type of dorsal-horn neuron recorded, that is, low-threshold, high-threshold (nociceptive specific), or wide-dynamic range by characterizing the neuronal response to a variety of stimuli.

2. Materials

2.1. Surgical Preparation of the Animal

1. Halothane anesthetic system consisting of halothane vaporizer, O_2 and N_2O supply with flow meters, anesthesia mask, anesthetizing box.
2. Tracheal cannula (~ 5 cm length of fine-bore polythene tubing 2 mm outer diameter), thread (3-0 silk thread) and Y-connector to connect cannula to anesthetic tubing.
3. Homeothermic animal blanket system.
4. Surgical instruments including scissors, scalpel, range of forceps (including tissue, small curved, and watchmakers) and delicate bone rongeurs (we use Friedman rongeurs from Harvard Apparatus).
5. Frame with ear bars and vertebrae clamps to support the animal during electrophysiological recording, such as the small animal spinal unit and vertebrae clamps produced by David Kopf Instruments (Tujunga, CA).

2.2. Electrophysiological Recording

1. AC recording system with spike discrimination and audio monitoring. We use the NeuroLog system (Digitimer, UK); *see* **Fig. 1** for details.
2. Oscilloscope.

→

Fig. 1. Diagram illustrating the neuronal recording system using Neurolog modules (Digitimer). Note that the gray connections between the modules are via the rear panel connectors.

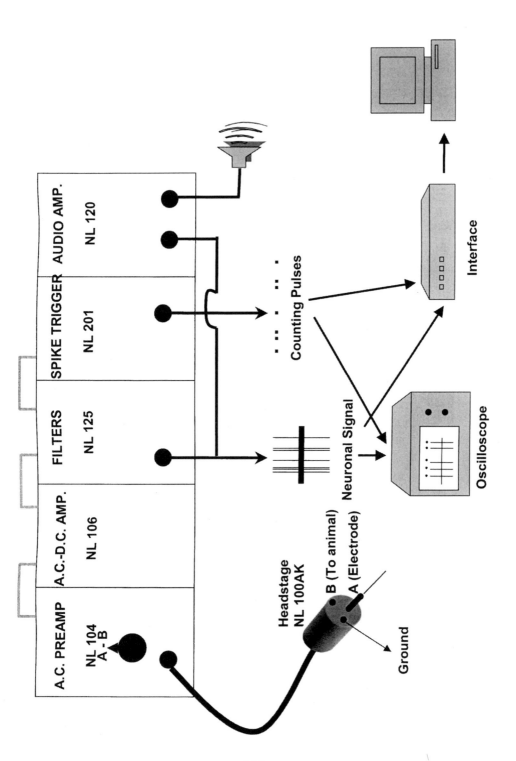

141

3. Data acquisition interface and computer with data capture and analysis software (we use micro 1401 interface with Spike 2 software from Cambridge Electronic Design, UK).
4. Three axis micromanipulator with programmable stepper (optional, e.g., SCAT-01 computer controlled stepper; Digitimer).
5. Electrodes (Parylene-C insulated tungsten microelectrodes, 125 μm diameter, 2 M Ohms, A-M Systems Inc.)

2.3. Characterization of the Neuronal Response

Equipment needed for characterization of the neuronal response depends on the stimulus modalities required.

1. Mechanical stimulation: Von Frey filaments.
2. Thermal stimulation: water bath, 50 mL syringe with 21-G needle.
3. Electrical stimulation: constant current stimulator (we use the Neurolog System from Digitimer, consisting of Period Generator NL 304, Digital Width NL 401, Pulse Buffer NL 510, Counter NL 603, and Stimulus Isolator NL 800) and transcutaneous stimulating electrodes (we use 27-G syringe needles soldered to fine insulated wire).

3. Methods

The methods described here outline: (1) the surgical preparation of the animal, (2) neuronal recording, including searching for and isolating the response of a single dorsal-horn neuron; (3) characterizing the neuronal response; (4) pharmacological evaluation; and (5) application of this technique in animal models of persistent pain.

3.1. Surgical Preparation of the Animal

The aim of this section is to get the animal anesthetised and to expose and support the lumbar spinal cord in preparation for electrophysiological recording. This stage will take approx 30 min.

1. Anesthetize the rat in anesthetizing box using 3% halothane in a 33% O_2 (150 cm^3/min) 66% N_2O (300 cm^3/min) mixture (*see* **Note 1**). Once the animal has lost consciousness, place the animal on its back in the anesthesia mask or nose cone and reduce the level of anesthesia to 2%, or whatever is required to maintain areflexia.
2. Once the animal is areflexic, make an incision in the skin of the throat and use blunt dissection to expose the trachea. Use a scalpel to open the trachea between the cartilage rings, taking care not to cut all the way through, and insert the cannula 1 cm. Tie the cannula securely in place and connect to the anesthetic system using a Y-connector (*see* **Note 2**).
3. Secure the rat in the ear bars of the frame and ensure that heating blanket is in place to maintain the body temperature of the animal at $37 \pm 0.5°C$. Make a rostro-caudal

incision through the skin on the animal's back and locate the lumbar enlargement. Make parallel incisions through the muscle either side of lumbar enlargement to allow the fixing of spinal clamps. Position the first spinal clamp on the frame just rostral to vertebra L1 (*see* **Note 3**), lift the vertebral column into the jaws of the clamp and tighten securely, taking care not to crush the vertebrae. After positioning the first clamp, gently pull back the clamp on the frame to straighten the torso of the animal and aid breathing.

4. Cut and scrape away the connective tissue and muscle (*see* **Note 4**) overlying the vertebrae to be removed until the joins between the vertebrae can be seen. Insert the tip of the rongeurs between the vertebrae and perform a laminectomy by nibbling off the dorsal surface of the vertebrae, working in a rostral direction and keeping the jaws of the rongeurs parallel to the spinal cord to avoid damaging the cord.

5. Once the laminectomy is completed, position the second spinal clamp caudally to the exposed cord and tighten (*see* **Note 5**). If the dura remains on the spinal cord (the surface of the cord should look smooth and shiny; if it has a wrinkled appearance this indicates the presence of the dura) following the laminectomy, this can be removed with fine watchmaker's forceps. The pia should be left intact. In most cases, a flow of cerebrospinal fluid (CSF) will keep the exposed cord moist; if the cord appears dry, a small volume (50 µL) of physiological saline (0.9%) can be applied (this does not need to be warmed).

6. Prior to commencement of the electrophysiological recording, reduce level of halothane to 1% (or the minimum level required to keep the rats areflexic; this should be checked regularly throughout the experiment, although in practice once a suitable level of anesthesia has been established this rarely changes during the experiment).

We do not routinely monitor parameters such as blood pressure and heart rate because we have previously shown that the blood pressure of the animal and end-expiratory CO_2 levels remain constant under these anesthetic conditions, even during the application of noxious stimuli *(4)*. However, these parameters can be measured to check the physiological condition of the animal and the depth of anesthesia if required. If not monitoring externally, the "pinkness" of the animal's paws and the abolition of reflexes to strong noxious stimuli are good indicators of the physiological well-being and adequate anesthesia of the animal, respectively.

3.2. Recording

3.2.1. Recording Neuronal Responses

Using the recording system shown in **Fig. 1,** parylene-coated tungsten electrodes are used to record the activity of single dorsal-horn neurons. The recording system is grounded through the animal frame, and the headstage receives an input from both the electrode (signal A) and from a clip attached to the animal (signal B) allowing differential recording to remove much of the interference from the neuronal signal. Subsequently, the neuronal signal is amplified, filtered, and displayed on an oscilloscope and also fed to an audio amplifier. The filtered signal is also fed to a window discriminator to allow spike discrimination. Quantification of the neuronal activity is made with a data-acquisition interface and data-capture and -analysis software such as the micro1401 interface and Spike2 software from Cambridge Electronic Design.

3.2.2. Isolating a Single Neuron

Insert electrode into the spinal cord (*see* **Note 6**) as close to the central vessel as possible and withdraw slowly until surface of cord is reached (if the electrode is withdrawn while tapping the ipsilateral hindpaw, the signal will go quiet as the electrode leaves the dorsal horn). Once the surface of the cord has been reached, slowly advance the electrode through the spinal cord using either a manual micromanipulator or stepper (10 μm steps) while tapping the plantar surface of the hindpaw (*see* **Note 7**). Care should be taken during prolonged searching not to sensitize the tissues of the foot through over-vigorous tapping. Once a neuron has been identified by spikes that are distinguishable from background activity, the signal-to-noise ratio can be optimized by carefully moving the electrode up and down the tract (10 μm steps) until the signal to noise ratio is maximal. In practice, a signal-to-noise ratio of at least 4:1 is desirable, although larger ratios in the order 8:1 of are usually achieved (*see* **Note 8**). Once isolated, the neuronal response of a single neuron will have a uniform spike amplitude; a collection of spikes of different amplitudes indicates the activity of more than one neuron is being recorded. In this case, the neurons can often be separated by moving the electrode (~ 10–50 μm in either direction) in order to increase the neuronal separation, and the window discriminator can be set to count only the larger neuron.

The laminar localization of the neuron can be estimated by its depth from the surface of the dorsal horn. In the lumbar spinal cord of adult rats, the highest concentration of lamina I-type neurons is located approx 0–100 μm from the surface of the dorsal horn and the neurons of the substantia gelatinosa, which are predominantly interneurons, at depths of 100–250 μm. Wide-dynamic range or convergent neurons, which are the main type of neuron encoding stimulus intensity in the dorsal horn, are found in highest concentrations in the deeper laminae (V–VI) *(5)* which is found approx 500–1000 μm from the surface. These depths are approximate, and the characteristics of the neuronal response provide an additional guide to the type of neuron recorded (*see* **Subheading 3.3.**).

Although the majority of projection neurons transmitting nociceptive information supraspinally are found in laminae I and V/VI, the technique described here does not distinguish between intrinsic and projection neurons. It is possible to establish whether a dorsal-horn neuron projects supraspinally by showing antidromic activation of that neuron (meeting the three classical criteria of: (1) constant latency of the evoked spike; (2) ability to follow high-frequency (200–500 Hz) stimulation; (3) collision between the antidromically and ortho-dromically evoked spikes) from the relevant brain region, e.g., the contralateral thalamus for spinothalamic tract neurons *(6)* or the parabrachial area for spin-oparabrachial neurons *(7)*. This will not be described further here.

3.3. Characterizing the Neuronal Response

Once the neuron has been isolated, and the receptive field on the hindpaw mapped, the characteristics of the neuronal response can be used to broadly classify the type of dorsal-horn neuron being recorded.

3.3.1. Low-Threshold Neurons

These neurons respond (in some cases quite vigorously) to low-intensity stimuli such as brush and light touch, but will not give a sustained response to a noxious stimulus such as pinch. Low-threshold neurones only receive A-fiber input, and transcutaneous electrical stimulation of their peripheral receptive field (*see* **Subheading 3.3.5.**) will evoke only a short latency Aβ- and/or Aδ-fiber response. They are found primarily in laminae II, III, and IV *(5)* but may be encountered at any depth. Neurons responding to flexion of joints are known as proprioceptive neurons.

3.3.2. Wide-Dynamic Range Neurons

Wide-dynamic range (WDR) neurons receive input from both A- and C-fibers and hence respond to both innocuous (such as light touch and brush) and noxious (such as pinch) stimuli. These neurons code stimulus intensity well, so will give a graded response to a stimulus increasing in intensity from innocuous to noxious (*see* **Fig. 2**). Unlike low-threshold neurons, WDR neurons will give a sustained response to noxious pinch, with the firing often con-tinuing for some seconds following cessation of the stimulus. Transcutaneous electrical stimulation (*see* **Subheading 3.3.5.** and **Fig. 3**) of the peripheral receptive field of WDR neurons evokes both a low-threshold, short-latency, A-fiber-evoked response and a longer-latency, higher-threshold, C-fiber response. WDR neurons are found predominantly in lamina V, but also in laminae I, II$_o$, IV, VI, and X *(5)*.

It is worth pointing out that if you are able to evoke both a short-latency (A-fiber) and longer-latency (C-fiber) response following a single electrical stimu-lus, then you must be recording from a postsynaptic neuron; there is no possibility you are recording a single fiber. In the case of low-threshold stimuli, fibers can be distinguished from neurons by the former having broad action potentials and generally being recorded in the zone above lamina I.

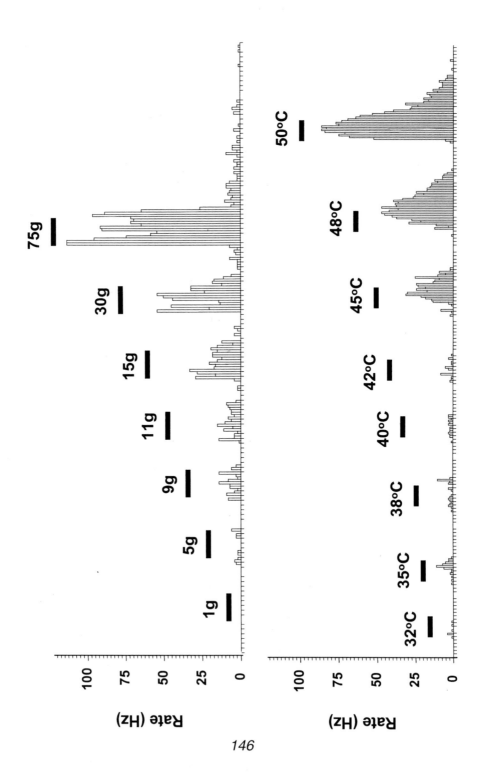

3.3.3. Nociceptive-Specific Neurons

These neurons respond only to high-intensity noxious stimuli, and so are rarely encountered in this preparation because of the non-noxious search stimulus used (*see* **Note 7**). They do not respond to touch, only stimuli such as strong pinch, although transcutaneous electrical stimulation will often evoke a short-latency, A-fiber response. Nociceptive specific neurons are found predominantly in lamina I of the dorsal horn *(5)*.

3.3.4. Characterizing and Quantifying Responses to Natural Stimuli

1. Mechanical stimuli. The response of the neuron to a range of intensities of mechanical stimuli can be assessed by applying a series of graded von Frey filaments to the most sensitive area of the receptive field for a period of 10 s and counting the response evoked using the rate function of the data-analysis software (*see* **Fig. 2**). The response to dynamic stimuli can be assessed by uniform brushing of the receptive field (with a small artist's paintbrush) for a period of time and counting the response evoked.
2. Thermal stimuli. A straightforward and effective way to test the thermal responsiveness of the neuron is by quantifying the response evoked by a jet of water squirted onto the receptive field for a period of 10 s using a syringe (*see* **Fig. 2**); this is easily achievable within the confines of the frame. The use of water as a heating medium ensures good contact with the skin of the receptive field and provides rapid heating to the desired temperature, which can be adjusted over the range required. The mechanical component to the stimulus can be corrected for by first applying a jet of water at 32°C and then subtracting this response from the response to subsequent thermal stimuli. Alternatively, other thermal stimulators such as radiant lamps (slow rate of cutaneous heating), contact thermodes (relatively slow, and require good thermode-skin contact), or CO_2 lasers (expensive and complex) can be used if preferred *(8)*.

3.3.5. Transcutaneous Electrical Stimulation

Transcutaneous electrical stimulation of the peripheral receptive field of the neuron using a constant current stimulator can be a very useful method of stimulation. It is well-controlled, so very stable reproducible responses of the dorsal-horn neuron can be obtained, and the responses evoked in the dorsal-horn neuron by the different peripheral-fiber types can be clearly separated on the basis of

---

Fig. 2. Rate recordings of the response of a wide-dynamic range neuron to a graded series of von-Frey filaments (1–75 g, top) or thermal stimuli (32–50°C, bottom) applied to the peripheral receptive field for a period of 10 s (shown by the horizontal bars). These neurons show the encoding of stimulus intensity typical of wide-dynamic range neurons.

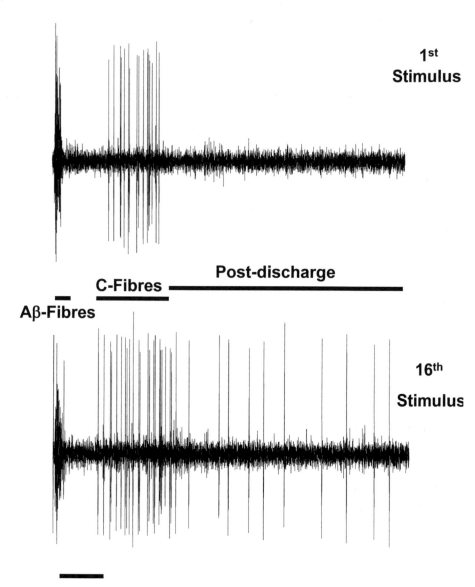

Fig. 3. Responses evoked in a single wide-dynamic range neuron by transcutaneous electrical stimulation. Traces show the response of the neuron to the first and the last stimulus in a train of 16 stimuli delivered at 0.5 Hz and three times the threshold current required to evoke a C-fiber response. The first stimulus evokes a short-latency Aβ-fiber response and a longer-latency, clearly separate, C-fiber-evoked response (this neuron shows no clear Aδ-fiber-evoked response). With repeated stimulation, this neuron displays the phenomenon of wind-up, which results in the increased C-fiber-evoked response and prolonged firing (known as the post-discharge) seen in response to the 16th stimulus.

both threshold and poststimulus latency. In addition, it allows a suprathreshold noxious stimulus to be administered repeatedly without tissue damage. Electrical stimulation directly activates the peripheral endings of the fibers, bypassing the transduction mechanism, which can be an advantage because it allows us to be sure that any changes seen are the result of changes in the central processing, rather than the peripheral transduction, of nociceptive information.

1. Locate the most sensitive area of receptive field and insert stimulating needles intradermally, e.g., on adjacent toes, ensuring that the needles are not touching.
2. Set the stimulus intensity to 0–1 mA range and stimulate while gradually increasing the intensity until a short latency (<20 ms poststimulus) neuronal response is evoked; this is the Aβ-fiber-evoked response. The average threshold current required to evoke this response is ~0.12 mA. Increase the range on the stimulator to 1–10 mA and increase the current until the longer latency response evoked by the slower conducting C-fibers is seen (**Fig. 3**); the latency for this response is between 90–300 ms poststimulus for 200–250 g rats, but the range for this response will be earlier or later in smaller or larger rats, respectively (see below). The average threshold current required to evoke a C-fiber response in the dorsal-horn neuron is approx 1.5 mA
3. The stimulator (we use Neurolog modules) can then be set as required to deliver a train of stimuli at the desired intensity. We use a train of 16 stimuli (square wave pulse, 2 ms pulse width) delivered at 3 times the threshold current required to evoke a C-fiber response at a frequency of 0.5 Hz, which is sufficient to evoke the phenomenon of wind-up (*see* ref. *9*). Reducing the intensity and/or frequency of stimulation to 0.1 Hz eliminates the development of wind-up (*9*).
4. Use a data-capture and -analysis program such as Spike2 (Cambridge Electronic Design) to display the neuronal responses as a poststimulus time histogram (PSTH) (**Fig. 4**) from which the responses evoked by Aβ-fibers (0–20 ms poststimulus), Aδ-fibers (20–90 ms), and C-fibers (90–300 ms) can be separated on the basis of latency and quantified. Activity evoked more than 300 ms after the stimulus is termed the post-discharge (300–800 ms poststimulus) and is generated as a result of the mechanisms underlying wind-up. These latencies are based on a 200–250 g rat and will need to be adjusted as required for larger or smaller animals. In rats weighing 350 g, the C-fiber latency band will extend to 350 ms, with the postdischarge taken between 350 and 800 ms (the A-fiber latency bands are unchanged). In rat pups (P14–P28, weighing 35–100 g) and mice, A-fibers are recorded between 0 and 50 ms poststimulus, C-fibers 50 and 250 ms and postdischarge 250 and 800 ms. In the smaller animals, it is not possible to separate the Aβ- and Aδ-fiber evoked activity.

3.4. Evaluation of Drug Effects on the Evoked Neuronal Responses

Once stable control responses have been established (*see* **Note 9**) (<10% variation in the natural or C-fiber-evoked response) the ability of drugs to modulate the various components of the evoked response can be tested. Drugs can be administered systemically (subcutaneously [sc] or via an intravenous [iv] cannula), locally

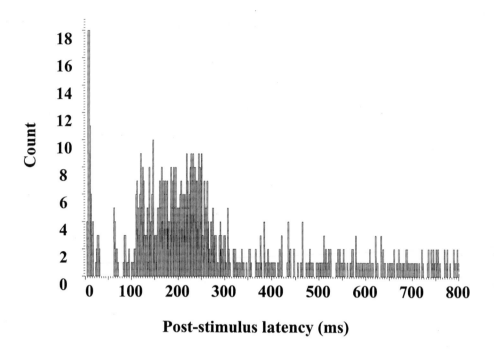

Fig. 4. Poststimulus time histogram showing the cumulative response of a wide-dynamic range neuron (recorded in a 250 g rat) to a train of 16 stimuli (0.5 Hz) delivered at three times the threshold current required to activate C-fibers. The responses evoked by the different fiber types can be separated on the basis of latency: Aβ-fibers (0–20 ms), Aδ-fibers (20–90 ms), and C-fibers (90–300 ms). The post-discharge (the neuronal activity generated as a result of wind-up) is counted from 300–800 ms poststimulus.

into the peripheral receptive field of the neuron (in a volume of 20 μL) or topically onto the exposed spinal cord akin to an intrathecal (it) injection. Administration of drugs directly onto the exposed spinal cord is performed by using a Hamilton syringe to gently place 50 μL of drug solution into the well formed by the laminectomy (*see* **Note 10**). Following administration of the drug, the testing cycle can be repeated at 10-min (or 15-min) intervals for an appropriate time-course (usually 40–90 min, depending on the drug and route of administration).

3.5. Use of this Technique to Study Animal Models of Acute and Persistent Nociception

In addition to studying the evoked responses of dorsal-horn neurons recorded in naïve, noninjured animals, this technique can also be used to study changes in the spinal transmission and modulation of sensory messages in animals with an inflammatory or neuropathic insult. Examples of acute pain models include carrageenan-induced inflammation *(2)* and the formalin response *(10)*, which, because of their short (h) time-course, are induced while recording the neuronal response. In more persistent pain models, such as the L5/L6 spinal nerve ligation described in this volume by Chung, the electrophysiological recordings are made days or weeks after the initial nerve injury *(11)*.

4. Notes

1. We use adult male rats weighing 200–250 g, although the technique can be adapted to younger rats (as young as P14; *see* **ref.** *12*) or mice *(13)*. Anesthetics other than halothane can also be used. For convenience of administration, we use urethane rather than halothane anesthesia for the younger rats (P14–P28, 2.4 g/kg ip) and mice (3 g/kg ip). In adult rats, urethane *(12,14)*, pentobarbital sodium *(15)*, and α-chloralose *(16)* have been used as an alternative to halothane during similar electrophysiological procedures.

2. We insert a tracheal cannula because this provides a convenient and secure way to deliver anesthetic throughout the experiment; however, a rodent anesthetic mask could also be used.

3. For neurons receiving input from the hindpaw, expose the region of cord receiving input from spinal nerves L4–L5; this can be located by feeling for the point where the animal's ribs meet the vertebral column and removing one vertebra above and one below this point.

4. It is best to remove only the narrow center strip of tissue, leaving the edges of the vertebrae covered, because this will form the walls of a "pool" over the exposed spinal cord in the completed preparation, which will hold CSF, drugs, and so on.

5. Stability. To ensure that the completed preparation is as stable as possible during the electrophysiological recording, it is advisable to keep the laminectomy as narrow and short as possible (approx 3 × 13 mm), to position the spinal clamps close to either end of the exposed spinal cord, and to place the exposed cord under a small degree of tension by pulling back on the second clamp.

6. If the electrode has been inserted into L4–L5 insertion region, then neuronal activity will be heard while tapping the ipsilateral hindpaw; if activity is heard while tapping the base of the tail, the electrode should be repositioned rostrally, while activity from the flank indicates that the electrode needs to move caudally.

7. The use of a non-noxious search stimulus is preferable to avoid tissue damage, but will only activate low-threshold afferents, thereby only identifying low-threshold or convergent/WDR spinal neurons. If high-threshold neurons are required, a correspondingly higher intensity of search stimulus will have to be used.

8. Occasionally during the course of an experiment, instability of the preparation (e.g., owing to respiratory movements) can cause the amplitude of the neuron to become smaller; this can often be rectified by moving the electrode up or down 10–40 μm to bring it closer to the neuron. This is not always successful and the experiment may have to be terminated if it is not possible to clearly separate the

neuron from the background activity/other neurons. Sometimes neurons are lost during the course of an experiment because they are burst by the tip of the electrode; this has a distinctive sound resulting from a short period of frantic neuronal firing as the neuron dies, followed by an inability to evoke a response.

9. Control (and post-drug administration) responses are usually performed at 10-min intervals, but if many modalities of stimuli are being tested, e.g., electrical, mechanical, and thermal, this may need to be extended to 15 min to allow the testing cycle to be completed without the neuron being over-stimulated. (This is particularly important when using high-intensity noxious heat, which can evoke prolonged firing in the dorsal-horn neurons.)

10. If spinal administration of drugs is to be performed, care should be taken during the laminectomy to leave as much of the muscle surrounding the exposed spinal cord as possible to form a good "well" to hold the drug solution in place and once the initial surgical procedure is completed, to check that the spinal cord is held level in the clamps such that saline placed onto the cord does not run off.

References

1. Matthews, E. A. and Dickenson, A. H. (2001) Effects of spinally delivered N- and P-type voltage-dependent calcium channel antagonists on dorsal horn neuronal responses in a rat model of neuropathy. *Pain* **92**, 235–246.

2. Stanfa, L. C., Sullivan, A. F., and Dickenson, A. H. (1992) Alterations in neuronal excitability and the potency of spinal mu, delta and kappa opioids after carrageenan-induced inflammation. *Pain* **50**, 345–354.

3. Woolf, C. J., Shortland, P., and Coggeshall, R. E. (1992) Peripheral nerve injury triggers central sprouting of myelinated afferents. *Nature* **355**, 75–78.

4. Dickenson, A. H. and Le Bars, D. (1987) Supraspinal morphine and descending inhibitions acting on the dorsal horn of the rat. *J. Physiol.* **384**, 81–107.

5. Millan, M. J. (1999) The induction of pain: an integrative review. *Prog. Neurobiol.* **57**, 1–164.

6. Dickenson, A. H. and Le Bars, D. (1983) Diffuse noxious inhibitory controls (DNIC) involve trigeminothalamic and spinothalamic neurones in the rat. *Exp. Brain Res.* **49**, 174–180.

7. Bester, H., Chapman, V., Besson, J.-M., and Bernard, J.-F. (2000) Physiological properties of the lamina I spinoparabrachial neurones in the rat. *J. Neurophysiol.* **83**, 2239–2259.

8. Le Bars, D. Gozariu, M., and Cadden, S. W. (2001) Animal models of nociception. *Pharmacol. Rev.* **53**, 597–652.

9. Dickenson, A. H. and Sullivan, A. F. (1987) Evidence for a role of the NMDA receptor in the frequency dependent potentiation of deep dorsal horn neurones following C-fibre stimulation. *Neuropharmacology* **26**, 1235–1238.

10. Dickenson, A. H. and Sullivan, A. F. (1987) Subcutaneous formalin-induced activity of dorsal horn neurones in the rat: differential response to an intrathecal opioid administered pre or post formalin. *Pain* **30**, 349–360.

11. Chapman, V., Suzuki, R., and Dickenson, A. H. (1998) Electrophysiological characterisation of spinal neuronal response properties in anaesthetized rats after ligation of spinal nerves L5–L6. *J. Physiol.* **507,** 881–894.
12. Urch, C. E., Rahman, W., and Dickenson, A. H. (2001) Electrophysiological studies on the role of the NMDA receptor in nociception in the developing rat spinal cord. *Dev. Brain Res.* **126,** 81–89.
13. Souslova, V., Cesare, P., Ding, Y., et al. (2000) Warm-coding defects and aberrant inflammatory pain in mice lacking P2X$_3$ receptors. *Nature* **407,** 1015–1017.
14. Rygh, L. J., Svendsen, F., Hole, K., and Tjølsen, A. (2001) Increased spinal *N*-methyl-D-aspartate receptor function after 20 h of carrageenan-induced inflammation. *Pain* **93,** 15–21.
15. Jinks, S. L. and Carstens, E. (2000) Superficial dorsal horn neurons identified by intracutaneous histamine: chemonociceptive responses and modulation by morphine. *J. Neurophysiol.* **84,** 616–627.
16. Chizh, B. A., Cumberbatch, M. J., Herrero, J. F., et al. (1997) Stimulus intensity, cell excitation and the *N*-methyl-D-aspartate receptor component of sensory responses in the rat spinal cord *in vivo. Neuroscience* **80,** 251–265.

13

Single-Fiber Recording

In Vivo and In Vitro Preparations

Maria Schäfers and David Cain

Summary

This chapter focuses on in vivo and in vitro recording setups of extracellular single-unit recordings of peripheral sensory nerve or dorsal root fibers in rodents. Extracellular single-unit recording methods have been used to obtain a wealth of data about the properties of peripheral nervous system (PNS) and central nervous system (CNS) structures. The rationale for studying the activity of single-unit primary afferent fibers is predicated on the significance of relatively fine variations of fiber responsiveness to mechanical, chemical, and/or thermal stimuli. It involves microdissection of nerve fiber bundles until the electrical activity of a single fiber is isolated. Electrophysiological changes in thresholds and discharge rates of peripheral nociceptors to polymodal stimuli can provide neurophysiological correlation to behavioral hyperalgesia and allodynia as well as to cellular differences observable with immunohistochemistry. This chapter gives an overview about the necessary general and special equipment, details about the different setups and tissue preparations. Additionally, the chapter informs about the procedure of recording from single units, data acquisition and analysis including unit isolation criteria and techniques for spike discrimination techniques and fiber classification. It describes criteria for the classification of nociceptors and identification of cutaneous afferent units.

Key Words: Extracellular recording, in vivo setup, in vitro setup, teased-fiber microdissection, nociceptor, single unit.

1. Introduction

Since their refinement in the early 1950s, extracellular, single-unit recording methods have been used to obtain a wealth of data about the properties of peripheral nervous system (PNS) and central nervous system (CNS) structures *(1–3)*. The most practical approach to this form of electrophysiology for the PNS is known as the teased-fiber technique, which has been described as delicate, tedious, and time-consuming *(4)*. The rationale for studying the

From: *Methods in Molecular Medicine, Vol. 99: Pain Research: Methods and Protocols*
Edited by: Z. D. Luo © Humana Press Inc., Totowa, NJ

activity of single-unit primary afferent fibers is predicated on the significance of relatively fine variations of fiber responsiveness to mechanical, chemical, and/or thermal stimuli. It involves microdissection of nerve-fiber bundles until the electrical activity of a single fiber is isolated. Although such recordings do not give information about the inputs to a particular cell (excitatory and inhibitory postsynaptic potentials or currents) as intracellular recordings would, they can provide a wealth of information about the functional properties of single cells and neuronal connectivity in the intact and injured nervous system. Electrophysiological changes in thresholds and discharge rates of peripheral nociceptors to polymodal stimuli can provide neurophysiological correlation to behavioral hyperalgesia and allodynia as well as to cellular differences observable with immunohistochemistry *(5)*. Elaborate methods have been developed to study such activity in anesthetized or awake animals or in in vitro preparations. This chapter will focus on in vivo and in vitro recording setups of extracellular single-unit recording of peripheral sensory-nerve or dorsal-root fibers in rodents.

2. Materials

In most extracellular studies, it is the frequency of neuronal spikes that is of most interest. Therefore, the recordings are usually done with an AC amplifier, with which most irrelevant signals such as DC shifts and high-frequency noise can be filtered out. These amplifiers usually have filters to cut off frequencies below and above a particular range (band-pass filters) and allow an amplification of at least 10,000 times the actual signal. The signal is normally visualized on an oscilloscope. Action potentials of the spikes of interest are separated from other activity by means of a window discriminator. The output of the amplifier or the output of the window discriminator is also fed into a loudspeaker, so that the experimenter can "listen" to the electrical activity picked up by the microelectrode.

2.1. General Equipment

1. Silver wire recording electrode and connector (connections to the headstage should be coaxial cables; *see* also **Note 5**).
2. Stimulation electrodes (*see* **Note 6**).
3. Ground electrode.
4. Stimulator.
5. AC differential amplifier.
6. Filters (60 Hz notch filter, band pass filter).
7. Digital oscilloscope (sometimes a second oscilloscope is used to look at the unfiltered signal).
8. Computer board.
9. PC computer and data aquisition software.

10. Antivibration table.
11. Faraday cage with metal surface plate with screwed holes for vertical rods and screw clamps (all tubes from equipment with motors should be long enough so that the motor is outside the cage).
12. Headstage/preamplifier (set up within the cage as close to recording electrode as possible).
13. Ground wires (to connect equipment to each other and to the building ground).
14. Dissecting fiber optic lights (with neck long enough so that the motor can be outside the cage).
15. Dissecting microscope.
16. Microdissection tools: microscissors, jewelers forceps (size 55).
17. Micromanipulator.
18. Light mineral oil.

2.2. Additional Equipment for In Vivo Recording (Fig. 1)

1. Customized ring with metal arm (ring should have holes or slots around its circumference to aid in sewing the skin to stable points).
2. Customized mirrored platform with metal arm.
3. Dental impression material (e.g., Reprosil®, Dentsply, or Coe-Flex®, GC America Inc. Chicago, IL).
4. Peltier-controlled thermode, radiant heat or CO_2-laser (feedback-controlled).
5. von Frey monofilaments.
6. Polyethylene tubing (PE50) with three-way stopcocks, 30-G needles.
7. Pancuronmium bromide (bolus 1 mg/kg iv).
8. Perfusion cocktail: urethane 50 mg/h, pancuronium 0.1 mL/h, ringer lactate 0.2 mL/h, total 0.5 mL/h (rat).
9. Heparin: 1000 IU/1 mL saline.
10. Rodent ventilator with attached tubes: inspiration/exspiration ratio 1:2, tidal volume $0.0062 \times$ body weight in grams, frequency 70–100/min.
11. Blood pressure monitor.
12. Electrocardiogram (ECG) monitor.
13. End-tidal CO_2 monitor (for rats).
14. Rectal temperature probe.
15. Water or electric heating blanket (feedback-controlled; if electric, it must be grounded).

2.3. Additional Equipment for In Vitro Recording (Fig. 2)

1. Recording chamber with mirror plate and ground electrode (**Fig. 2**).
2. Suction stimulation electrode.
3. Oxygenated artificial cerebrospinal fluid (ACSF): 130 mM NaCl, 3.5 mM KCl, 1.25 mM NaH$_2$PO$_4$, 24 mM NaHCO$_3$, 10 mM dextrose, 1.2 mM MgCl$_2$, 1.2 mM CaCl$_2$, oxygenate with 5% CO_2 and 95% O_2 for 5 min, then adjust pH to 7.3, continue to oxygenate during the experiment.
4. Vaseline®.

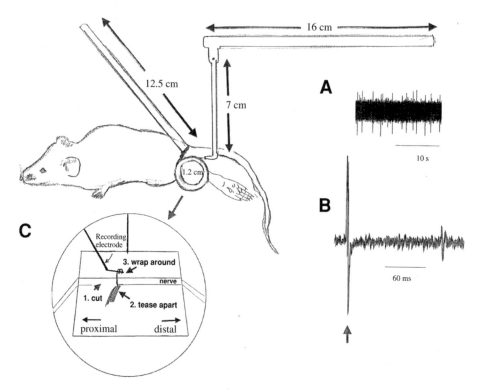

Fig. 1. In vivo recording of primary afferent fiber activity in the mouse. The record-ing electrode is lowered by micromanipulator through the ring opening. The indifferent (ground) electrode may be attached by alligator clip to the descending pole (with swivel joint) that supports the mirrored platform. (**A**) Raw data trace showing spontaneous activity in a C-fiber response. (**B**) Three superimposed traces of raw data indicating stimulus artifact (arrow) and the constant latency of a C-fiber response to electrical stimulation of the receptive field. (**C**) The nerve is cut and teased into small fiber bun-dles. A single bundle is wrapped over the recording electrode.

3. Methods

3.1. In Vivo Recording Preparations

3.1.1. Animal Preparation

1. In acute animal preparations, the animals are anesthetized during the entire proce-dure and it is important that stable levels of anesthesia and an excellent physiologi-cal state are maintained to enable relevant unit recordings.
2. Rats can be anesthetized with, e.g., urethane 1.25 g/kg or pentobarbital 60 mg/kg ip and supplemental halothane in an air/O_2 mixture as needed. If urethane is used, rats should not be stimulated immediately after injection to achieve optimal sedation.

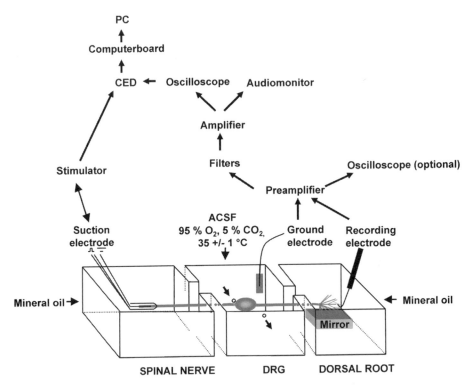

Fig. 2. Schematic of the preparation for in vitro microfilament recording from the dorsal root. The DRG is positioned into the middle chamber, which is continously perfused with oxygenated ACSF. The dorsal root and spinal nerve are led into the adjacent mineral oil-filled chambers for recording and stimulation. ACSF, artifical cerebrospinal fluid; DRG, dorsal-root ganglion

3. Usually, the animals are also paralyzed so that controlled artificial ventilation can be undertaken. Concentration of carbon dioxide in the expired air can be continously monitored to help adjusting the rate and tidal volume of ventilation and stabilize recording conditions as increased end-tidal CO_2 (lowered pH) will enhance excitability. The expired CO_2 is usually kept between 3.5 and 4.5% to provide optimal alveolar ventilation.

4. The ECG, rectal temperature (maintained between 37.5 ± 1.0°C by feedback control to the heating blanket), and blood pressure can provide important feedbacks regarding the adequacy of anesthesia. For blood pressure monitoring, the carotid or tail artery is cannulated with a heparinized catheter. A continous infusion of urethane, muscle relaxants, and ringer lactate solution (0.5 mL/h) is also maintained during recording.

5. In mice, recording has to be done without intravenous (iv) anesthesia because of the small diameter and fragile nature of blood vessels. In addition, the tracheotomy performed routinely in the rat for artificial respiration can easily lead to damage of the much more delicate mouse trachea. As an alternative, the mouse can be positioned on a square piece of plexiglass so that its chin extends slightly over the edge of a square platform and is resting on a supporting object to allow for unobstructed ventilation. For maintaining adequate body temperature in the mouse, a heating lamp may suffice, although a heating blanket is preferred. Again, feedback control is essential. Mice can be sedated with a pre-anesthetic dose of, e.g., acepromazine maleate (20 mg/kg, ip, *see* **Note 1**) 10 min prior to anesthesia with sodium pentobarbital (e.g., Nembutal, 48 mg/kg, ip). Supplemental doses of sodium pentobarbital (15 mg/kg) can be given ip as needed to maintain areflexia and surgical levels of anesthesia.

3.1.2. Recording Setup

1. To minimize respiration associated movements during recording, the animal can be suspended so that the chest can expand freely.
2. For recording of a peripheral nerve, the desired nerve is exposed and the skin at the incision is sewn to a customized metal ring (e.g., inner diameter 1.2 cm for a mouse; 2.5 cm for a rat) attached to a vertical metal rod firmly secured to the recording table (*see* **Fig. 1**). The metal ring is gently lifted to form a basin so that a small, mirrored platform can be positioned within the basin and the nerve placed on it. To prevent leakage of oil from the recording basin, the limb can be encased with a paste-like polysulfide impression material; this is rarely necessary for rats (*see* **Note 2**). The epineurium of the nerve is opened with a miniature scalpel and then with fine forceps pulled distally along the nerve like a sleeve if looking at receptive fields in skin. Small fascicles are cut to allow the proximal ends to be spread out on the mirrored platform for separation with fine forceps. Fine fascicles are teased apart.
3. For recording of the dorsal roots in rats, the animal is mounted on a spinal investigation frame. The spinal cord is exposed by laminectomy of the L1 to L6 vertebrae. The advantage of this approach is that the recording is in continuity with both the skin and the fibers' cell bodies, whereas in peripheral nerve recording a choice must be made. A heated mineral oil pool is constructed over the exposed tissue to prevent it from drying. The dura mater is opened and the dorsal root of interest is cut close to the spinal cord. In addition, the dorsal ramus of the L5 spinal nerve can be cut to prevent having intact afferent inputs from the dorsal parts of the skin and muscle. The dorsal root can directly be teased into small bundels until single unit activity can be recorded.

3.2. In Vitro Recording Preparations

3.2.1. Tissue Preparation

1. On the day of the recording, the rat is anesthetized with, e.g., urethane (1.25 g/kg) and supplemental halothane in an air/O_2 mixture.

2. For recording of the dorsal roots or spinal nerve, a laminectomy is performed (vertebral segments L1–L6) and the desired dorsal-root ganglion (DRG) and its dorsal root are identified. The spinal nerve is transsected as distally as possible. Once the DRG is exposed, oxygenated (95% O_2, 5% CO_2) ACSF is dripped onto its surface occasionally during the surgical procedure to prevent drying and hypoxia.

3. The ganglion and the attached peripheral nerve and ventral and dorsal roots are carefully but quickly removed and positioned in a petri dish filled with oxygenated ACSF at room temperature. After removing the perineurium and epineurium that form the ganglionic capsule, the whole ganglion is freed of the surrounding tissues and the ventral root is cut as short as possible.

4. The ganglion with the attached nerve and roots is then transferred into an incubation chamber filled with continously oxygenated ACSF kept at room temperature. Incubation should be done for at least 60 min before recording. Multiple DRGs can be harvested from a single animal.

3.2.2. Recording Setup

The ganglion with attached nerve and dorsal root is mounted in a recording chamber consisting of three compartments **(Fig. 2)**. The DRG is positioned into the central chamber, which is continuously perfused with oxygenated ACSF at a rate of 5–6 mL/min (*see* **Note 3**). The temperature in this chamber is kept at $35 \pm 1°C$ by running the tube with the perfusion fluid through a temperature-controlled water bath. The element to be recorded from (e.g., the dorsal root) is led out of this chamber into an adjacent mineral-oil filled chamber where microfilament recording will be performed. In this chamber, a mirror is mounted on the bottom for nerve splitting. The element to be stimulated (e.g., the spinal nerve) is put into a suction electrode or positioned across a pair of hook electrodes in another chamber filled with mineral oil. Fluid in each chamber is kept separate by a wall of Vaseline with the nerve or dorsal root running through.

3.3. Recording

On the mirror, the peripheral nerve or dorsal root is teased into small fiber bundles (*see* **Note 4**). A single bundle is wrapped over a silver hook recording electrode. Smaller fascicles continue to be dissected from the bundle until activity from only a few units is seen upon stimulation through the stimulation electrode. Extracellular recordings from single fibers are discriminated according to amplitude, polarity, and waveform. Action potentials are amplified, band-pass filtered (300 Hz low filter, 3 kHz high filter), audio-monitored, and displayed on an oscilloscope, before being sent to a PC computer for data acquisition and analysis.

4. Data Analysis

4.1. Unit Isolation Criteria

First, the evoked potential is probably from a single unit if it has the all-or-none amplitude with near-threshold levels of stimulation, i.e., the amplitude is not graded as stimulus intensity from the stimulating electrode is raised.

A second criterion is that of constancy of potential amplitude and shape, while the recording electrode remains at a single recording position. If the electrode picks up the activity of more than one unit, they can still be discriminated and analyzed separately by exploiting the fact that spikes from different neuronal elements frequently have different heights and shapes.

4.2. Spike Discrimination Techniques

The simplest method of separating single-unit spike trains is with the use of a simple window discriminator. In such a device, the input signal is fed to two voltage comparators, whose reference inputs define the upper and lower limits of a "voltage window." Circuitry is arranged so that the device generates an output pulse only if a voltage signal exceeds the lower limit of the window and does not also exceed the upper limit. By having several such windows, whose upper and lower limits are adjustable, it is possible to separate the response from several simultanously recorded units. Proper discrimination is verified by displaying the entire waveform of each accepted spike on a storage oscilloscope. The storage scope is triggered from the acceptance pulse of the discriminator or by an internal trigger regarding the amplitude of the spike so that only selected spikes are displayed.

The more sophisticated spike-discrimination device is one that operates on the configuration of the entire waveform. Computer programs are available that can identify spike templates for each of the units in a multi-unit recording and process separately the response of each unit (e.g., Spike2, Cambridge Electronic Design).

5. Fiber Classification

5.1. Conduction Velocity

1. The basic criterion for classifying a unit according to fiber type is the conduction velocity. Square-wave pulses (duration 0.2 ms, 0.5 Hz) are delivered at a stimulating voltage 1.5 times the voltage required to evoke a threshold response.
2. The stimulation electrode can be installed proximally or distally on the nerve (for ortho- or antidromic stimulation, respectively) or, as in mice owing to the limitations imposed by their small size of the animal, in or on adjacent tissues such as skin. In general, the stimulation electrode should be positioned as far away from the recording site as possible to minimize artifacts. The millimeter distance between the stimulating electrodes and the recording electrode is divided by the latency to

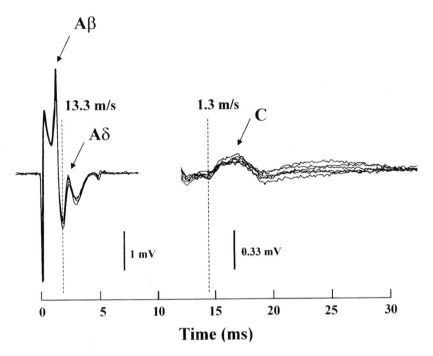

Fig. 3. Examples of six overlays of Aβ, Aδ, and C components of compound action potentials evoked by electrical stimulation (time 0) recorded from the same mouse. Dashed lines indicate conduction velocity cutoffs for differentiation between Aβ and Aδ fibers as well as the maximal conduction velocity cutoff for C fibers. Abscissa indicates real time from the beginning of the stimulus artifact. Note difference in vertical scales for A and C components: Aβ-Aδ components were evoked by a 100-μA stimulus; C fibers' response evoked by a 6-mA stimulus.

obtain the conduction velocity of the fiber according to the formula: velocity (v) = Δd/Δt, where Δd is the distance (mm) from the receptive field to the recording electrode, and Δt is the constant latency (ms) of action potentials propagating over the same distance.

3. In rats, Aβ fibers are defined as fibers with conduction velocities greater than 24 m/s, those conducting from 2.5 to 24 m/s as Aδ-units, and those conducting at less than 2.5 m/s as C-units (*6*).

4. In mice, units with conduction velocities greater than 1.3 m/s are classed as myelinated and subdivided into Aδ fibers (1.3–13.6 m/s) and Aβ fibers (>13.6 m/s). Fibers with conduction velocities less than 1.3 m/s are identified as C fibers (*7*, Fig. 3). Of course, different species have different limits. In addition, if the preparation is cold (if the mineral oil is not heated in the in vivo or in vitro system) it conducts more slowly.

5.2. Stimulus-Evoked Response

5.2.1. Classification of Nociceptors

Nociceptors are characterized according to responses evoked by noxious mechanical, thermal, and chemical stimuli.

1. Mechanoreceptors are considered rapidly adapting if they exhibit an abrupt response to the onset (and offset) of mechanical stimuli but fail to maintain discharge during a 10-s continous application of the stimulus. Slowly adapting mechanoreceptors are those that discharge throughout a 10-s period of stimulation. Aδ- and C-fibers that respond maximally to noxious levels of mechanical stimulation, but do not repond to the applied range of thermal stimuli, are classed as mechanonociceptors (AM, CM, respectively).
2. Nociceptors excited by heat, but not cold, are classed as mechanoheat nociceptors (AMH or CMH), and those responding to cold but not heat are classed as mechanocold nociceptors (AMC or CMC).
3. Nociceptors excited by both types of thermal stimuli, mechanoheatcold nociceptors, are designated AMHC or CMHC. AMH nociceptors exhibiting response thresholds less than or equal to 53°C are subclassed as AMH Type II fibers *(8)*. Those Aδ-nociceptors not responsive during initial heat trials can be exposed (up to three times) to 53°C for 30 s to induce sensitization to heat. If these nociceptors subsequently respond to heat, they can be classified as AMH Type I.

5.2.2. Identification of Cutaneous Afferent Units

After documenting the basal discharge activity, a series of search stimuli can be applied to the cutaneous receptive field (RF) to identify the receptor type *(6)*.

1. Very gentle stimuli are used initially (e.g., for Aβ-mechanoreceptor units, brushing or stroking with a camel-hair brush or tapping with the smooth tip of a glass rod; for Pacinian corpuscles, vibration with a tuning fork (256 Hz); for cold and warm units, contact with a test tube filled with warm or cold water).
2. If these stimuli fail to excite the unit, the stronger stimuli are used for nociceptive units. The RFs of units have to be located initially: for mechanically responsive units, von Frey filaments at a strength twice threshold or a glass rod can be used; for thermally responsive units, with a test tube filled with cold, hot, ice, or warm water; or for cold units, with an ether-soaked cotton ball.
3. For analysis of mechanical properties of low-threshold mechanoreceptors, constant force and vibratory stimuli can be applied with a feedback-controlled mechanical stimulator (up to 400 mN). For high-threshold mechanoreceptors, a hand-held stimulator can be devised with the use of forceps, stimuli (up to 14 Newton) can be delivered for 10 s at 2-min intervals.
4. Thermal thresholds can be determined with a feedback-controlled Peltier thermal stimulator, which can produce rapid heating (8°C/s) and cooling (4°C/s) of the skin. Thermal pulses with 20 s duration can be delivered in steps of 5°C. Nocicep-

tive units are not responsive to a range of pulses within 12°C to 47°C and can be identified by thermal pulses up to 52°C. Thermal threshold can be expressed as the temperature necessary to evoke two impulses over the background activity during the 20 s stimulus.

5. When mechanical and thermal stimuli fail to evoke activity of the desired unit, electrical stimuli can be applied to the skin to locate and map the RF. A saline-soaked cotton ball stimulating electrode is then moved over the surface of the skin innervated by the nerve under study to see if activity of the unit can be evoked. Constant current pulses of 0.5–3 mA in amplitude and 0.5–2 ms in duration can be delivered at a frequency of 0.5 Hz for cutaneous stimulation.

6. Notes

1. Acepromazine maleate reduces the occurrence of spinal reflexes often observed in mice during pentobarbital anesthesia. It is also suggested that for mice, the injected Nembutal dose be obtained from a concentration diluted to 5 mg/mL instead of the 50 mg/mL commercially supplied. For the rat, sodium pentobarbital (50–60 mg/kg, ip) or urethane (1.3 gm/kg, ip) can be used for initial anesthesia.

2. The skin of the mouse is utterly permeable to mineral oil. If the hindlimb region is not completely sealed with dental impression material, the oil drains immediately from the pool and is absorbed by the entire pelt over the whole animal. It is also important that the seal includes the underside of the hindlimb. A dollop of wet impression material should be placed on a thin piece of plastic (e.g., cut from a weighing boat) and gently inserted under the hindlimb so that the entire recording region up to the edge of the ring is sealed to prevent leakage of mineral oil from the basin.

3. A constant nonpulsitile flow is prefered for perfusion of the DRG chamber to avoid electrical noise caused by the movement of the DRG. Gravity-induced flow controlled by a conventional flowmeter or pressure-regulated perfusion systems can be useful. The inflow of the ACSF should be at the bottom, the outflow at the top of the chamber to guarantee even distribution of the perfusate within the chamber. In our system we use an open canal instead of a limited channel (drilled hole) to improve steady outflow of the DRG chamber.

4. The tibial nerve, along with the sural and the common peroneal nerves, is a distal branch of the sciatic nerve. Because the tibial nerve innervates primarily glabrous skin on the hindpaw, it provides a good target for the study of nociceptors, which can be particularly useful in correlating pain behavior with specific neurophysiological activity. Others prefer the sural or saphenous nerve for their recordings. The larger sciatic nerve also contains the same primary afferent fibers as the tibial nerve, but it also innervates a much larger cutaneous region and includes a larger number of deeper (i.e., noncutaneous sensory fibers) units as well.

5. Spigelman et al. (9) have suggested that platinum-iridium electrodes are preferable to Ag-AgCl electrodes because the latter are known to be toxic to excitable tissue over long-term exposure. We have found no discernibly deleterious effect by silver

wire electrodes on primary afferent fiber responses, even while recording activity for 2 h or more.

6. Smaller stimulating thermodes (Yale University) with contact areas of 2–3 mm^2 compared to the thermode described earlier (1 cm^2) can be used. The advantage of stimulating a smaller region of skin lessens the chance of thermal sensitization of other cutaneous nociceptors, but it can be more difficult to position correctly.

Acknowledgments

The authors thank L.S. Sorkin and D.A. Simone for helpful suggestions during the preparation of the manuscript

References

1. Humphrey, D. R. and Schmidt, E. M. (1990) Extracellular single-unit recording methods, in *Neuromethods* (Boulton, A. A., Baker, G. B., Vanderwolf, C. H., eds.), Humana Press, Totowa, NJ, pp. 1–59.
2. Millar, J. (1991) Extracellular single and multiple unit recording with microelectrodes, in *Monitoring Neuronal Activity: A Practical Approach* (Stamford, J. A., ed.), University Press, Oxford, pp. 1–26.
3. Viudyasagar, T. R. (1997) Extracellular single neuronal recording in the whole animal, in *Neuroscience Methods* (Martin, R. ed.), Harwood Academic Publishers, London, pp. 25–33.
4. Perl, E. R. (1996) Cutaneous polymodal receptors: characteristics and plasticity. *Prog. Brain Res.* **113,** 21–37.
5. Cain, D. M., Wacnik, P. W., Turner, M., et al. (2001b) Functional interactions between tumor and peripheral nerve: changes in excitability and morphology of primary afferent fibers in a murine model of cancer pain. *J. Neurosci.* **21,** 9367–9376.
6. Leem, J. W., Willis, W. D., and Chung, J. M. (1993) Cutaneous sensory receptors in the rat foot. *J. Neurophysiol.* **69,** 1684–1691.
7. Cain, D. M., Khasabov, S. G., and Simone, D. A. (2001a) Response properties of mechanoreceptors and nociceptors in mouse glabrous skin: an in vivo study. *J. Neurophysiol.* **85,** 1561–1574.
8. Treede, R. D., Meyer, R. A., and Campbell, J. N. (1998) Myelinated mechanically insensitive afferents from monkey hairy skin: heat-response properties *J. Neurophysiol.* **80,** 1082–1093.
9. Spigelman, I., Gold, M. S., and Light, A. R. (2001) Electrophysiological recording techniques in pain research, in *Methods in Pain Research* (Kruger, L., ed.), CRC Press, Boca Raton, FL, pp. 147–168.

14

Anatomical Identification of Neurons Responsive to Nociceptive Stimuli

Luc Jasmin and Peter T. Ohara

Summary

We describe methods for labeling and identifying neurons within the central nervous system involved in the transmission of nociceptive stimuli. The most reliable methods are physiological identification followed by intracellular injection or immunocytochemical detection of stimulus-induced markers such as Fos. These latter strategies are used with appropriate controls to distinguish neurons activated secondarily (e.g., motor response or inhibitory neurons) by the nociceptive stimuli. Other methods include location and morphology as determined by standard cytological and tracing methods and/or the presence of specific neurochemical markers such as substance P determined by immunocytochemistry.

Key Words: Tract tracing; pain; immunocytochemistry; Fos; stereotaxis; microscopy; morphology.

1. Introduction

The most parsimonious definition of a nociceptive neuron is "a neuron responsive to nociceptive stimuli delivered to a somatic or visceral structure." A more comprehensive description is that it is a "neuron that produces, is associated with, or alters nociceptive responses." The latter definition is based on the understanding that nociception is more than just a withdrawal reflex, and includes autonomic responses, emotional responses such as fear and anxiety, and changes in the inflammatory and immune responses. Although the second definition is intellectually preferable, for the sake of brevity, we limit ourselves to the first, more simple, definition and describe labeling neurons more directly responsible for transmitting or modulating of peripheral nociceptive stimuli.

From: *Methods in Molecular Medicine, Vol. 99: Pain Research: Methods and Protocols*
Edited by: Z. D. Luo © Humana Press Inc., Totowa, NJ

Table 1
Common Anatomical Markers Induced by Nociceptive Stimuli

Marker, location	Maximal signal	Typical nociceptive stimulus[a]	Disadvantages
NK1 receptor internalization, cytoplasmic *(67)*	2–15 min	Formalin, 100 μL of 5%. Carrageenan, 100 μL of 2% + noxious mechanical stimulus. Complete Freund's adjuvant, 100 μL of 50% + noxious mechanical stimulus	Difficult to quantify accurately
Erk, nuclear and cytoplasmic *(9,10)*	5–180 min	Hot plate (<1 min, 46 to 52°C)	High normal baseline (especially in cathechol-aminergic nuclei)
Fos, nuclear *(2–8)*	1–6 h	Formalin test *(8,16)* Nitroglycerine *(4)* Noxious mechanical or thermal stimulation of the skin *(6)*	High baseline in the forebrain of many strains of mice
NK1 receptor levels, cytoplasmic *(49)*	At least 48 h	Nerve injury or peripheral inflammation	Quantifiable only by densitometry, which requires standardized immunocyto-chemistry

[a] All chemicals are injected sc in the footpad or dorsum of the foot.

1.1. Identification of Nociceptive Neurons by Monitoring Activity (Table 1)

The most reliable way of identifying a nociceptive neuron is by directly recording its activity using electrophysiological methods and then intracellularly injecting a tracer such as biotin dextran or horseradish peroxidase (HRP) in order to characterize the neuron histologically *(1)*. Alternatively, one can monitor increase in activity of populations of neurons following a nociceptive stimulus by using inducible markers such as the *c-fos* proto-oncogene **(Fig. 1A)** *(2–8)*; extracellular signal-regulated kinase, *Erk (9,10)*; the zinc finger transcription factor gene, Krox-24 *(11)*; or the cAMP response element-binding protein, CREB *(5)* **(Table 1)**. These markers are used to identify second order activated nociceptive neurons in the terminal area of primary spinal, trigeminal, and vagal nerve afferents. With the exception of Erk, they are of limited value to monitor stimulus-induced activity in the soma of primary afferent neurons (first-order nociceptive neurons).

On a cautionary note, we would like to emphasize that none of these inducible markers are specific to nociception, and the increase in a marker in a given cell after a nociceptive stimulus does not necessarily mean that this cell is nociceptive. For instance, increased Fos in motor areas of the lumbar spinal cord after a nociceptive stimulus to the hindpaw most probably results from the grooming/protective behavior directed towards that paw as a consequence of the nociceptive stimulus (11,12). Strictly speaking, such motor-related neurons are not nociceptive even though their activation results from the nociceptive stimulus. Also, neurons can be activated by a nociceptive stimulus in the absence of nociceptive behavior in experiments where high doses of morphine are given prior to the stimulus (8), indicating that behavior and neural activation can be dissociated. To avoid these, and other, errors of interpretation, it is necessary to include controls exposed to the same experimental conditions with the exception of the nociceptive stimulus. Such sham controls are necessary to determine basal levels of expression in various regions of the brain and spinal cord.

1.2. Identification of Nociceptive Neurons Based on Location (Table 2)

The location of a retrogradely labeled neuron in an area where nociceptive neurons are concentrated is often used to infer that the labeled neuron is nociceptive (**Fig. 1B,C**). The superficial dorsal horn of the spinal cord and the nucleus caudalis of the trigeminal nuclear complex (4,8,13–16) are generally considered to contain mostly nociceptive neurons. Other brain areas containing nociceptive relay neurons include the nucleus of the solitary tract (17), the parabrachial nuclear area (5,14,18,19), the PAG (4), and many thalamic nuclei (20,21).

1.3. Identification of Nociceptive Neurons Based on Morphology and Specific Neurochemical Markers (Table 2)

Morphological criteria specific to nociceptive neurons are few and usually it is necessary to rely on other parameters to identify the nociceptive nature of the neuron. In the dorsal-root ganglion (DRG), many nociceptive neurons have small diameter perikarya (dark neurons or C cells, diameter < 35 μm), small myelinated or unmyelinated axons and contain specific neuropeptides such as substance P (SP) and calcitonin gene-related peptide (CGRP) (**Table 2**). Unfortunately, these two parameters, size and peptide content, alone or combined, cannot be used to uniquely identify nociceptive neurons, because not all the small-diameter neurons in the DRG are nociceptive and many large diameter neurons (light neurons or A cells) contain SP, CGRP, and other peptides (22,23). In addition, about 40% of the small-diameter primary sensory neurons

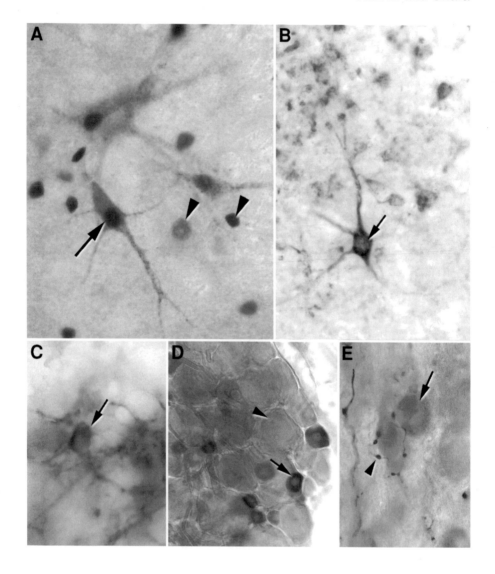

are nonpeptidergic *(24,25)* and they selectively bind the agglutinin isolectin B4 (IB4) as well as other lectins and express a fluoride-resistant acid phosphatase in their central terminals *(24,26,27)*. Like peptidergic primary sensory neurons, IB4-positive fibers innervate many peripheral tissue types including skin, cornea, muscle, abdominal, and pelvic viscera, and the olfactory bulb *(24,28–30)*.

IB4-positive neurons express several genes that suggest that their involvement in nociception is different from that of peptidergic neurons. For instance,

Fig. 1. Labeled nociceptive neurons, nonfluorescence. (**A**) Dorsal horn of the rat spinal cord following a formalin injection in the plantar aspect of the hindpaw. Nuclei showing increased Fos protein expression demonstrated by immunocytochemistry (arrowheads) appear gray to black following visualization with Ni-DAB. The cell indicated by the arrow is double-labeled with Fluoro-Gold injected into the parabrachial nucleus and visualized immunocytochemically using DAB alone to yield a light reaction product. (**B**) A neuron in the trigeminal nucleus caudalis double-labeled with pseudorabies viras (PRV) injected into the amygdala and B subunit of cholera toxin (CTB) injected into the parabrachial nucleus. The PRV is visualized immunocytochemically with DAB and produces a light flocculent label in the cytoplasm and nucleus and leaves dendrites unlabeled. The B subunit of cholera toxin (CTB) is visualized immunocytochemically using Ni-DAB and gives a gray/black labeling of the cytoplasm and dendrites. (**C**). An example of a neuron identified as nociceptive by its location in the superficial spinal dorsal horn and by the expression of NK1 receptors demonstrated immunocytochemically with Ni-DAB. The "ghost-like" appearance is typical staining for a membrane-located antigen. (**D**) In the dorsal-root ganglion, small size and the presence of specific markers such as VR1 (arrow) are suggestive, but not conclusive, indicators of nociceptive neurons. In this 100 μm section prepared for EM, the VR1 immunopositive neurons are dark brown following reaction with DAB. Unlabeled neurons (arrowhead) are lightly stained from the osmium tetroxide fixation. (**E**) Biotin-dextran labeled thalamic mediodorsal nucleus afferents visualized with Ni-DAB (bead-like profiles, arrowheads) in close apposition to lightly labeled GABAb receptor expressing neurons in the infralimbic cortex (arrow) visualized with a red chromogen (Nova red, Vector). Neurons in the infralimbic cortex are known to respond to noxious visceral stimuli (*66*). See http://anatomy.ucsf.edu/ohara for color version of figure.

IB4 neurons uniquely express the P2X3 receptor (*31*), which is responsible for the nociceptive inducing actions of ATP (*32*). Also preferentially expressed by IB4 primary afferent neurons are the NR2B subunit of the *N*-methyl-D-aspartate (NMDA) receptor (*33*), the bradykinin B1 receptor (*34*), and the tetrodotoxin-resistant sodium channel (TTX) (*35*), all of which are linked to nociception. In contrast, except during the early postnatal period, the trkA receptor is expressed almost exclusively by peptidergic afferents (*25*). Finally, some proteins involved in nociceptive behavior such as the enzyme cyclooxygenase-1 (COX-1) or the vanilloid receptor 1 (VR1; **Fig. 1D**) are equally express by IB4 and peptidergic primary sensory neurons (*36,37*).

Most small-diameter DRG neurons project to the superficial dorsal horn (*38*), an area where most neurons respond to noxious or thermal stimulation (*39–41*). In the superficial dorsal horn, the morphology of neurons has been used by a few investigators as a marker of their nociceptive nature (*42,43*). Electrophysiological recordings in cats have revealed that fusiform cells are exclusively nociceptive, whereas multipolar cells are either nociceptive-specific or polymodal, i.e.,

Table 2
Markers of Nociceptive Neurons in Specific CNS Areas

Location and morphology	Markers
Dorsal root and trigeminal ganglia, small diameter	Substance P *(27,68,69)*
	TTX resistant channels *(35)*
	CGRP *(27,69)*
	Somatostatin receptor *(70)*
	GluR5 subunit of the kainate receptor
	CCK *(5,69)*
	VR1 *(71,72)*
	IB4 *(35,36,73)*
Superficial dorsal horn of the trigeminal n. caudalis and spinal cord (lamina I and outer II). Pyramidal, fusiform, multipolar neurons *(6,13–15)*	Substance P *(68)*
	NK1 receptor *(17,43,74–77)*
	μ-opioid receptor *(78)*
	Fos *(2,6)*
	TrkA *(46)*
Neck dorsal horn of the trigeminal n. caudalis *(16,79)* and spinal cord (lamina V and adjacent parts of lamina IV and VI).	Fos *(16,79)*
Brainstem A1 group	Fos *(80)*
Parabrachial area *(14)*	μ-opioid receptor *(81)*
	Substance P *(82)*
Cerebral cortex	μ-opioid receptor *(83)*

responding to heat, pinch, and cold *(44)*. Similar cell types are found in the primate spinal cord and most of them express the NK1 receptor and one-third to one-half of them project to the thalamus *(43)*.

In the spinal cord and more rostrally in the CNS, neurons can be identified as nociceptive if they are contacted by nociceptive afferents **(Fig. 1E)**. For example, spino-parabrachial neurons have been identified as nociceptive because they were contacted by CGRP afferents *(45)*, spinoreticular neurons by SP and CGRP afferents *(46)*, and spino-thalamic neurons by enkephalin afferents *(47)*.

After peripheral or CNS injury many neurons that were previously associated with innocuous stimuli can become involved in pathologic pain sensation. Clearly in these circumstances the anatomical criteria for identifying nociceptive neurons have to be expanded. Similarly, as the expression and synthesis of transmitters and their receptors can be up- or downregulated trans-synaptically in the spinal cord and brain in various pain conditions, neurochemical markers also might have to be reassessed *(48,49)*.

2. Materials

From the anatomical point of view, the investigator needs the following equipment and reagents.

2.1. Stereotaxic Injection

1. Micropipet glass without an internal filament (OD 1.2 mm, ID 0.68 mm; WPI, Sarasota, FL, www.wpiinc.com).
2. Micropipet puller. The characteristics of the pulled pipets are not as critical as those needed for electrophysiology therefore any commercial pipet puller will suffice. We use one manufactured by Kopf instruments (Tujunga, CA, www.kopfinstruments.com).
3. 1 μL microliter Hamilton syringe (model 7101; www.hamiltonco. thomasregister.com).
4. Mineral Oil (Sigma, St. Louis, MO; Cat. no. M 1180; www.sigma-aldrich.com).
5. Dental wax (Sticky wax, Patterson Dental Supplies, Cat. no. 07-226-0354; www.patterson.com).
6. A stereotaxic apparatus equipped with a pipet or syringe holder (Kopf Instruments).

2.2. Tracers

1. A retrograde tracer (**Table 3** and *see* **ref.** [*50*]).
2. Diluent for tracer, usually distilled water or 0.1 M phosphate-buffered saline (PBS).
3. 100 μL Eppendorf tubes. Diluted tracers can be aliquoted and frozen for long-term storage.

2.3. Perfusion, Fixation, Sectioning

1. Tyrode's solution for pre-perfusion: 140 mM NaCl, 4.5 mM KCl, 2.5 mM CaCl$_2$, 1.0 mM MgCl$_2$, 10 mM glucose, 20 mM HEPES, pH 7.4.
2. Paraformaldehyde-lysine-periodate (fixative): 200 mL 0.1 M phosphate buffer, 200 mL 8% paraformaldehyde, 1.77 g L-lysine, 0.22 g sodium-m-periodate. Adjust pH to 7.4 with 10 N NaOH or 6 N HCl (*see* **Note 1**).
3. Feeding needle for transcardiac perfusion, 18-G for a 300-g rat (Fisher Scientific Cat. no. 0129010B, www1.fishersci.com).
4. Peristaltic pump for perfusion, capable of delivering at least 30–50 mL/min (Barnant Co, Barrington, IL, Manostat Simon pump; www.barnant.com/manostat/simon.htm).
5. Cryoprotectant: 30% sucrose in 0.1 M phosphate buffer (*see* **Note 2**).
6. Tissue-sectioning apparatus: freezing microtome (Richard-Allan Scientific, Kalamazoo, MI, Cat. no. HM400R; www.rallansci.com).

2.4. Immunocytochemistry

1. Primary (**Tables 1** and **2**) and secondary antibodies to detect tracer or neuropeptides.
2. Tris-buffer, pH 7.4.
3. Serum appropriate for the secondary antibody used, e.g., if a secondary antibody raised in goat is used, then a goat serum is preferable for blocking.
4. Triton X-100 (Sigma, Cat. no. T 8787).

Table 3
Retrograde Tracers Used for Double-Labeling Nociceptive Neurons

Tracer	Advantages	Disadvantages
Fluoro-Gold, (hydroxystilba-midine) 4% Molecular Probes, www.probes.com *(6,7,16)*	Fluorescent, stable, immuno[a]	Lesion at injection site, not visible in many confocal microscopes
Cholera toxin B, 1% (Cat. no. 104; www.listlabs.com)	Minimal uptake by PNS unmyelinated fibers, immuno,[a] glutaraldehyde OK	Big injection site, moderate transneuronal transport if survival >36 h
Rhodamine 10% (Cat. no. A 1318; *(84)* www.probes.com)	Fluorescent, restricted injection site, immuno[a]	Mostly an anterograde tracer
Diamidino Yellow (www.sigma-aldrich.com)	Easily used with Fast Blue	
HRP, type VI (Cat. no. P 8375; www.sigma-aldrich.com)	Strong signal with TMB histochemistry	Nonspecific uptake
WGA-HRP (Sigma, Cat. no. L 3892)	Strong signal with TMB histochemistry Good anterograde	Transneuronal transport if survival >36 h
WGA-Apo-HRP-gold *(3,13)*	Restricted injection site, no uptake by fibers of passage	Not commercially available.
HSV-1 or PRV *(14)*	Transneuronal transport, immuno[a]	Live tracer, biosafety II hood required, increases expression of genes such as Fos
Fluorescent Latex Microspheres (www.lumafluor.com)	Restricted injection site, fade-resistant	Coverslip with nonglycerol containing medium
Biotin Dextran, 10,000 MW, 10% (Cat. no. D-1956; www.probes.com)	Restricted injection site	Mostly anterograde transport
Fast Blue (Sigma, Cat. no. F5756)	Contrasts with other dyes	Fades, dye leakage

[a] Can be visualized with immunocytochemistry using the appropriate antibody

5. Liver powder (Pel-Freez Bio, Cat. no. 56123-2, www.pelfreez-bio.com).
6. Affinity purified secondary antibodies according to the species in which the primary antibody was raised (Jackson Immunolaboratories Research Inc., www.jacksonimmuno.com). The antibodies should be labeled with a fluorescent tag or biotinylated if the DAB reaction is used.

7. ABC Elite® kit (Vector labs, Cat. no. PK-6100; www.vectorlabs.com) or peroxidase conjugated ExtrAvidin® (Sigma, Cat. no. E-2886).
8. TSA-Plus Cyanine 3/Fluorescein System® (Perkin Elmer, Cat. no. NEL701001KT, http://las.perkinelmer.com/
9. 3,3′-Diaminobenzidine tetrahydrochloride (DAB). DAB can be purchased in powder form or as 10 mg tablets (Sigma, Cat. no. D5905).
10. DePeX® mounting medium (EMS, Cat. no. 13514; www.emsdiasum.com).
11. Antifade mounting medium such as Vectashield (Vector labs, Cat. no. H-1000, www.vectorlabs.com) or ProLong®, (Molecular Probes, Cat. no. P-7481; www.probes.com) is recommended if using fluorescence.
12. Transmission, epifluorescent, or confocal microscope.

3. Methods

3.1. Tracer Injection

1. The most straightforward injection method that is reliable, accurate and requires minimal equipment is to attach a glass micropipet to a Hamilton syringe. A glass micropipet without an internal filament is pulled on a pipet puller and the tip is cut to obtain a diameter of 20–50-µm, depending on the viscosity of the tracer.
2. The glass pipet is filled with mineral oil and then fixed to a 1-µL Hamilton syringe also filled with mineral oil, using melted dental wax (*see* **Note 3**).
3. The micropipet is then filled with tracer, the syringe is attached to a stereotaxic apparatus, and the tracer is injected in the brain at the required coordinates. Initial coordinates can be obtained from an atlas such as Paxinos and Watson *(51)*.
4. An alternative method of injection is to use compressed air to eject tracer from a micropipet using a commercial device such as a picospritzer (General Valve Corp., Fairfield, NJ). The length and pressure of the injection pulse can be varied to control the amount of tracer delivered. When using the picospritzer, the micropipet should contain a microfilament to facilitate filling either by capillary action of backfilling. Whichever method is used for injecting, in most rat CNS targets we would begin with volumes between 50–100 nanoliters of tracer.
5. Iontophoresis can also be used provided the tracers are polar and dissolved in a ion-containing solution *(52)*. Typically 2 *M* KCl is used as the vehicle with a tracer concentration of 4% and a positive injection current. The specific parameters for injection must be determined empirically but 7 µA for 10 min using a 20-µm tip pipet is a good starting point. The advantages of iontophoresis is minimal tissue damage at the injection site, less leakage from the pipet if a holding current is used, and uptake at the injection site is increased for some tracers such as Phaseolus vulgaris leucoagglutinin (PHAL). Disadvantages include long injection times and smaller choice of tracers.

3.1.1. Choice of Tracer

1. To visualize retrogradely labeled neurons as nociceptive, one usually needs to double-label the neurons with either a marker of activity (e.g., Fos; **Fig. 1A**) or for a

Fig. 2. Labeled nociceptive neurons, fluorescence. (a_1–a_4) Fluorescent dyes lend themselves well to multiple-labeling techniques. A neuron in the ventral tegmental area with a True Blue labeled nucleus (a_1, arrowhead) from a prefrontal cortex injection, with granular cytoplasmic rhodamine labeling (a_2, arrowhead) from a rostral insular cortex injection, and with tyrosine hydroxylase (a_3, arrowhead) immunocytochemistry labeling the cytoplasm using an FITC fluorophore. The merged image is shown in a_4 (arrowhead). (**B**) A cell in the ventral tegmental area retrogradely labeled with True Blue from the rostral insular cortex and for tyrosine hydroxylase with CY3 fluorophore (arrow). Cells not retrogradely labeled are clearly distinguished by the unstained nucleus (arrowhead). (**C**) A confocal image showing the granular labeling (arrow) in an A5 catecholaminergic neuron following injection of green beads into the spinal dorsal horn. Fluorescent beads give a granular label that contrasts well with the diffuse label, usually resulting from cellular antigen labeling. The neuron is also immunolabeled for tyrosine hydroxylase using CY3 fluorophore (light gray staining of perinuclear cytoplasm and dendrites). A neuron containing only green beads is also present (arrowhead). See http://anatomy.ucsf.edu/ohara for color version of figure.

neurotransmitter or its receptor (e.g., substance P and NK1). For this purpose, fluorescent or nonfluorescent techniques both allow satisfactory results. Nonfluorescent methods have the advantage of permanence and do not require special microscopes, but are rarely used to view more than two signals (**Fig. 1a,b,e**). Fluorescent tracers are prone to fading but provide a wider choice of labels and can be used for triple-labeling (**Fig. 2a$_1$–a$_4$**). Investigators should be aware that some fluorescent tracers such as Fluoro-Gold, can be visualized and made permanent by nonfluorescent methods using anti-Fluoro-Gold antisera (**Fig. 1B**) (*8*). We recommend the use of fluorescent techniques in the initial experiments for ease of use and rapid results. When doing double-label immunocytochemistry, we follow the steps enumerated in **Table 4**. We habitually do the complete protocol for the first antibody and then redo the entire protocol on the same tissue but with a different chromogen or fluorophore for the second antigen. All antibodies should be tested first on control tissue to determine the optimal conditions of use (*see* **Note 4**).

2. Double labeling with an inducible marker such as Fos (**Fig. 1A**) involves choosing an appropriate stimulus as determined by preliminary experiments and perfusing at a time when induction of the marker is maximum (**Table 1**). In these experiments, it is important to be aware of, and control, as many variables as possible in addition to the stimulus. For example, when doing a 1-h long nociceptive test, we found increased Fos induction in the inferior colliculi of rats showing pain behavior. The Fos expression was caused by a tone emitted during the scoring key press and the increase was because the animals heard the tone, rather than as direct result of the intensity of the nociceptive stimulus.

3. Ideally one should combine fluorophores that have emission signals that are far apart (**Table 5**), but strongly excited by the light source. Four epifluorescence

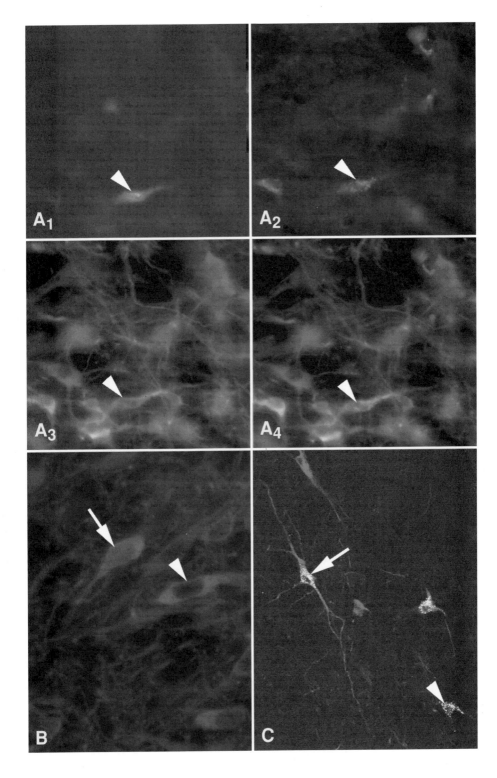

Table 4
Standard Immunolabeling Protocol

Steps	Fluorescence and amplified fluorescence	Nonfluorescent
1	Wash[a] × 2	Wash[a] × 2
2	Permeabilize[b] and wash × 4	Permeabilize[b] and wash × 4
3	10% Normal serum[c] × 60 min	10% Normal serum[c] × 60 min
4	Primary Ab[d] × 18–48 h	Primary Ab[d] × 18–48 h
5	Wash × 4	Wash × 4
	For amplified fluorescence go to step 7	
6	Fluorescent secondary Ab[e], 1 h Proceed to step 10	Biotinylated secondary Ab × 1–18 h
7	Biotinylated secondary Ab, 1 h	Wash × 4
8	Wash × 4	ABC reaction
9	ABC reaction	Wash × 4
10	Wash × 4	DAB reaction, with or without nickel[h] (*see* **Note 7**)
11	Tyramine fluorescent solution[f]	Wash × 4
12	Wash × 4	Mount on gelatinized slides
13	Mount on gelatinized slides	Dry overnight at 37°C
14	Dry for 10 min	Dehydrate, coverslip with DePex
15	Coverslip with Vectashield medium and seal.[g] Store in the dark at 4°C.	

[a] Tris-buffer pH 7.4. For steps 1–5, the wash buffer also contains 0.1–5% serum and 0.1–0.3% Triton X-100

[b] Use Triton X-100 (0.1–1%) for 1 h or 50% ethanol in ddH$_2$O for 30 min

[c] Serum from the same species as the secondary Ab in buffer to decrease background labeling.

[d] The optimal dilution should be pre-determined for each Ab. Some polyclonal Ab should be affinity purified or pre-adsorbed with liver powder from the same species as the tissue. Low signal can result if the Ab concentration is too high or too low. Mouse Ab can be used on mouse tissue using the MOM kit from Vector Labs (Cat. nos. BMK-2202 or PK-2200 or FMK-2201; www.vectorlabs.com)

[e] Affinity purified secondary antibodies are preferable for double-labeling.

[f] TSA-Plus Cyanine 3/Fluorescein System®,

[g] Sealing the edges of the slide with nail varnish prevents the tissue drying.

[h] Nickel-DAB gives a black label, non-nickel-DAB give a brown label (8). For red or blue labeling, use Cat. no. SK-5100 or SK-5300; www.vectorlabs.com.

microscopy light sources are available: tungsten, mercury, xenon, and cesium, all which have different emission spectra. The choice of a given source is based on a pairing the emission of the source with the absorption wavelength of the fluorophore(s). Customarily mercury lamps are used because they emit in both the ultraviolet (UV) as well as the visible spectrum, allowing, with the appropriate fil-

Table 5
A Few of the Commonly Used Fluorophores and Their Parameters

Fluorophore	Excitation (nm)	Emission (nm)	Color
Fluoro-Gold (Molecular Probes)	323	408	Gold at pH 7.4; Blue at pH 3.3
Alexa Fluor 350 (Molecular Probes, Cat. no. S-11249)	346	442	Blue
Hoechst 33342 (Sigma, Cat. no. B 2261)	343	483	Blue
Cy2[a]	489	505	Green
Fluorescein (FITC)[a]	495	519	Green at pH 7.4
Alexa Fluor 488 (Molecular Probes)	495	519	Green
Cy3[a]	552	565	Scarlet
Alexa Fluor 546 (Molecular Probes)	556	575	Red
Rhodamine[a]	570	590	Red
Texas Red[a]	595	615	Red
Alexa Fluor 594 (Molecular Probes)	590	617	Red
Cy5[a]	650	670	Far-red

[a] Conjugated to various carriers (*see* www.jacksonimmuno.com).

ter set, the use of the most common fluorophores (*see* **Note 5**). However, microscopes can be configured with easily interchangeable light sources to permit a wider range of fluorophores to be used, particularly those with absorption spectra in the longer wavelengths, such as using a cesium source with red fluorochromes.
4. When possible, fluorophores with clearly separated absorption and emission spectrum should be used for multiple-labeling studies. Using a mercury lamp, Fluoro-Gold and Cy3 have virtually no overlap and the signals from both fluorophores are easily distinguished. However, Fluoro-Gold and FITC, and FITC and CY3 have emission spectra that are close enough together that some bleed-through can occur between these combinations, making it appear as though cells are double-labeled when this is not actually the case. A technical error should be suspected when all cells are double-labeled. A number of strategies can be adopted to reduce the possibility of falsely identifying double-labeled cells. The combination of a cytoplasmic marker and a nuclear marker greatly simplifies the recognition of double-labeled neurons (**Fig. 2B**). Using fluorophores of approximately equivalent brightness also aids in unambiguously recognizing double-labeled cells. When using two

fluorophores of unequal strength, the one with the weak signal, should be use to identify the antigen with the highest expression. Single-labeled cells should be identified and the intensity and pattern of labeling in these cells should be compared with the double-labeled cells. For example, Fluoro-Gold produces a very granular label and if FITC label in the same cell has the same granular appearance and distribution in the cytoplasm, then one should suspect the FITC label results from bleed-through of the Fluoro-Gold signal.

5. Depending on the transport distance, a delay of 1–3 d is usually sufficient for the transport to occur from the injection site to the cell body of the projecting neuron. Some tracers such as HRP are degraded quickly within the cell, whereas others such as Fluoro-Gold will stay in the cell for months after retrograde transport.

3.2. Fixation

1. Great care should be taken to achieve optimal fixation of the nervous tissue as a prerequisite to good immunocytochemistry.
2. Anesthesia is done with pentobarbital because it causes vasodilation and thus results in better fixative penetration. After a swift thoracotomy, transcardiac perfusion is done with a round-ended feeding needle inserted in the ascending aorta through the apex of the heart. The time from the initial incision to insertion of the needle should be less than 15 s. Perfusion of Tyrode's solution is started immediately and the left auricle is cut open (*see* **Note 6**). Once the blood is cleared from the liver (approx 20 s), periodate-lysine-Paraformaldehyde (PLP) fixative is immediately started and perfused for not less than 5 min.
3. The brain, spinal cord, and DRG (if needed) are quickly removed and immersed in the same fixative for 4 h at 4°C, before being transferred to buffered 30% sucrose for 48 h at 4°C.
4. The tissue is then sectioned 40–60 µm on a freezing microtome and freely floated in Tris-saline buffer (pH 7.4).

3.3. Analysis

1. Prior to analyzing the distribution of retrogradely labeled cells, the extent of the injection site should be determined and the possibility of tracer being taken up by axons of passage must be considered. First, one must estimate the "effective" uptake site of the tracer, which is usually smaller than the visible extent of the injection site. The effective site is determined by doing control injections around the target injection site, assuming that these surrounding regions have unique afferent projections. By a process of subtraction, one should be able to evaluate the limits of uptake around the intended injections. Vanderhorst and colleagues (*53*) used such a strategy when they retrogradely labeled the spino-periaqueductal neurons. It is also necessary to determine if retrogradely filled neurons result from uptake of fibers of passage or by collateral terminal fields in the injection site (**Fig. 3**). In this case, using two different tracers injected in different locations or using an anterograde tracer such as 10% biotin-dextran (**Table 3**) injected into the location of the retrogradely labeled neurons might be required to further confirm the existence of a

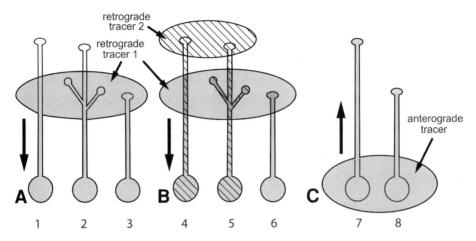

Fig. 3. Illustration of problems in retrograde labeling. (**A**) Retrograde labeling can result from uptake of a tracer from fibers of passage (cell 1), from en passant or collateral projections (cell 2), or from a terminal projection (cell 3). (**B**) To distinguish between these possibilities, a second tracer injected at a more distal site will help to determine if a neuron has a single terminal field as shown in cell 6. (**C**) Injecting an anterograde tracer into the cell body region will positively identify the terminal fields of those neurons. See httpsa://anatomy.ucsf.edu/ohara for color version of figure.

projection (**Fig. 3C**). If labeled terminals are not present in the target site, this would suggest that cells retrogradely labeled from that site are the result of tracer uptake by fibers of passage (*54–56*).

2. Establishing simply the existence of a projection or location of a particular transmitter might be achieved by demonstration of a few labeled neurons. However, usually one would like more information regarding the robustness of a projection or the percentage of cells that contain a particular neurotransmitter. In the latter case, some quantification is needed. The most accurate method is to count every cell in all sections without counting the same cell in adjacent sections. This is usually a labor-intensive and time-consuming task and a number of sampling techniques have been used to facilitate quantification. Stereological quantification methods (*57–59*) can be done by hand or by one of a number of computer-aided systems (e.g., Stereo Investigator, MicroBrightField Inc., VT; www.microbrightfield.com). In these methods, a grid is superimposed over the region of interest and cells within counting frames of that grid are counted. Various mechanical and statistical methods are used to ensure that sampling is random, cells are not counted twice, and that the number counted will give a reasonable estimate of the total number of labeled or unlabeled cells. Additional analysis can be carried out by measuring the distance between cells or from a reference point to determine whether the distribution of the cells is random or concentrated in particular regions.

3. As in any quantitative evaluation, one must pay attention to the number of experiments needed to yield statistical significance when data from each animal is pooled for comparison of groups according to time and treatment. Standard tests such as analysis of variance (ANOVA), Scheffé's F test, and serial *t*-tests, which are corrected for multiple comparisons using the method of Bonferroni should be used to ensure statistical significance ($p < 0.05$).

4. Notes

1. The original description of the fixative *(60)* recommends that a 2% paraformaldehyde solution gives the best balance between fixation and retention of antigenicity. In our experience, a 4% solution is a good starting point, because tissue preservation is better. However, if poor retention of antigenicity occurs, then lower percentages of paraformaldehyde should be tried.
2. For long-term freezing/storage of tissue or sections, use 500 mL 0.1 M phosphate buffer, pH 7.2; 9.0 g NaCl; 300 g sucrose, 10 g polyvinylpyrrolidine (PVP-40, Sigma); 300 mL ethylene glycol, and bring to 1 L with distilled water *(61)*.
3. Micropipets without an internal microfilament are easier to seal onto the syringe needle. Care should be taken so that no air bubbles are introduced into the system, because this makes it almost impossible to eject the tracer.
4. It is difficult to provide precise dilutions or protocols for particular antigens, because there is a large variation between antibodies, even from the same supplier, and between conditions in laboratories. As a general guide, it is best to begin with an antibody that has been used in a published study and begin with that protocol. Common problems such as high background or poor antibody specificity can usually be traced to poor fixation, lack of blocking, contaminated components, or poor tissue handling. Always running positive and negative controls will aid in troubleshooting the most common problems. There are also available a number of excellent references for detailed protocols and troubleshooting *(62–65)*.
5. Most spectra show a gap in the emission of Mercury lamps in the FITC range. In practice, however, FITC is adequately visualized with a mercury source.
6. Some methods use heparin in the fixation solutions to help clear the blood from the vasculature. We have found that a rapid perfusion with adequate pressure is the most important step for a good perfusion.
7. DAB is considered possibly carcinogenic therefore care should be taken in handling. The use of DAB in 10 mg tablet form reduces the exposure to the powder; however, the resulting solution tends to contain undissolved solids and must be filtered before use.

Acknowledgments

We would like to thank the following for supplying antibodies: NK1, Dr. S. Vigna, Duke University; VR1, Dr D. Julius, UCSF; GABAb, Dr. M. Margeta-Mitrovic, UCSF. This work was supported by the American Fibromyalgia Syndrome Association and by NIH.

References

1. Sugiyama, K., Ryu, H., and Uemura, K. (1992) Identification of nociceptive neurons in the medial thalamus: morphological studies of nociceptive neurons with intracellular injection of horseradish peroxidase. *Brain Res.* **586**, 36–43.
2. Li, J. L., Li, Y. Q., Kaneko, T., and Mizuno, N. (1999) Preprodynorphin-like immunoreactivity in medullary dorsal horn neurons projecting to the thalamic regions in the rat. *Neurosci. Lett.* **264**, 13–16.
3. Li, T., Gao, W., and Rao, Z. R. (1998) Noxious somatic stimulation-induced expression of Fos-like immunoreactivity in catecholaminergic neurons with habenular nucleus projection in the medullary visceral zone of rat. *Brain Res.* **783**, 51–56.
4. Tassorelli, C., Joseph, S. A., and Nappi, G. (1999) Reciprocal circuits involved in nitroglycerin-induced neuronal activation of autonomic regions and pain pathways: a double immunolabeling and tract-tracing study. *Brain Res.* **842**, 294–310.
5. Hermanson, O., Larhammar, D., and Blomqvist, A. (1998) Preprocholecystokinin mRNA-expressing neurons in the rat parabrachial nucleus: subnuclear localization, efferent projection, and expression of nociceptive-related intracellular signaling substances. *J. Comp. Neurol.* **400**, 255–270.
6. Tavares, I., Lima, D., and Coimbra, A. (1993) Neurons in the superficial dorsal horn of the rat spinal cord projecting to the medullary ventrolateral reticular formation express c- fos after noxious stimulation of the skin. *Brain Res.* **623**, 278–286.
7. Lee, J. H., Price, R. H., Williams, F. G., Mayer, B., and Beitz, A. J. (1993) Nitric oxide synthase is found in some spinothalamic neurons and in neuronal processes that appose spinal neurons that express Fos induced by noxious stimulation. *Brain Res.* **608**, 324–333.
8. Jasmin, L., Wang, H., Tarczy-Hornoch, K., Levine, J. D., and Basbaum, A. I. (1994) Differential effects of morphine on noxious stimulus-evoked fos-like immunoreactivity in subpopulations of spinoparabrachial neurons. *J. Neurosci.* **14**, 7252–7260.
9. Ji, R. R., Baba, H., Brenner, G. J., and Woolf, C. J. (1999) Nociceptive-specific activation of ERK in spinal neurons contributes to pain hypersensitivity. *Nat. Neurosci.* **2**, 1114–1119.
10. Karim, F., Wang, C. C., and Gereau, R. I. (2001) Metabotropic Glutamate receptor subtypes 1 and 5 are activators of extracellular signal-regulated kinase signaling required for inflammatory pain in mice. *J. Neurosci.* **21**, 3771–3779.
11. Herdegen, T., Kovary, K., Leah, J., and Bravo, R. (1991) Specific temporal and spatial distribution of JUN, FOS, and KROX-24 proteins in spinal neurons following noxious transsynaptic stimulation. *J. Comp. Neurol.* **313**, 178–191.
12. Jasmin, L., Gogas, K. R., Ahlgren, S. C., et al. (1994) Walking evokes a distinctive pattern of Fos-like immunoreactivity in the caudal brainstem and spinal cord of the rat. *Neuroscience* **58**, 275–286.
13. Matsushita, M. (1998) Ascending propriospinal afferents to area X (substantia grisea centralis) of the spinal cord in the rat. *Exp. Brain Res.* **119**, 356–366.

14. Jasmin, L., Burkey, A. R., Card, J. P., and Basbaum, A. I. (1997) Transneuronal labeling of a nociceptive pathway, the spino-(trigemino-) parabrachio-amygdaloid, in the rat. *J. Neurosci.* **17,** 3751–3765.

15. Zhang, E. T. and Craig, A. D. (1997) Morphology and distribution of spinothalamic lamina I neurons in the monkey. *J. Neurosci.* **17,** 3274–3284.

16. Wang, L. G., Li, H. M., and Li, J. S. (1994) Formalin induced FOS-like immunoreactive neurons in the trigeminal spinal caudal subnucleus project to contralateral parabrachial nucleus in the rat. *Brain Res.* **649,** 62–70.

17. Guan, Z. L., Ding, Y. Q., Li, J. L., and Lu, B. Z. (1998) Substance P receptor-expressing neurons in the medullary and spinal dorsal horns projecting to the nucleus of the solitary tract in the rat. *Neurosci. Res.* **30,** 213–218.

18. Krout, K. E. and Loewy, A. D. (2000) Parabrachial nucleus projections to midline and intralaminar thalamic nuclei of the rat. *J. Comp. Neurol.* **428,** 475–494.

19. Gauriau, C. and Bernard, J. F. (2002) Pain pathways and parabrachial circuits in the rat. *Exp. Physiol.* **87,** 251–258.

20. Craig, A. D., Bushnell, M. C., Zhang, E. T., and Blomqvist, A. (1994) A thalamic nucleus specific for pain and temperature sensation. *Nature* **372,** 770–773.

21. Willis, W. D., Jr., Zhang, X., Honda, C. N., and Giesler, G. J., Jr. (2001) Projections from the marginal zone and deep dorsal horn to the ventrobasal nuclei of the primate thalamus. *Pain* **92,** 267–276.

22. Lawson, S. (1992) Morphological and biochemical cell types of sensory neurons, in *Sensory Neurons* (Scott, S., ed.), Oxford University Press, Oxford, pp. 27–59.

23. Lee, K. H., Chung, K., Chung, J. M., and Coggeshall, R. E. (1986) Correlation of cell body size, axon size, and signal conduction velocity for individually labelled dorsal root ganglion cells in the cat. *J. Comp. Neurol.* **243,** 335–346.

24. Silverman, J. D. and Kruger, L. (1990) Selective neuronal glycoconjugate expression in sensory and autonomic ganglia: relation of lectin reactivity to peptide and enzyme markers. *J. Neurocytol.* **19,** 789–801.

25. Bennett, D. L., Averill, S., Clary, D. O., et al. (1996) Postnatal changes in the expression of the trkA high-affinity NGF receptor in primary sensory neurons. *Eur. J. Neurosci.* **8,** 2204–2208.

26. Kitchener, P. D., Wilson, P., and Snow, P. J. (1993) Selective labelling of primary sensory afferent terminals in lamina II of the dorsal horn by injection of Bandeiraea simplicifolia isolectin B4 into peripheral nerves. *Neuroscience* **54,** 545–551.

27. Fried, K., Arvidsson, J., Robertson, B., et al. (1989) Combined retrograde tracing and enzyme/immunohistochemistry of trigeminal ganglion cell bodies innervating tooth pulps in the rat. *Neuroscience* **33,** 101–109.

28. Petruska, J. C., Streit, W. J., and Johnson, R. D. (1997) Localization of unmyelinated axons in rat skin and mucocutaneous tissue utilizing the isolectin GS-I-B4. *Somatosens. Mot. Res.* **14,** 17–26.

29. Li, H., Nomura, S., and Mizuno, N. (1997) Binding of the isolectin I-B4 from Griffonia simplicifolia to the general visceral afferents in the vagus nerve: a light- and electron- microscope study in the rat. *Neurosci. Lett.* **222,** 53–56.

30. Wang, H. F., Shortland, P., Park, M. J., and Grant, G. (1998) Retrograde and transganglionic transport of horseradish peroxidase- conjugated cholera toxin B subunit, wheatgerm agglutinin and isolectin B4 from Griffonia simplicifolia I in primary afferent neurons innervating the rat urinary bladder. *Neuroscience* **87,** 275–288.

31. Bradbury, E. J., Burnstock, G., and McMahon, S. B. (1998) The expression of P2X3 purinoreceptors in sensory neurons: effects of axotomy and glial-derived neurotrophic factor. *Mol. Cell Neurosci.* **12,** 256–268.

32. Burnstock, G. (2000) P2X receptors in sensory neurones. *Br. J. Anaesth.* **84,** 476–488.

33. Ma, Q. P. and Hargreaves, R. J. (2000) Localization of N-methyl-D-aspartate NR2B subunits on primary sensory neurons that give rise to small-caliber sciatic nerve fibers in rats. *Neuroscience* **101,** 699–707.

34. Wotherspoon, G. and Winter, J. (2000) Bradykinin B1 receptor is constitutively expressed in the rat sensory nervous system. *Neurosci. Lett.* **294,** 175–178.

35. Fjell, J., Hjelmstrom, P., Hormuzdiar, W., et al. (2000) Localization of the tetrodotoxin-resistant sodium channel NaN in nociceptors. *Neuroreport* **11,** 199–202.

36. Chopra, B., Giblett, S., Little, J. G., et al. (2000) Cyclooxygenase-1 is a marker for a subpopulation of putative nociceptive neurons in rat dorsal root ganglia. *Eur. J. Neurosci.* **12,** 911–920.

37. Michael, G. J. and Priestley, J. V. (1999) Differential expression of the mRNA for the vanilloid receptor subtype 1 in cells of the adult rat dorsal root and nodose ganglia and its downregulation by axotomy. *J. Neurosci.* **19,** 1844–1854.

38. Woodbury, C. J., Ritter, A. M., and Koerber, H. R. (2000) On the problem of lamination in the superficial dorsal horn of mammals: a reappraisal of the substantia gelatinosa in postnatal life. *J. Comp. Neurol.* **417,** 88–102.

39. Light, A. R., Trevino, D. L., and Perl, E. R. (1979) Morphological features of functionally defined neurons in the marginal zone and substantia gelatinosa of the spinal dorsal horn. *J. Comp. Neurol.* **186,** 151–171.

40. Bennett, G. J., Abdelmoumene, M., Hayashi, H., and Dubner, R. (1980) Physiology and morphology of substantia gelatinosa neurons intracellularly stained with horseradish peroxidase. *J. Comp. Neurol.* **194,** 809–827.

41. Woolf, C. J. and Fitzgerald, M. (1983) The properties of neurones recorded in the superficial dorsal horn of the rat spinal cord. *J. Comp. Neurol.* **221,** 313–328.

42. Gamboa-Esteves, F. O., Kaye, J. C., McWilliam, P. N., et al. (2001) Immunohistochemical profiles of spinal lamina I neurones retrogradely labelled from the nucleus tractus solitarii in rat suggest excitatory projectiosn. *Neuroscience* **104,** 523–538.

43. Yu, X. H., Zhang, E. T., Craig, A. D., et al. (1999) NK-1 receptor immunoreactivity in distinct morphological types of lamina I neurons of the primate spinal cord. *J. Neurosci.* **19,** 3545–3555.

44. Han, Z. S., Zhang, E. T., and Craig, A. D. (1998) Nociceptive and thermoreceptive lamina I neurons are anatomically distinct. *Nat. Neurosci.* **1,** 218–225.

45. Nahin, R. L., Humphrey, E., and Hylden, J. L. (1991) Evidence for calcitonin gene-related peptide contacts on a population of lamina I projection neurons. *J. Chem. Neuroanat.* **4,** 123–129.
46. Pezet, S., Onteniente, B., Grannec, G., and Calvino, B. (1999) Chronic pain is associated with increased TrkA immunoreactivity in spinoreticular neurons. *J. Neurosci.* **19,** 5482–5492.
47. Ruda, M. A., Coffield, J., and Dubner, R. (1984) Demonstration of postsynaptic opioid modulation of thalamic projection neurons by the combined techniques of retrograde horseradish peroxidase and enkephalin immunocytochemistry. *J. Neurosci.* **4,** 2117–2132.
48. Coderre, T. J., Katz, J., Vaccarino, A. L., and Melzack, R. (1993) Contribution of central neuroplasticity to pathological pain: review of clinical and experimental evidence. *Pain* **52,** 259–285.
49. Goff, J. R., Burkey, A. R., Goff, D. J., and Jasmin, L. (1998) Reorganization of the spinal dorsal horn in models of chronic pain: correlation with behaviour. *Neuroscience* **82,** 559–574.
50. Kobbert, C., Apps, R., Bechmann, I., et al. (2000) Current concepts in neuroanatomical tracing. *Prog. Neurobiol.* **62,** 327–351.
51. Paxinos, G. and Watson C. (1998) *The Rat Brain in Stereotaxic Coordinates,* 4th ed. Academic Press, New York.
52. Yu, D. and Gordon, F. J. (1994) A simple method to improve the reliability of iontophoretic administration of tracer substances. *J. Neurosci. Methods* **52,** 161–164.
53. Vanderhorst, V. G., Mouton, L. J., Blok, B. F., and Holstege, G. (1996) Distinct cell groups in the lumbosacral cord of the cat project to different areas in the periaqueductal gray. *J. Comp. Neurol.* **376,** 361–385.
54. Chen, S. and Aston-Jones, G. (1995) Evidence that cholera toxin B subunit (CTb) can be avidly taken up and transported by fibers of passage. *Brain Res.* **674,** 107–111.
55. Dado, R. J., Burstein, R., Cliffer, K. D., and Giesler, G. J., Jr. (1990) Evidence that Fluoro-Gold can be transported avidly through fibers of passage. *Brain Res.* **533,** 329–333.
56. Cechetto, D. F., Standaert, D. G., and Saper, C. B. (1985) Spinal and trigeminal dorsal horn projections to the parabrachial nucleus in the rat. *J. Comp. Neurol.* **240,** 153–160.
57. Bjugn, R. and Gundersen, H. J. (1993) Estimate of the total number of neurons and glial and endothelial cells in the rat spinal cord by means of the optical disector. *J. Comp. Neurol.* **328,** 406–414.
58. West, M. J. and Gundersen, H. J. (1990) Unbiased stereological estimation of the number of neurons in the human hippocampus. *J. Comp. Neurol.* **296,** 1–22.
59. West, M. J., Slomianka, L., and Gundersen, H. J. (1991) Unbiased stereological estimation of the total number of neurons in thesubdivisions of the rat hippocampus using the optical fractionator. *Anat. Rec.* **231,** 482–497.
60. McLean, I. W. and Nakane, P. K. (1974) Periodate-lysine-paraformaldehyde fixative. A new fixation for immunoelectron microscopy. *J. Histochem. Cytochem.* **22,** 1077–1083.

61. Watson, R. E., Jr., Wiegand, S. J., Clough, R. W., and Hoffman, G. E. (1986) Use of cryoprotectant to maintain long-term peptide immunoreactivity and tissue morphology. *Peptides* **7,** 155–159.

62. Hockfield, S., Carlson, S., Evans, C., et al. (1993) *Selected Methods for Antibody and Nucleic Acid Probes.* Cold Spring Harbor Laboratory Press, Cold Spring Harbor, NY.

63. Harlow, E. and Lane, D. (1999) *Using Antibodies.* Cold Spring Harbor Laboratory Press, Cold Spring Harbor, NY.

64. Javois, L. (1999) *Immunocytochemical Methods and Protocols.* Humana Press, Totowa, NJ.

65. Polak, J. (1997) *Introduction to Immunocytochemistry.* Bios Scientific Publishers, Oxford, UK.

66. Traub, R. J., Silva, E., Gebhart, G. F., and Solodkin, A. (1996) Noxious colorectal distention induced-c-Fos protein in limbic brain structures in the rat. *Neurosci. Lett.* **215,** 165–168.

67. Honoré, P., Menning, P. M., Rogers, S. D., et al. (1999) Spinal substance P receptor expression and internalization in acute, short-term, and long-term inflammatory pain states. *J. Neurosci.* **19,** 7670–7678.

68. Conti, F., De Biasi, S., Giuffrida, R., and Rustioni, A. (1990) Substance P-containing projections in the dorsal columns of rats and cats. *Neuroscience* **34,** 607–221.

69. Bortolami, R., Calza, L., Lucchi, M. L., et al. (1991) Peripheral territory and neuropeptides of the trigeminal ganglion neurons centrally projecting through the oculomotor nerve demonstrated by fluorescent retrograde double-labeling combined with immunocytochemistry. *Brain Res.* **547,** 82–88.

70. Carlton, S. M., Du, J., Zhou, S., and Coggeshall, R. E. (2001) Tonic control of peripheral cutaneous nociceptors by somatostatin receptors. *J. Neurosci.* **21,** 4042–4029.

71. Itoh, M., Takasaki, I., Andoh, T., et al. (2001) Induction by carrageenan inflammation of prepronociceptin mRNA in VR1- immunoreactive neurons in rat dorsal root ganglia. *Neurosci. Res.* **40,** 227–233.

72. Ahluwalia, J., Urban, L., Capogna, M., et al. (2000) Cannabinoid 1 receptors are expressed in nociceptive primary sensory neurons. *Neuroscience* **100,** 685–688.

73. Petruska, J. C., Cooper, B. Y., Johnson, R. D., and Gu, J. G. (2000) Distribution patterns of different P2x receptor phenotypes in acutely dissociated dorsal root ganglion neurons of adult rats. *Exp. Brain Res.* **134,** 126–132.

74. Li, Y. Q. (1999) Substance P receptor-like immunoreactive neurons in the caudal spinal trigeminal nucleus send axons to the gelatinosus thalamic nucleus in the rat. *J. Hirnforsch.* **39,** 277–282.

75. Ding, Y. Q., Takada, M., Shigemoto, R., and Mizumo, N. (1995) Spinoparabrachial tract neurons showing substance P receptor-like immunoreactivity in the lumbar spinal cord of the rat. *Brain Res.* **674,** 336–340.

76. Li, H. and Li, Y. Q. (2000) Collateral projection of substance P receptor expressing neurons in the medullary dorsal horn to bilateral parabrachial nuclei of the rat. *Brain Res. Bull.* **53,** 163–169.

77. Marshall, G. E., Shehab, S. A., Spike, R. C., and Todd, A. J. (1996) Neurokinin-1 receptors on lumbar spinothalamic neurons in the rat. *Neuroscience* **72,** 255–263.
78. Wang, X. M., Zhang, K. M., Long, L. O., et al. (2000) Endomorphin-1 and endomorphin-2 modulate responses of trigeminal neurons evoked by *N*-methyl-D-aspartic acid and somatosensory stimuli. *J. Neurophysiol.* **83,** 3570–3574.
79. Carstens, E., Saxe, I., and Ralph, R. (1995) Brainstem neurons expressing c-Fos immunoreactivity following irritant chemical stimulation of the rat's tongue. *Neuroscience* **69,** 939–953.
80. Pan, B., Castro-Lopes, J. M., and Coimbra, A. (1999) Central afferent pathways conveying nociceptive input to the hypothalamic paraventricular nucleus as revealed by a combination of retrograde labeling and c-fos activation. *J. Comp. Neurol.* **413,** 129–145.
81. Chamberlin, N. L., Mansour, A., Watson, S. J., and Saper, C. B. (1999) Localization of mu-opioid receptors on amygdaloid projection neurons in the parabrachial nucleus of the rat. *Brain Res.* **827,** 198–204.
82. Yamano, M., Hillyard, C. J., Girgis, S., et al. (1988) Presence of a substance P-like immunoreactive neurone system from the parabrachial area to the central amygdaloid nucleus of the rat with reference to coexistence with calcitonin gene-related peptide. *Brain Res.* **451,** 179–188.
83. Burkey, A. R., Carstens, E., Wenniger, J. J., et al. (1996) An opioidergic cortical antinociception triggering site in the agranular insular cortex of the rat that contributes to morphine antinociception. *J. Neurosci.* **16,** 6612–6623.
84. Li, J. L., Li, Y. Q., Li, J. S., et al. (1999) Calcium-binding protein-immunoreactive projection neurons in the caudal subnucleus of the spinal trigeminal nucleus of the rat. *Neurosci. Res.* **35,** 225–240.

15

Isolation and Culture of Sensory Neurons From the Dorsal-Root Ganglia of Embryonic or Adult Rats

Thomas H. Burkey, Cynthia M. Hingtgen, and Michael R. Vasko

Summary

There is increasing use of isolated sensory neuronal preparations to examine the cellular mechanisms involved in pain signaling. Indeed, these in viro preparations have several advantages that make them beneficial for examining physiological and/or pathological processes affecting neuronal function. With isolated cells it can be determined whether various inflammatory mediators and algogenic agents have direct actions on sensory neurons. Additionally, the intracellular signaling pathways for agents that modulate the excitability and sensitization of sensory neurons can be examined. Finally, the concentrations of mediators and drugs that are used to alter cell function can be well controlled. The purpose of this chapter is to provide the reader with detailed methods for the harvest and growth of embryonic and adult rat sensory neurons (dorsal root ganglia neurons) in culture. Because numerous methods for growing sensory neurons exist, the rationale for certain aspects of the protocols described in the chapter are included, as are discussions of potential pitfalls.

Key Words: Cell dissociation; cell culture; dorsal-root ganglia; nerve growth factor; rat; sensory neurons; growth medium.

1. Introduction

An increasing number of studies are being performed using isolated sensory neuronal preparations in an attempt to understand cellular mechanisms regulating neuronal excitability and neurotransmitter release. In some instances, these studies are performed on cells after acute dissociation, but the majority of this work is done using primary cultures of these neurons. Although controversy exists as to which of these methods most accurately reflects the in vivo condition, the protocols outlined here are useful for both procedures because they discuss both isolation and dissociation of dorsal-root ganglia (DRG) neurons as well as the procedures necessary to maintain sensory neurons in culture.

From: *Methods in Molecular Medicine, Vol. 99: Pain Research: Methods and Protocols*
Edited by: Z. D. Luo © Humana Press Inc., Totowa, NJ

There are several advantages of using primary sensory neuronal cultures to examine physiological or pathological processes affecting neuronal function. First, the use of sensory neurons in culture allows one to determine whether a given compound has a direct action on these cells. This advantage is especially important when examining inflammatory mediators because a number of these compounds can act on multiple cellular targets in tissue preparations and often these targets generate other inflammatory mediators. Thus, with in vivo preparations, it is difficult to interpret whether a compound has a direct action on sensory neurons or whether the compound acts indirectly through generating other agents. The use of isolated neuronal preparations readily resolves this issue. A second advantage of using cells in culture is the ability to closely monitor the concentrations of compounds that reach the target cells. As a result, one can examine the effects of different drug concentrations without having to deal with the pharmacokinetic variables that can occur in vivo or during administration of drugs in isolated tissue preparations. The third major advantage of using primary cultures of sensory neurons is the ability to study cellular mechanisms that mediate excitability and release, a task that is extremely difficult in vivo or in isolated tissues. Indeed, the more homogenous the cell population, the more amiable the system is for determination of critical pathways involved in regulating function.

It should be pointed out that the use of primary culture has limitations, including the lack of ability to ascertain the physiological functions of sensory neurons. Indeed, this can only be accomplished in vivo. Furthermore, culture conditions offer additional variables that can alter expression of proteins or transmitters. These variables do not limit performing studies with sensory neurons in culture; rather, they limit extrapolation of results to the in vivo condition. Overall, much knowledge about neuronal excitability, neurotransmitter release, and the cellular mechanisms regulating these processes can be gained by utilizing primary sensory neuron cultures as a model as long as the cells behave in a manner analogous to their in vivo counterparts.

The purpose of this chapter is to provide the reader with the methods utilized in our laboratory for the harvest and growth of embryonic and adult rat sensory neurons (DRG neurons). The protocols discussed here are modifications of methods from a number of laboratories, including the techniques for isolating and growing chick DRG neurons (1), and techniques for adult sensory neurons (2,3). The modifications that we have implemented and the potential pitfalls in the techniques are outlined here. We have used these same procedures to isolate and grow sensory neurons from the mouse, so the techniques are applicable to this species as well as the rat.

2. Materials

2.1. Animals

1. Male Sprague-Dawley rats (150–175 g, Harlan Sprague-Dawley, Indianapolis, IN).
2. Timed pregnant (E15-E17) Sprague-Dawley rats (Harlan Sprague- Dawley).

2.2. Supplies

1. Dulbecco's Modified Eagle's Medium (DMEM) (Invitrogen, San Diego, CA, Cat. no. 31600-034) reconstituted in deionized and filtered water. Add sodium bicarbonate and pH as per packet instructions (*see* **Notes 1** and **2**).
2. F12 medium (Invitrogen, Cat. no. 21700-075) reconstituted in deionized and filtered water. Add sodium bicarbonate and pH as per packet instructions (*see* **Notes 1** and **2**).
3. Dulbecco's phosphate-buffered saline (PBS; Invitrogen, Cat. no. 21600-010).
4. Fetal bovine serum (FBS), heat-inactivated (Invitrogen, Cat. no. 10082-147).
5. Horse serum (HS), heat-inactivated (Invitrogen, Cat. no. 26050-088).
6. Nerve growth factor 7S (NGF) (Harlan Sprague-Dawley, Cat. no. BT-5023).
7. L-glutamine (200 m*M,* Invitrogen, Cat. no. 25030-081).
8. Penicillin G (5000 U/mL)/Streptomycin sulfate (5 mg/mL, Invitrogen, Cat. no. 15070-063).
9. 5-fluoro-2′-deoxyuridine (Sigma Chemical Co., St. Louis, MO, Cat. no. F-0503).
10. Uridine (Sigma, Cat. no. U-3750).
11. Sodium bicarbonate (Sigma, Cat. no. S-5761).
12. Normocin™O (InvivoGen, San Diego, CA, Cat. no. ant-nr-o).
13. Fungizone® (Invitrogen, Cat. no. 15295-017).
14. Trypsin Type IX (Sigma, Cat. no. T0134).
15. Trypsin inhibitor (Sigma, Cat. no. T9003).
16. Collagenase Type 1A (Sigma, Cat. no. C9891).
17. Laminin (Sigma, Cat. no. L-2020).
18. Poly-D-lysine (Sigma, Cat. no. P-6407).
19. Deoxyribonuclease I (Sigma, Cat. no. D-5025).
20. Bottle top and syringe fitting 0.22-μm filters (Millipore, Bedford, MA).
21. Dumont forceps (no. 5, Fine Science Tools, Foster City, CA).
22. Dissecting scissors.
23. Dissecting pins.
24. Scalpel with a no. 10 blade.
25. Dissecting wax (Fisher Scientific, Pittsburgh, PA, Cat. no. S17432).
26. Trypan Blue Stain 0.4% (Invitrogen, Cat. no. 15250-061).
27. 70% ethanol.
28. Sterile 4-mL culture tubes (FisherBrand, Fisher Scientific, 14-956-3D).
29. Tissue culture dishes from Falcon (Corning, Corning, NY; 24-well, Cat. no. 351147; 6-well, Cat. no. 353046; 35-mm dish, Cat. no. 35300; 60-mm dish, Cat. no. 353002; 10-cm plate, Cat. no. 353003).

Table 1
Growth Medium Preparations[a]

	Adult Growth Medium	Embryonic Growth Medium
F12	880 mL	–
DMEM	–	880 mL
Horse serum	100 mL (10%)	–
Fetal bovine serum	–	100 mL (10%)
Penicillin/streptomycin	10 ml (50 U/mL 50 µg/mL)	10 ml (50 U/mL, 50 µg/mL)
L-glutamine	10 mL (2 mM)	10 mL (2 mM)
5-fluro-2′-deoxyuridine	300 mg (50 µM)	300 mg (50 µM)
Uridine	700 mg (150 µM)	700 mg (150 µM)

[a] Both NGF and normocin are added to the media after it is prepared.

2.3. Preparation of Media and Reagents

1. Growth Medium: **Table 1** shows the components of adult and embryonic growth media. The components are mixed and the pH is adjusted to 7.2. The media is filtered through a 0.22-µm filter and frozen in aliquots at –20°C until used (*see* **Notes 3** and **4**).
2. Nerve growth factor:
   a. NGF (1 mg) is resuspended in 10 mL deionized water then filtered through a 0.22-µm filter.
   b. The NGF solution (100 µg/mL) is divided into 50 or 100 µL aliquots (5 or 10 µg, respectively) in sterile 4-mL tubes, frozen at –70°C, then lyophilized. Tubes are loosely capped during lyophilization to allow a vacuum within the tubes while maintaining the sterility of the NGF.
   c. After lyophilization, NGF is stored at –20°C. Aliquots of NGF prepared in this manner are stable for at least 3 wk (*see* **Note 5**).
   d. Aliquots are resuspended in growth medium to a concentration of 250 ng/mL immediately prior to use (*see* **Notes 6** and **7**).
3. Modified Hank's balanced salt solution (HBSS): A Ca^{2+}- and Mg^{2+}-free HBSS is made consisting of: 171 mM NaCl, 6.7 mM KCl, 1.6 mM Na_2 PO_4, 0.5 mM KH_2PO_4, 6 mM D-glucose, and 0.01% phenol red. The pH is adjusted to 7.3. The solution is filter-sterilized through 0.22-µm filters into autoclaved glass bottles for storage at 4°C.
4. Fungizone® (Amphotericin B): Fungizone® is diluted to 250 µg/mL in sterile deionized water and frozen as aliquots at –20°C. Fungizone aliquots are added to HBSS at 1.6 µg/mL and used to inhibit fungal contaminants on the spinal column during the adult rat DRG preparation.
5. Normocin O™: Stock Normocin O™ (50 mg/mL) is frozen as aliquots at –20°C until needed.

6. Collagenase: Collagenase type 1A is dissolved in ice-cold Adult Growth Medium (**Table 1**) at 1.25 mg/mL (0.125%) and filter-sterilized through a 0.22-μm filter. The collagenase solution is divided into aliquots, frozen, and stored at –20°C until needed.
7. Trypsin: Trypsin type IX is prepared as a 0.025% solution in HBSS. The solution is sterilized by filtration through a 0.22-μm filter and aliquots are stored at –20°C.
8. Trypsin inhibitor: Trypsin inhibitor is prepared as a 0.25% solution in HBSS. The solution is sterilized by filtration through a 0.22-μm filter and aliquots are stored at –20°C.
9. Laminin: Laminin is diluted to 250 μg/mL in sterile PBS and aliquots are frozen at –70°C.
10. Poly-D-lysine: Poly-D-lysine is resuspended at 100 μg/mL in normal saline and sterilized through a 0.22-μm filter. Aliquots are frozen at –20°C until used.

3. Methods

3.1. Preparation of Wells

1. Tissue-culture wells are covered completely with a poly-D-lysine solution (100 μg/mL) and this solution is left in the wells for 20 min at room temperature (*see* **Note 8**).
2. The poly-D-lysine solution is removed and saved for reuse. It may be reused up to three times if stored at 4°C between uses.
3. The wells are rinsed three times with sterile deionized water and allowed to dry in a laminar flow hood.
4. If wells are used for culture of adult sensory neurons, dry poly-D-lysine coated plates are also coated with laminin. Laminin stock solution (*see* **Subheading 2.3., item 9**) is diluted to 5 μg/mL in sterile PBS and added to the wells for a minimum 2-h incubation at 37°C.
5. Laminin is removed and discarded immediately before adding adult sensory neurons to the wells.

3.2. Preparation of Instruments

Dissecting instruments are disinfected by soaking in 70% ethanol for at least 30 min. Instruments are then rinsed in sterile HBSS prior to use.

3.3. Preparation and Culture of Adult DRG Neurons

3.3.1. Harvesting DRG From Adult Male Sprague-Dawley Rats

1. Adult male Sprague-Dawley rats (150–170 g) are sacrificed by CO_2 asphyxiation. Each animal is placed in an airtight box containing a small amount of dry ice. The dry ice is covered with towels to prevent burning the animal. The animal is left in the box until respiration ceases (approx 5 min) (*see* **Notes 9** and **10**).
2. The rat is removed from the airtight box and the fur is disinfected by spraying with 70% ethanol.
3. The skin on the back of the rat is removed with dissecting scissors.

4. A transverse cut of the spinal column is made immediately rostral to the hind legs.

5. The spinal column is dissected from the animal by cutting toward the head on each side of the spinal column and another transverse cut of the spinal column is made at the base of the skull. It may be necessary to cut the internal organs away from the spinal column during removal.

6. The spinal column is washed under running tap water and excess tissue is trimmed away.

7. A blunt 18-G needle (0.5 in. long), attached to a 10-mL syringe containing HBSS, is inserted into the caudal end of the spinal canal and the HBSS rapidly injected into the spinal canal to extrude the spinal cord.

8. The spinal column is rinsed in ice-cold HBSS containing 1.6 µg/mL Fungizone (*see* **Note 11**).

9. The spinal column is pinned with the vertical side up to a dissecting surface.

10. The pointed end of dissecting scissors is inserted into the caudal end of the spinal canal and the canal opened by cutting toward the rostral end. The spinal column is turned over and cut through the dorsal surface.

11. Each half of the spinal column is pinned on a dissecting surface with the interior surface of the spinal canal facing up. Using a dissecting microscope, the DRG are identified. They are regularly spaced ball-like structures that are creamy in appearance (*see* **Fig. 1**).

12. The DRG are removed by grasping them with number 5 Dumont forceps and pulling gently upward.

13. The DRG are collected in a 35-mm Petri dish containing sterile ice-cold HBSS.

14. When all DRG are collected, the nerve trunks (the parts that look like white strings) are cut away using a no. 10 scalpel blade and the DRG are transferred to another 35-mm tissue Petri dish containing sterile ice-cold HBSS.

15. The HBSS is carefully aspirated from the dish with a Pasteur pipet and replaced by 3 mL of collagenase solution. The DRG are incubated for 1 h at 37°C (*see* **Note 12** and **13**).

16. The collagenase then is replaced with a fresh 3-mL aliquot and the incubation continued for an additional hour at 37°C.

17. At the conclusion of the incubation, the DRG in the collagenase solution is transferred to a sterile centrifuge tube containing 3 mg of Deoxyribonuclease I and the tube centrifuged (500*g*, 1 min).

18. The supernatant is aspirated and the DRG pellet resuspended in 3 mL of Adult Growth Medium (**Table 1**). The cells are dissociated by mechanical agitation through a fire-polished glass Pasteur pipet until the suspension of dissociated cells is homogeneous (the mixture is cloudy with no chunks of tissue).

3.3.2. Culture of Adult Sensory Neurons

1. Sensory neurons isolated from adult rats are cultured in Adult Growth Medium. NGF (250 ng/mL final concentration) and normocin O (100 µg/mL final concentration) are added to the medium immediately prior to use.

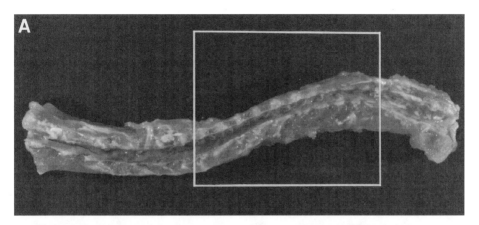

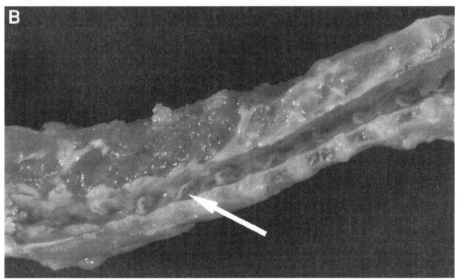

Fig. 1. (**A**) shows the adult rat spinal column bisected as described in **Subheading 3.3.1.** In this figure, the rostal end of the vertebral column is on the right and the dorsal surface is on the top. (**B**) is a magnified view of the spinal canal and the arrow indicates one of the DRG within the spinal canal.

2. After mechanical dissociation, an aliquot of the cell suspension is mixed 1:1 with trypan blue and counted immediately using a hemocytometer. Viable cells appear light against a blue background, whereas dead cells appear dark blue. Sensory neurons are plated at 10,000–15,000 cells per well in 24-well tissue-culture plates. Cells are plated at 40,000–50,000 cells/well in 6-well plates. In 24-well plates, 500

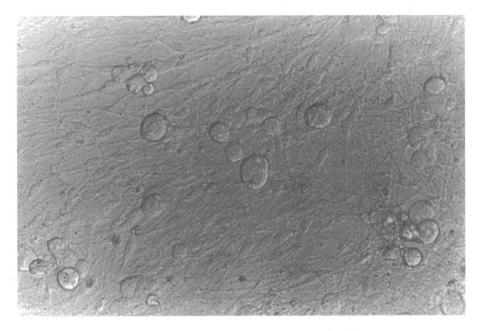

Fig. 2. This photomicrograph is a representative view of adult rat sensory neurons grown in culture for 8 d (magnification 30×).

µL of medium is sufficient for each well, whereas 2 mL of medium/well is used in the 6-well plate format (*see* **Note 14**).

3. Cells are maintained at 37°C under a 3% CO_2 atmosphere. Medium is replaced every 2–3 d. **Figure 2** shows a photomicrograph of cells after 8 d in culture (*see* **Note 15**).

3.4. Preparation and Culture of DRG Neurons From Embryonic (d 15–17) Rats

1. A timed pregnant (d 15–17) Sprague-Dawley rat is sacrificed by CO_2 asphyxiation (*see* **Subheading 3.3.1.**) and cervical dislocation (*see* **Note 16**).
2. The fur on the ventral surface of the mother rat is disinfected by application of 70% ethanol.
3. The abdomen of the mother rat is cut open, the uterus dissected out and transferred to a 10 cm Petri dish containing sterile ice-cold HBSS. The abdominal cavity is examined carefully to avoid missing parts of the uterus.
4. The embryos are dissected from the uterus using small pointed surgical scissors and transferred to a second sterile HBSS-filled Petri dish to wash away excess blood.
5. Embryos are placed in a third Petri dish containing sterile ice-cold HBSS and placed on ice.

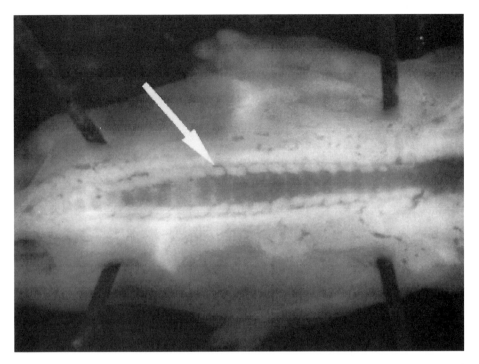

Fig. 3. This photomicrograph shows the view through a dissecting microscope of E16 rat embryo with the DRG exposed as described in **Subheading 3.4.** The rostral end of the animal is on the right and the animal is pinned ventral side down. The overlying skin and spinal cord have been removed as described in **Subheading 3.4.** The arrow indicates one DRG in a line of DRG lining the spinal canal.

6. Individual embryos are transferred to a glass Petri plate previously coated with dissecting wax and filled with sterile ice-cold HBSS.
7. The head of each embryo is pinched off using forceps and the remainder of the body is pinned to the wax-coated glass Petri dish, dorsal side up.
8. The translucent skin on the back of the embryo is broken by lightly scraping with the tips of the Dumont forceps (*see* **Note 17**).
9. The tips of the forceps are used to separate the cord from the side walls of the spinal canal (*see* **Note 18**).
10. One tip of the forceps is hooked under the caudal end of the spinal cord to dislodge it.
11. The cord is lifted from the embryo with the Dumont forceps.
12. At this point, the DRG appear as two rows of white ball-like structures lining the spinal canal **(Fig. 3)**. DRG are removed by grasping them with the forceps below the enlarged section and gently pulling the DRG from the animal.
13. The DRG are collected in a 15-mL conical tube containing sterile ice-cold HBSS (*see* **Note 19**).

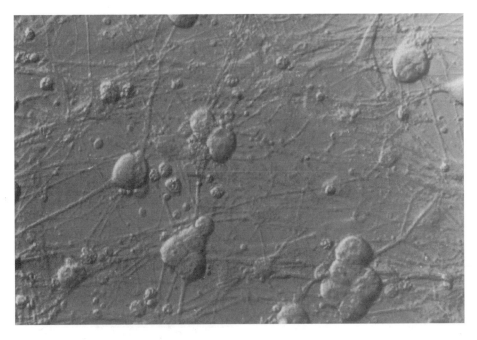

Fig. 4. This photomicrograph is a representative view of embryonic rat sensory neurons grown in culture for 14 d (magnification 75×).

14. When all the DRG from one embryo have been removed, another embryo is pinned to the Petri dish and the procedure is repeated.
15. After all the ganglia are dissected, they are centrifuged (500g, 1 min) and the supernatant is decanted (*see* **Note 20**).
16. The DRG are resuspended in 3 mL of trypsin solution and incubated for 20–25 min at 37°C (*see* **Note 21**).
17. At the end of the incubation, 3 mg of Deoxyribonuclease I is added and the DRG are centrifuged as in **step 15.**
18. Supernatant is aspirated, the DRG pellet is rinsed once with 3 mL of sterile HBSS containing trypsin inhibitor and the DRG are again centrifuged in as in **step 15.**
19. The resulting pellet is resuspended by mechanical agitation through a fire-polished glass Pasteur pipet in 3 mL of Embryonic Growth Medium containing NGF until a homogeneous suspension is obtained.
20. After mechanical dissociation, 100 µL of the cell suspension is mixed 1:1 with trypan blue and counted immediately on a hemocytometer. Viable cells appear light against a blue background, whereas dead cells appear dark blue.
21. The cell suspension is diluted with Embryonic Growth Medium **(Table 1)** containing NGF so that 150,000 viable cells in 0.5 mL are plated per well in 24-well plates or 450,000 cells in 2 mL are plated per well in 6-well plates (*see* **Note 22**).

22. Cultures are maintained at 37°C under a 5% CO_2 atmosphere. Embryonic Growth Medium is replaced every 2–3 d. **Figure 4** shows a photomicrograph of cells after 14 d in culture (*see* **Note 13**).

4. Notes

1. The catalog numbers listed for DMEM and F12 are for the powder formulations. For DMEM or F12, 7.7, or 1.18 g of sodium bicarbonate must be added (final concentration 44 or 14 m*M*, respectively) prior to adjusting the pH.
2. The water used for reconstituting DMEM and F12 must be deionized and filter-purified. We use a Barnstead Nanopure water purification system with a final filter of 0.2 μm.
3. Neurons grown in culture require L-glutamine *(4)*. It is essential that the 200 m*M* stock solution of L-glutamine be warmed and mixed so that all of the solid is in solution before addition to the media mixture. Always check the expiration date of the L-glutamine to assure that it has not expired.
4. Fetal bovine and horse sera are undefined products that vary among suppliers and even between lots from the same supplier. Consequently, variations between batches of serum have the potential to alter the biochemistry of cultured cells. If possible, orders should be placed for a number of bottles of serum from the same batch. When it is necessary to buy a new batch of serum with a different lot number, the new serum should be tested to assure that the culture conditions have not changed.
5. NGF is very labile in solution. By lyophilizing aliquots, the NGF remains stable at –20°C for at least 3 wk.
6. NGF is essential for the survival of embryonic sensory neurons *(5,6)*. Although 250 ng/mL NGF is typically used for these preparations, lower concentrations may be used. As shown in **Table 2,** there is no significant difference in the content of substance P or calcitonin gene-related peptide (CGRP) in embryonic sensory neurons grown for 10–12 d in the presence of 100–1000 ng/mL NGF. The concentration of NGF to which the cells are exposed also does not alter the release of CGRP evoked by 30 m*M* KCl. In contrast, the potassium-evoked release of substance P is significantly higher in cells treated with 500–1000 ng/mL NGF in comparison to those treated with 100 ng/mL *(8–11)*.
7. NGF is not essential for the survival of DRG neurons isolated from adult rats. However, peptide contents are higher and capsaicin sensitivity is augmented if the neurons are grown with NGF.
8. There are a number of different matrices that have been used to provide a surface for the adherence of sensory neurons in culture. In past work, we used rat-tail collagen. Although it is possible that the matrix used to grow cells can alter protein expression, we have not seen a significant difference in excitability or neuropeptide release using either collagen or poly-D-lysine. Because the use of poly-D-lysine or poly-D-lysine and laminin is efficient, we recommend these substances for coating wells.
9. We use animals that are 150–175 g. Although it is possible to do the preparation with larger animals, it becomes more difficult to cut through the spinal column to expose the DRG.

Table 2
The Effect of Nerve Growth Factor on Peptide Content
and Peptide Release From Embryonic Sensory Neurons[a]

		Substance P[b]			CGRP[b]		
NGF (ng/mL)	Wells	Basal Release	30 mM KCl	Content	Basal Release	30 mM KCl	Content
100	4	6 ± 2	17 ± 5	13 ± 2.4	215 ± 99	667 ± 309	120 ± 7.1
250	4	7 ± 1	42 ± 7	16 ± 1.8	141 ± 26	440 ± 148	120 ± 1.7
500	4	7 ± 1	68 ± 18^c	14 ± 3.2	164 ± 2	526 ± 148	110 ± 9.4
1000	4	17 ± 5	66 ± 8^c	17 ± 1.5	166 ± 12	513 ± 90	130 ± 22

[a] Neuropeptide release and content were measured as previously published (7).
[b] Mean ± standard error of the mean in fmol/well/10 min for release and pmol/well for content.
[c] Indicates a statistically significant difference from 100 ng/mL as determined by an analysis of variance and the Bonferroni-Dunn all means test ($p < 0.05$).

10. Adult rats are sacrificed by CO_2 asphyxiation. Cervical dislocation is not used on these animals because the break in the spinal column makes hydraulic extrusion of the spinal cord from the spinal canal difficult.
11. Adult DRG preparations seem prone to bacterial and fungal overgrowth. The antibiotic mixture Fungizone greatly reduces this problem.
12. During the isolation of sensory neurons from DRG, 3 mL of collagenase solution is sufficient to digest the connective tissue in the DRG isolated from one or two rats. When isolating DRG from three or more rats concurrently, increase the volume of collagenase solution accordingly.
13. Recently, members of our group have adapted the method of Eckert et al. *(14)* for the dissociation of sensory neurons from adult rats. With this procedure, DRG are incubated for 20 min at 37°C with papain (20 U/mL). After this incubation, the supernatant is removed and replaced with collagenase (0.3%)/dispase (0.4%) for an additional 20 min as above. At the conclusion of the incubation, the DRG are centrifuged (500*g*, 1 min), the supernatant aspirated, and the pellet resuspended in 3 mL of Adult Growth Medium. The sensory neurons are resuspended and plated according to our usual protocol (*see* **Subheading 3.3.2.**). Sensory neurons prepared by this protocol are well-suited for patch-clamp electrophysiology.
14. An experienced technician can isolate sensory neurons from two rats in approx 3.5 h using this preparation. The spinal column from the second rat can be stored in sterile ice-cold HBSS containing Fungizone without detrimental effect during the removal of DRG from the spinal column of the first rat. We typically isolate sufficient cells to plate 16 wells of a 24-well plate or four to six wells of a 6-well plate per rat.
15. A potential problem with sensory neuron isolation is that cells harvested from DRG include cells other than sensory neurons. This problem is further compounded by the fact that the neurons do not divide in culture, but the non-neuronal cells can. For this reason, it is necessary to include mitotic inhibitors such as 5-fluoro-2′-

Table 3
Enzyme Treatment Used for Cell Dissociation Does Not Alter Basal or Stimulated Peptide Release From Sensory Neurons

Enzyme	n	Substance P[a]			CGRP[a]		
		Basal	30 mM KCl	100 nM Capsaicin	Basal	30 mM KCl	100 nM Capsaicin
Collagenase	6–10	7 ± 1	22 ± 2	171 ± 9	60 ± 10	171 ± 32	644 ± 38
Trypsin	5–10	7 ± 1	27 ± 3	143 ± 16	67 ± 7	117 ± 26	512 ± 114

[a] fmol/well/10 min, mean $\pm$ S.E.M.

deoxyuridine and uridine in the medium. Previously, 5-fluoro-2′-deoxyuridine has been reported to kill Schwann cells and fibroblasts at a lower concentration than used in the medium outlined here *(12)*. However, we find that 5-fluoro-2′-deoxyuridine (50 μM) and uridine (150 μM) prevent replication of the non-neuronal cells but do not eliminate them from the culture. Other investigators have used the mitotic inhibitor cytosine arabinoside to eliminate dividing cells from neuronal cultures *(3,8,9)*. However, we do not use cytosine arabinoside because it is reported to be toxic to sensory neurons *(13)*.

16. We use E15–17 embryos for the preparation of sensory neurons. Younger embryos are poorly formed, making removal of the DRG difficult. Conversely, older embryos have more completely formed vertebrae, increasing the difficulty in removing the DRG. Both situations lead to reduced cell yields.

17. It is essential to have well-maintained Dumont forceps with sharp tips. The tips are used to cut the skin of the embryo, and blunted forceps result in tearing of the tissue with the loss of the morphology necessary to identify the DRG.

18. DRG are frequently attached to the spinal cord of the embryonic rat when it is removed. This is particularly true for DRG at the caudal end of the cord. Thus, it is necessary to examine the spinal cord under a dissecting microscope and remove the attached DRG before discarding the spinal cord.

19. Embryos and DRG should be kept in sterile HBSS on ice as much as possible to improve viable cell yield.

20. The percentage of viable cells declines if more than 2 h elapses between removing the embryos from the mother and completing the removal of DRG from all of the embryos. Experienced personnel require approx 10 min to remove all the DRG from one embryo.

21. We compared the effect of collagenase (3 mL of 0.01% collagenase in HBSS for 30 min at 37°C) and trypsin dissociation of embryonic sensory neurons on basal and stimulated neuropeptide release. There was no difference in basal, capsaicin-stimulated or KCl-stimulated release of substance P and CGRP between neurons initially dissociated with collagenase or trypsin (**Table 3**). However, the use of trypsin and trypsin inhibitor results in a qualitatively higher yield of viable cells.

22. Experienced personnel average approx 450,000 cells per rat pup using this protocol.

References

1. Dichter, M. A. and Fischbach, G. D. (1977) The action potential of chick dorsal root ganglion neurons maintained in culture. *J. Physiol.* **267,** 281–298.
2. Scott, B. S. (1977) Adult mouse dorsal root ganglia neurons in cell culture. *J. Neurobiol.* **8,** 417–427.
3. Lindsay, R. M. (1988) Nerve growth factors (NGF, BDNF) enhance axonal regeneration but are not required for survival of adult sensory neurons. *J. Neurosci.* **8,** 2394–2405.
4. Aruffo, C., Ferszt, R., Hildebrandt, A. G., and Cervos-Navarro, J. (1987) Low doses of L-monosodium glutamate promote neuronal growth and differentiation in vitro. *Dev. Neurosci.* **9,** 228–239.
4. Barde, Y.-A. (1989) Trophic factors and neuronal survival. *Neuron* **2,** 1525–1534.
5. Ruit, K. G., Elliott, J. L., Osborne, P. A., et al. (1992) Selective dependence of mammalian dorsal root ganglia neurons on nerve growth factor during embryonic development. *Neuron* **8,** 573–587.
6. Hingtgen, C. M. and Vasko, M. R. (1994) Prostacyclin enhances the evoked-release of substance P and calcitonin gene-related peptide from rat sensory neurons. *Brain Res.* **655,** 51–60.
7. Lindsay, R. M., Lockett, C., Sternberg, J., and Winter, J. (1989) Neuropeptide expression in cultures of adult sensory neurons: modulation of substance P and calcitonin gene-related peptide levels by nerve growth factor. *Neuroscience* **33,** 53–65.
8. Muldberry, P. K. (1994) Neuropeptide expression by newborn and adult rat sensory neurons in culture: effects of nerve growth factor and other neurotrophic factors. *Neuroscience* **59,** 673–688.
9. Shu, X. and Mendell, L. M. (1999) Nerve growth factor sensitizes the response of adult rat sensory neurons to capsaicin. *Neurosci. Lett.* **274,** 159–162.
10. Aguayo, L. G. and White, G. (1992) Effects of nerve growth factor on TTX- and capsaicin-sensitivity in adult rat sensory neurons. *Brain Res.* **570,** 61–67.
12. Martin, D. P., Wallace, T. L., and Johnson, E. M. Jr. (1990) Cytosine arabinoside kills postmitotic neurons in a fashion resembling trophic factor deprivation: evidence that a deoxycytidine-dependent process may be required for nerve growth factor signal transduction. *J. Neurosci.* **10,** 184–193.
13. Wallace, T. L. and Johnson, E. M. Jr. (1989) Cytosine arabinoside kills postmitotic neurons: evidence that deoxycytidine may have a role in neuronal survival that is independent of DNA synthesis. *J. Neurosci.* **9,** 115–124.
14. Eckert, S. P., Taddese, A., and McCleskey E. W. (1997) Isolation and culture of rat sensory neurons having distinct sensory modalities. *J. Neurosci. Methods* **77,** 183–190.

16

Primary Cultures of Neonatal Rat Spinal Cord

Virginia S. Seybold and Lia G. Abrahams

Summary

Primary cultures of neurons provide opportunities to study the cell biology of neurons under controlled conditions. Because differences exist in cellular properties among populations of neurons in the brain, survival requirements for neurons among these regions differ as well. This chapter outlines protocols for the preparation of primary cultures of spinal cord from 2-d-old neonatal rats. One protocol prepares cultures enriched in neurons and an alternative procedure prepares cultures enriched in non-neuronal cells. Comparison of biochemical data between these two culture preparations allows deductions of effects of treatments on neurons in the cultures. Limitations in interpretation of data obtained from cultured neurons are discussed.

Key Words: Cell culture; neuron; glia; serum; culture media; rat; neonate.

1. Introduction

Molecular biology has facilitated the discovery of many receptors and ion channels that participate in neurotransmission. Manipulation of cell lines to express these proteins has provided insights into signal transduction pathways activated by receptors and membrane properties controlled by ion channels. However, differences in expression of complementary proteins by different cell types can alter the properties of a receptor or ion channel. For example, G protein coupled receptors can couple to multiple G proteins, such that the relative abundance of different G proteins can alter the apparent second messengers generated in cells in response to receptor activation. Chinese hamster ovary (CHO) cells transfected with neurokinin 1 (NK1) receptors generate adenosine-cyclic monophosphate (cAMP) and inositol phosphates in response to tachykinins *(1)*, but NK1 receptors on neonatal rat spinal neurons only couple to generation of inositol phosphates *(2)*. Diversity in expression of G proteins among different populations of cells, including different populations of

From: *Methods in Molecular Medicine, Vol. 99: Pain Research: Methods and Protocols*
Edited by: Z. D. Luo © Humana Press Inc., Totowa, NJ

neurons, underscores the importance of understanding receptor signaling within defined populations of neurons in order to understand regulation of neurotransmission along pathways. Studies on acute preparations of regions of the adult nervous system have provided limited data. Although in vitro preparations have the advantage of controlling the concentration of ligands and blocking secondary effects of agonists (e.g., inhibition of neurotransmission with tetrodotoxin), data from acutely isolated tissues may be confounded by desensitization of receptors following dissection of the tissue. Also, the volume of the tissue slice used in the experiments may compromise the number of living cells within the tissue. These factors may contribute to a larger effective concentration for an agonist determined on adult brain in vitro *(3)* compared to primary cultures of neonatal neurons *(2)*. Primary cultures of neurons from selected regions of the nervous system provide the opportunity to study receptors and membrane properties of neurons under controlled conditions.

This chapter addresses preparation of primary cultures of neonatal rat spinal cord. For additional background on culturing neurons, the book *Culturing Nerve Cells (4)* is highly recommended.

1.1. Limitations of Primary Cultures

Primary cultures of neonatal rat spinal cord have been used in electrophysiological and immunohistochemical studies of single neurons as well as ligand binding and signal transduction studies of mixed samples of spinal cord cells. Despite the utility of the preparation, the investigator must be aware of several factors that affect the properties of the neurons in the cultures: (1) Age of animals from which spinal cord is obtained. Embryonic and early postnatal (1–2 d postnatal) nervous tissue generally exhibits better viability in culture, but the results may be biased by the developmental maturation of certain pathways. (2) Neurons may acquire different properties in culture. Plasticity is evident at early postnatal stages in neurons *(5,6)* as well as in glia *(7)*. The artificial conditions in cell culture, which include substrates to promote cell attachment of neurons to the culture wells (e.g., laminin is described here), inhibitors of cell division to prevent over-expression of non-neuronal cells (e.g., cytosine-arabinoside), volume of media/number of cells, and length of time in culture may all contribute to the properties of cultured neurons. Therefore, the possibility must be considered that the spinal cord cells acquire different properties than might be observed in vivo under normal conditions. Primary cultures of neonatal neurons are generally studied after 1 wk in vitro. This period coincides with the formation of synapses *(8)*. Whereas studies of acutely dissociated neurons offer some data for comparison *(9)*, these data may also be compromised by the acute injury of dissociation. (3) Different populations of neurons may have different requirements for survival. Embryonic hippocampal neurons appear to survive well in defined medium *(10)*, but we have not been able to get long-term survival of neonatal spinal neurons without horse serum. Consequently, the investigator needs to consider the extent to which undefined factors in serum contribute to the expression of proteins and the response of the neurons to agonists. In addition, some populations of neurons may not survive in culture. (4) The cultures contain mixed cell types. Populations of cells dissociated from whole spinal cord include projection neurons, interneurons, motor neurons, meningial fibroblasts, endothelial cells, and glia. If biochemical assays sample all of the cells in a culture well, the investigator needs to consider the extent to which non-neuronal cells contribute to the response. We have relied on comparative data from cultures enriched in non-neuronal cells. These cultures are prepared in parallel with the neuronal cultures. Preparation of cultures enriched in non-neuronal cells is possible because the non-neuronal cells settle faster and adhere more tightly to the substrate in a shorter period of time *(11)*. Consequently, neurons and a portion of non-neuronal cells can be removed from a well with a gentle rinse, leaving non-neuronal cells behind to multiply in vitro and a preparation enriched in neurons to be plated in separate wells.

2. Materials

2.1. Buffers and Media

Sera and Bacto-trypsin are shipped sterile. Therefore, except for media with serum and Bacto-trypsin, all buffers and media are sterilized after preparation of the stock by passing them through a 0.2-μm filter so that they are stored sterile. All reconstitutions and dilutions are made in distilled or MilliQ filtered water. All media and buffers are made in tissue-culture glassware (*see* **Note 1**).

1. Voller's Carbonate Buffer: 15 mM sodium carbonate, 34.9 mM sodium bicarbonate, and 3.08 mM sodium azide. Dissolve salts in H_2O and adjust pH to 9.6. Store at room temperature. Sterile filter before use (*see* **Note 2**).
2. Dulbecco's Modified Eagle's Medium (DMEM), low glucose (Sigma Aldrich Cat. no. D-5523). Stored at 4°C.
3. Horse serum (HS), heat-inactivated (Gibco BRL, Cat. no. 26050-088).
4. Fetal bovine serum (FBS), heat-inactivated (Gibco BRL, Cat. no. 10082-147).
5. Antibiotic-antimycotic (penicillin/streptomycin/fungizone) (Gibco BRL, Cat. no. 15240-062). The stock is 100X; it is diluted to 1X in DMEM. All references to DMEM refer to medium that includes antibiotic (*see* **Note 3**).
6. DMEM/HS: 90% DMEM, 10% HS. Store at 4°C (*see* **Note 4**).
7. DMEM/HS/FBS: 80% DMEM, 10% HS, 10% FBS. Store at 4°C.
8. Dulbecco's Phosphate-Buffered Saline without calcium and magnesium (DPBS) (10X), pH 7.4, at room temperature (Gibco BRL, Cat. no. 14200-075). Store at room temperature (*see* **Note 2**).

9. DPBS, pH 7.89 at room temperature. Increase pH of DPBS, pH 7.4, with NaOH. Store at 4°C.
10. Bacto-trypsin (Difco Laboratories, Cat. no. 015360-2). Store 300 µL aliquots in sterile, 6-mL polystyrene tubes at –20°C.
11. Cytosine-B-D-arabinoside (Ara-C) (Sigma Aldrich, Cat. no. C-1768).
12. 1–2-d-old rat pups (*see* **Note 5**).

2.2. Day Before Culturing:

1. Laminin (Sigma Aldrich, Cat. no. L-2020), store at –80°C (*see* **Note 6**).
2. Voller's Carbonate Buffer.
3. 24-Well culture plates, sterile (*see* **Note 7**).
4. 25-mm Acrodisc syringe filter, 0.2 µm.
5. 15-mL syringe.
6. 1-mL pipettor with appropriate tips.
7. 10-mL sterile serological pipets.
8. 15-mL sterile conical centrifuge tubes with caps.
9. Parafilm.

2.3. Day of Culturing

1. Bacto-Trypsin.
2. 9 in. Pasteur pipets.
3. 15-mL sterile conical tube with caps.
4. 50-mL sterile conical tubes with caps.
5. Fine scissors, 11 cm, straight, blunt/blunt.
6. Two pairs of fine forceps, Dumont no. 5, Biologie tip.
7. Spring scissors, 10 cm, straight, sharp/sharp.
8. Surgical scissors, 6 $^3/_4$ in.
9. Two plastic cups (100 mL).
10. Sterile field barrier.
11. 70% EtOH.
12. Hemacytometer.
13. 1-mL pipettor with appropriate tips.
14. 5-mL sterile serological pipets.
15. 10-mL sterile serological pipets.
16. 35 × 10 mm sterile tissue-culture dish.
17. Glass petri dish (100 × 10 mm), top and bottom.
18. 25-mm Acrodisc syringe filter, 0.2 µm.
19. 15-mL syringe.
20. Eight rat pups, 1–2 d old.
21. Laminin-coated culture plates.

3. Method

All procedures involved in preparation of primary tissue cultures are conducted in a laminar flow hood using sterile technique (*see* **Note 8**). The amounts listed below are sufficient to fill two 24-well plates with neuron-enriched preparations of neonatal rat spinal cord at a density of 160,000 cells/well and 12 wells enriched in non-neuronal spinal cord cells.

3.1. Day Before Culturing

1. Prepare a solution of 12.5 µg laminin/mL in Voller's Carbonate Buffer. 16 mL will coat two 24-well plates plus 12 wells on a separate plate to be used in the pre-plating procedure (250 µL/well).
2. Sterile-filter the laminin solution using the syringe and Acrodisc syringe filter.
3. Aliquot 250 µL of laminin solution into each well. When all of the wells on one plate have been filled, rotate the plate slowly to coat the bottom of the wells.
4. Place the lids on the plates, and seal the seams with stretched strips of parafilm.
5. Store plates with laminin solution at 4°C overnight (*see* **Note 9**).

3.2. Day of Culturing

3.2.1. Prepare Culture Wells

1. Work in groups of three wells so that the laminin coating does not dry between changes of solution. If you use a manifold pipettor, you can work in groups of six wells. Remove the laminin solution from the wells using a Pasteur pipet. Rinse each well two times with 500 µL of DMEM.
2. To wells that will be used in the final plating, remove DMEM and add 750 µL of DMEM/HS/FBS.
3. To wells that will be used for preplating, remove DMEM and add 400 µL DMEM/HS.
4. Place plates in 37°C incubator with a humidified mixture of air/CO_2 (90%/10%).
5. Put DMEM/HS, DMEM/HS/FBS, and DPBS, pH 7.89, in water bath to warm to 37°C.

3.2.2. Spinal Cord Dissection

1. Leave the sterile barrier field unfolded, and place it toward the front of the hood. Place tips of sterilized instruments on the barrier field.
2. Aliquot 2–3 mL of sterile DPBS, pH 7.4 into a 35 × 10 mm culture dish.
3. Anesthetize a rat pup by placing it in a closed container with a small amount of isoflurane for 1 min.
4. Decapitate the pup using the surgical scissors. Place the body in a cup of 70% EtOH (the body should be completely submerged) for 3–4 min to sterilize the surface.
5. Remove the body from the EtOH and place it on the bottom half of a glass petri dish.
6. Use a forceps to hold the rostral end of the pup at the midline with the dorsal surface of the animal facing up. Make longitudinal cuts on each side of the vertebral column with the fine scissors, separating the vertebral column from the rest of the body. It is important to avoid the stomach and intestines when cutting

in order to minimize contamination. Cut the skin, tissue, muscle, and ribs from the vertebral column.

7. Place the vertebral column on the top half of the petri dish with the ventral side facing up.
8. Use a forceps to anchor the vertebral column to the petri dish by placing the vertebral column beneath and between the open tips of a forceps mid-way along the vertebral column. Insert one tip of the fine scissors under the bone at the midline on the ventral surface of the vertebral column. Make a shallow, longitudinal cut through the vertebral column at the midline. The goal is to cut through the bone without cutting the spinal cord.
9. Without moving the forceps, make a second, longitudinal cut along the midline, on the dorsal surface of the vertebral column. You will end up with the vertebral column in two halves.
10. Using the fine forceps, remove the spinal cord tissue from each half of the vertebral column and place the tissue into the dish of DPBS.
11. Discard the carcass in a container inside the hood for disposal.
12. Remove the dura from the spinal cord by grasping one end of the spinal cord with the fine forcep and using the other forcep to push the spinal cord out of the dura (like decasing a sausage).
13. Discard the dura on a corner of the barrier field.
14. Repeat **steps 3–13** until eight spinal cords have been collected.

3.2.3. Preparation of Dissociated Cells

1. Add 4.7 mL DPBS, pH 7.89 to 300 µL Bacto-Trypsin. Mix by drawing the solution slowly up and down in the pipet to minimize creating bubbles.
2. Transfer trypsin solution to a 15-mL conical tube.
3. Using forceps, remove spinal cords from the DPBS and pile them on the lid of the 35×10 mm dish.
4. Using a Pasteur pipet, remove excess DPBS.
5. Mince the spinal cords with the spring scissors until the consistency of the preparation appears like molten gelatin.
6. To facilitate transfer of the spinal cord preparation to the 15-mL conical tube containing the trypsin, use a Pasteur pipet to add approx 1 mL of the trypsin solution to the minced spinal cords. The spinal cord preparation can then be aspirated into the Pasteur pipet and transferred to the tube containing the remainder of the trypsin solution.
7. Place the 15-mL conical tube in a 37°C water bath for 30 min.
8. Dissociate the spinal cords into cells by trituration: vigorously draw the tissue suspension in and out through Pasteur pipets that have a reduced bore (*see* **Note 10**) at least 20 times per pipet. Expel the suspension against the side of the tube to minimize foaming. The final spinal cord preparation will be cloudy and should not contain visible chunks of tissue.
9. Cap the tube and centrifuge the cell suspension at 1200 rpm for 10 min.
10. Using a Pasteur pipet, pull off the supernatant and discard (*see* **Note 11**).
11. Resuspend the cells in 6 mL DMEM/HS.

3.2.4. Plating Dissociated Cells

1. Remove media from six wells of the plate designated for preplating.
2. Divide the cell suspension evenly among six wells on the plate for preplating (~1 mL of the cell suspension/well).
3. Replace the lid on the culture plate, and place the plate in a 37°C incubator in a humidified mixture of air/CO_2(90%/10%) for 45 min. During this time the cells will settle to the bottom of the plate, and non-neuronal cells will attach.
4. Return the plate to the culture hood. Using a Pasteur pipet, draw up the cell suspension and gently expel it over the bottom of the well to dislodge settled but unattached cells.
5. Transfer the cell suspension to a 50-mL conical tube.
6. Add 1 mL of DMEM/HS to each of the preplate wells and repeat the rinse procedure. Add this media to the 50-mL tube.
7. Cap the tube and centrifuge the cell suspension at 1200 rpm for 10 min.
8. Using a Pasteur pipet, pull off the supernatant and discard.
9. Resuspend the cells in 6 mL DMEM/HS.
10. Repeat **steps 2–8** using the remaining six wells on the plate prepared for preplating.
11. Resuspend the pellet in 12 mL DMEM/HS/FBS.
12. Count the cells using a hemacytometer (*see* **Note 12**).
13. Add DMEM/HS/FBS to the cell suspension to dilute the cells to a concentration of 160,000 cells/250 µL (*see* **Note 13**).
14. Add 250 µL of cell suspension to each well prepared for primary culture.
15. Place cultures in a 37°C incubator in a humidified mixture of air/CO_2 (90%/10%).

3.3. Maintenance of Neuron-Enriched Cultures

3.3.1. Five Days In Vitro: Replenish Nutrients

1. Warm DMEM/HS/FBS to 37°C.
2. Remove 500 µL of medium from each well.
3. Add 500 µL of fresh medium to each well.

3.3.2. Seven Days In Vitro: Replenish Nutrients, Remove FBS, and Inhibit Growth of Non-Neuronal Cells

1. Warm DMEM/HS to 37°C.
2. Make a 10 mM solution of Ara-C in H_2O.
3. Sterilize the Ara-C solution by passing it through a Acrodisc syringe filter (0.2 µm).
4. Add Ara-C to DMEM/HS to a final concentration of 10 µM and mix.
5. Working in groups of three wells (or six wells if using a manifold pipettor), remove all media from a well and add 1 mL of DMEM/HS with 10 µM Ara-C to the well.

Cultures are ready for use in an experiment after 10–14 d in vitro. **Figure 1** is an example of cells present in the neonatal spinal cord cultures.

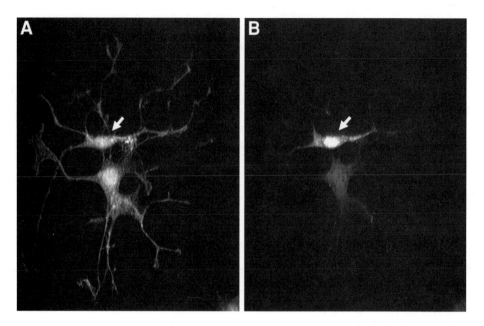

Fig. 1. Digitized images of a field from a spinal cord culture after 12 d in vitro. The culture was treated with forskolin (10 μ*M*) for 20 min prior to fixation with buffered 4% paraformaldehyde for 10 min. After rinsing, the culture was stained for the simultaneous visualization of two antigens by immunofluorescence. (**A**) Phosphorylated (p)-CREB immunoreactivity was visualized with rabbit anti-pCREB (Upstate Biotechnology) and lissamine-rhodamine conjugated to goat anti-rabbit antibody. Immunoreactivity occurred in multiple cell types. (**B**) A neuron (arrow) was identified in the same field using an antibody against the neuron-specific mRNA binding protein Hu *(13)*. Hu-immunoreactivity was visualized with mouse anti-Hu (Molecular Probes) and fluorescein-isothiocyanate conjugated to goat anti-mouse antibody.

3.4. Maintenance of Wells Seeded during Preplating as Cultures Enriched in Non-neuronal Cells

3.4.1. Day of Culture

1. After neurons have been recovered from the wells used in the preplating procedure (**Subheading 3.2.4., step 5**), add 1 mL of DMEM/HS/FBS to each well enriched in non-neuronal cells.
2. Keep cells in a 37°C incubator in a humidified mixture of air/CO_2 (90%/10%).

3.4.2. Five Days In Vitro: Replenish Nutrients

1. Warm DMEM/HS/FBS to 37°C.

2. Remove 500 μL of media from well.
3. Add 500 μL of fresh media to well.

3.4.3. Seven Days In Vitro: Remove FBS (see **Note 14**)

1. Warm DMEM/HS to 37°C.
2. Remove all media from well.
3. Add 1 mL of DMEM/HS to well.

3.4.4. Fourteen Days In Vitro: Replenish Nutrients

1. Warm DMEM/HS to 37°C.
2. Remove 500 μL of media from well.
3. Add 500 μL of fresh media to well.
4. Replenish nutrients at intervals of 7 d.

Non-neuronal cultures are used when there is a nearly confluent monolayer, typically 3–4 wk after initial culture.

4. Notes

1. Regular lab soap should not be used on glassware used for tissue culture. We use Linbro 7X cleaning solution diluted to 1X for cleaning culture labware and surgical instruments.
2. Because the stock of Voller's Carbonate buffer is shared by many, small volumes of this buffer are re-sterilized before use by using a syringe to pass the solution through a 25-mm Acrodisc syringe filter (0.2 μm).
3. An AcroCap filter unit with a Supor Membrane from Gelman Laboratory is used with a peristaltic pump to sterilize media when it is first made.
4. Because serum is undefined and variable in its composition, we have experimented with removing the serum from the cultures for 24 h to 4 d prior to using the cultures in biochemical experiments. Although the neurons in the cultures appeared healthy, neurochemical properties changed. Reducing the horse serum to 1% for 24 h prior to use in experiments has not had a detectable effect on biochemical responses currently being studied. Because of the undefined properties of serum, it is important to track lot numbers and note when serum of a different lot number is used in the protocol in the event that a change occurs in the control response. To minimize this confound, it is possible to reserve bottles of sera and request aliquots for testing in culture preparations before an order is placed.
5. At this age, dissection of the spinal cord into regions (dorsal, ventral) is not feasible. Some investigators can select the dorsal one-third in 3–4 d old pups *(12)*. Whereas late-term pregnant rats are generally available from suppliers, it is possible to order, for a higher price, timed-pregnant rats so that pups of a given age are available when desired.
6. Laminin pricing varies greatly among supplies. It pays to shop around. In addition, other substrates (collagen, poly-L-lysine) may be suitable depending on how the cultures will be used. In our hands, a laminin substrate optimized attachment of neurons.

7. Neonatal rat spinal neurons adhere to laminin-coated plastic much better than to laminin-coated glass. If cultures are being prepared on chambered slides, request plastic slides instead of glass slides.

8. The interior of the hood and all small equipment (e.g., pipettors) are routinely sprayed with a solution of 70% alcohol and then wiped dry with a chemwipe to sterilize them before initiating each procedure. Instruments are sterilized by placing them in a solution of 70% EtOH. Alternatively they may be autoclaved. Pasteur pipets, glass Petri dishes and disposable pipet tips are routinely autoclaved. Serological pipets, conical tubes and barrier fields are purchased sterile.

9. We have frozen the culture plates with the laminin solution in the wells after they sit for 24 h at 4°C. We have not noted a significant effect of freezing on the subsequent cultures, but we do not freeze the prepared plates on a routine basis.

10. The tip of sterile Pasteur pipets is decreased by fire-polishing the pipet tip in the hood using a Bunsen burner. Two pipets of graduated smaller bores are routinely prepared with the smallest bore no less than half of the initial diameter.

11. The pellet formed after treatment in trypsin is not firm. Be VERY careful when aspirating the supernatant. Do it slowly and gently, keeping close watch on the pellet. If the pellet begins to "stream" to one side, try to remove more supernatant by aspirating from the side opposite the stream.

12. On a standard hemacytometer, we use the grids of 16 squares at the corners. # of cells/16 squares = # $\times\ 10^4$ cells/mL.

13. The desired cell density will depend on how the cultures are used. When seeding wells on 8-chambered slides for immunohistochemistry, we use a density of 35,000 cells/well.

14. Because the goal is to increase the density of non-neuronal cells, the media in these cultures does not contain Ara-C.

References

1. Takeda, Y., Blount, P., Sachais, B. S., et al. (1992) Ligand binding kinetics of substance P and neurokinin A receptors stably expressed in Chinese hamster ovary cells and evidence for differential stimulation of inositol 1,4,5-triphosphate and cyclic AMP second messenger responses. *J. Neurochem.* **59,** 740–745.

2. Parsons, A. M., El-Fakahany, E. E., and Seybold, V. S. (1995) Tachykinins alter inositol phosphate formation, but not cyclic AMP levels, in primary cultures of neonatal rat spinal neurons through activation of neurokinin receptors. *Neuroscience* **68,** 855–865.

3. Watson, S. P. and Downes, C. P. (1983) Substance P induced hydrolysis of inositol phospholipids in guinea-pig ileum and rat hypothalamus. *Eur. J. Pharmacol.* **93,** 245–253.

4. Banker, G. and Goslin, K. (ed.) (1991) *Culturing Nerve Cells.* MIT Press, Cambridge, MA.

5. Ruda, M. A., Ling, Q.-D., Hohmann, A. G., et al. (2000) Altered nociceptive neuronal circuits after neonatal peripheral inflammation. *Science* **289,** 628–630.

6. Saporta, S. (1986) Loss of spinothalamic tract neurons following neonatal treatment of rats with the neurotoxin capsaicin. *Somatosensory Res.* **4,** 153–173.

7. Fok-Seang, J. and Miller, R. H. (1992) Astrocyte precursors in neonatal rat spinal cord cultures. *J. Neurosci.* **12,** 2751–2764.

8. Goslin, K. and Banker, G. (1991) Rat hippocampal neurons in low-density culture, in *Culturing Nerve Cells* (Banker, G. and Goslin, K., eds.), MIT Press, Cambridge, MA, pp. 251–281.

9. Arancio, O., Yoshimura, M., Murase, K., and MacDermott A. B. (1993) The distribution of excitatory amino acid receptors on acutely dissociated dorsal horn neurons from postnatal rats. *Neuroscience* **52,** 159–167.

10. Lu, B., Yokoyama, M., Dreyfus, C., and Black, I. B. (1991) NGF gene expression in actively growing brain glia. *J. Neurosci.* **11,** 318–326.

11. Bray, D. (1991) Isolated chick neurons for the study of axonal growth, in *Culturing Nerve Cells* (Banker, G. and Goslin, K., eds.), MIT Press, Cambridge, MA, pp. 119–135.

12. Jo, Y. H., Stoeckel, M. E., and Schlichter, R. (1998) Electrophysiological properties of cultured neonatal rat dorsal horn neurons containing GABA and Met-Enkephalin-like immunoreactivity. *J. Neurophysiol.* **79,** 1583–1586.

13. Ikano, H. J. and Darnell R. B. (1997) A hierarchy of Hu RNA binding proteins in developing and adult neurons. *J. Neurosci.* **17,** 3024–3037.

17

Single-Cell Laser-Capture Microdissection and RNA Amplification

Fredrik Kamme, Jessica Zhu, Lin Luo, Jingxue Yu, Da-Thao Tran, Bernhard Meurers, Anton Bittner, Karin Westlund, Susan Carlton, and Jackson Wan

Summary

Generating gene-expression profiles from laser-captured cells requires the successful combination of laser-capture microdissection, RNA extraction, RNA amplification, and microarray analysis. To permit single-cell gene-expression profiling, the RNA amplification method has to be sufficiently powerful to bridge the gap between the amount of RNA available from a single cell to what is required by the microarray, a gap that spans 5 to 6 orders of magnitude. This chapter focuses on the amplification of RNA using a two-round T7 RNA amplification method. The protocols described are adapted for laser-captured material and have been used to generate gene expression profiles from single laser-captured cells.

Key Words: Laser-capture microdissection; single cell; gene-expression profiling; LCM; microarray; RNA amplification.

1. Introduction

The combination of laser-capture microdissection and microarray technologies enables the expression analysis of thousands of genes in a defined cell population within a complex tissue, such as the central nervous system (CNS) *(1)*. To generate a sufficient amount of hybridization target from 1 to 1000 laser-captured cells for microarray hybridization, a powerful global RNA amplification method is required. This is usually done by the T7 aRNA amplification protocol *(2–7)*, invented by Eberwine in 1990 *(8)*. Once procedures for laser-capture microdissection and microarray processing have been established, the T7 aRNA amplification procedure is the most technically demanding and time-consuming step in the process. This chapter aims to describe a modified version of the T7 aRNA amplification method that requires 4–5 d to

From: *Methods in Molecular Medicine, Vol. 99: Pain Research: Methods and Protocols*
Edited by: Z. D. Luo © Humana Press Inc., Totowa, NJ

complete. This protocol provides sufficient amplification allowing single-cell gene-expression profiling using fluorescent labeling of the target and microarrays. A short discussion of laser-capture microdissection strategies is also included (*see* **Subheading 3.1.**).

2. Materials

1. Superscript II reverse transcriptase, *Escherichia coli* DNA polymerase I, *E. coli* DNA ligase, Rnase H, T4 DNA polymerase, T7 RNA polymerase (a high-yield kit such as the Ampliscribe kit from Epicentre), Rnase inhibitor.
2. Rneasy RNA extraction kit (Qiagen), polymerase chain reaction (PCR) purification kit (Qiagen), Microcon YM-100 (Millipore).
3. Polyinosinic acid, Cy3-dCTP.
4. $T7dT_{21}$ oligonucleotide.
5. Agarose gel equipment.
6. Optional: Real-time PCR equipment.

3. Methods

3.1. Laser-Capture Microdissection

There are basically two laser-capture microdissection technologies: (1) photo-mediated attachment of the cell of interest to a capture membrane using the Pix-Cell II or AutoPix instrument from Arcturus Engineering (Mountain View, CA), and (2) excision of the cell of interest using a finely focused ultraviolet (UV) laser beam and subsequent collection of the excised cell using the PALM instrument (PALM Gmbh, Bernried, Germany). An instrument similar to the PALM instrument is available from Leica. The Arcturus instrument can pick several cells individually with relative ease, whereas the PALM instrument is better at capturing cells with irregular shapes or when lifting of the cells is a problem. We have performed single-cell studies successfully using both systems. In **Fig. 1,** laser excision of retrogradely labeled spinothalamic tract (STT) neurons in lamina I in the rat spinal-cord dorsal horn is shown. Rats received thalamic injections of horseradish peroxidase (HRP) conjugated to wheat-germ agglutinin. Retrogradely labeled neurons in lamina I were detected using TMB (3.3′, 5,5′-tetramethylbenzidine) as the chromogen, and captured using the PALM capture instrument.

3.2. RNA Extraction

The following RNA extraction protocol is suitable for fresh-frozen CNS tissue that has been cryo-sectioned. For general staining, we use Nissl stain (*see* **Note 1**).

1. a. Arcturus: Under a dissection microscope, use a sterile scalpel and cut a small square in the film of the Capsure cap around the captured cell (**Fig. 2**). This is a precaution against nonspecific lifting of tissue at the rim of the cap, which is

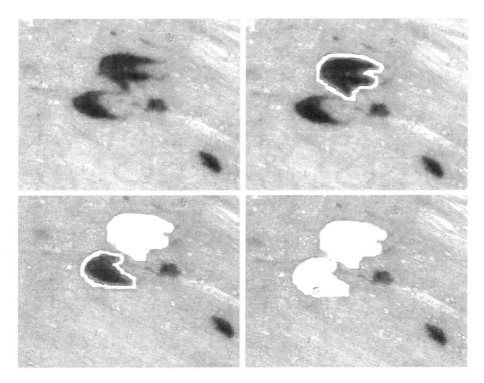

Fig. 1. Laser-capture microdissection of retrogradely labeled spinothalamic tract neurons in lamina I of the spinal cord in an adult rat. Cells were captured using the PALM laser-capture instrument. Note the ability of the PALM laser to outline irregular shapes.

slightly concave. (This step is circumvented by using the "CapSure HS LCM cap" from Arcturus, which requires a special extraction device. The extraction protocol described below can be followed, but the volume of RLT will be larger.) RNA is extracted by putting the piece of film into RLT buffer (Qiagen). The volume is adjusted depending on the size of the piece of film. The RLT buffer is supplemented with 250 ng polyinosinic acid (Sigma) to protect the extracted RNA from adsorption to plastics. For single cells, we use 8 µL of RLT buffer in a 500 µL PCR tube. Incubate the tube at 42°C for 20 min. Proceed to **step 2.**

b. PALM: Cells are catapulted directly into 35 µL RLT buffer and supplemented with 250 ng polyinosinic acid. Incubate the tube at 42°C for 20 min. Proceed to **step 2.**

2. Prepare a Microcon YM-100 (Millipore) by rinsing with 500 µL of H_2O containing 50 ng polyinosinic acid. (The purpose is to coat the interior of the microcon with polyinosinic acid.) Spin at 500g for 12 min. Add water to 500 µL in the microcon,

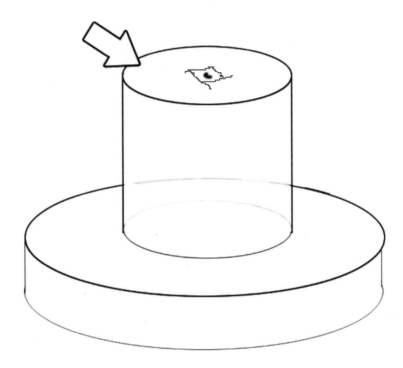

Fig. 2. Inverted Arcturus Capsure cap. Arrow indicates capture film with a captured cell in the middle. A small square is cut in the film around the cell under a dissection microscope and the piece of film carrying the cell is lifted using the tip of the scalpel into a tube with extraction buffer.

and then add the extracted RNA in RLT buffer. Spin at 500g until 10–20 µL remains in the microcon, which usually takes 12 min depending on the lot of microcons. Fill up to 500 µL with H_2O and spin until 10–20 µL remains. Repeat the process. Recover the final 10–20 µL by inverting the microcon into a 1.5-mL tube and spin 1 min at 3000g. Speed vac down to 10 µL.

3.3. T7 Amplification

3.3.1. First Round

1. Mix 0.5 µg of T7-cDNA synthesis primer (5′-TCTAGTACCTGCTTCACTGCATC-TAATACGACTCACTATAGGGAGATTTTTTTTTTTTTTTTTTTTTT-3′) (Operon, high-performance liquid chromatography [HPLC]-purified) and extracted RNA in a total volume of 11 µL. Denature for 10 min at 70°C and cool on ice. Spin to collect condensate.
2. Assemble the cDNA synthesis master mix: 4 µL 5X first-strand buffer (Invitrogen), 2 µL 0.1 M dithiothreitol (DTT), 1 µL RNase Block (Stratagene), 1 µL 10 mM

dNTPs (Amersham Biosciences), and 1 μL Superscript II (Invitrogen, 200U/μL) per reaction. Add 9 μL of master mix per sample and incubate at 42°C for 2 h, preferably in a hot-air oven.

3. Terminate cDNA synthesis by incubating at 70°C for 10 min.

4. Optional: Remove 1 μL and dilute in 3 μL of water. Use 2 μL for real-time PCR analysis to assess the yield of RNA from the tissue sample (*see* **Note 2**).

5. Assemble second-strand cDNA synthesis master mix: 92 μL water, 30 μL second-strand buffer (Invitrogen), 3 μL 10 m*M* dNTPs (Amersham Biosciences), 4 μL *E. coli* DNA pol. I (Invitrogen, 5U/μL), 1 μL Rnase H (invitrogen, 2U/μL), and 1 μL *E. coli* DNA ligase (Invitrogen, 10U/μL) per reaction. Add 131 μL mix per reaction. Incubate at 16°C for 2 h, then add 2 μL T4 DNA pol. (Invitrogen, 5 U/μL). Incubate at 16°C for 15 min and then heat-kill enzymes at 70°C for 15 min.

6. Purification of the transcription template: Add 1 μL of polyinosinic acid (Sigma; dissolved at 100 ng/μL). Then add 750 μL of PB buffer (Qiagen, PCR purification kit). Pipet to Qiaquick columns, spin at 13,000 rpm for 30–60 s. Wash with 750 μL PE buffer and spin as before. Spin 1 min at max speed to dry the column. Elute the DNA in 30 μL EB buffer diluted 1:10. Speed vac the eluate to yield 8 μL of sample.

7. T7 RNA polymerase transcription: Transcriptions are done using the Ampliscribe kit from Epicentre (Madison, WI). Assemble the reagents in the order described and be aware of precipitation: 2 μL 10X transcription buffer, 1.5 μL each of ATP, CTP, GTP, and UTP; 2 μL of DTT; and 2 μL of T7 RNA polymerase. Add 12 μL of transcription master mix to each sample. Incubate at 42°C for 3 h in a hot-air oven.

8. After incubation, add 1 μL DNase I (included in the transcription kit). Incubate an additional 15 min at 37°C.

9. Purification of transcription reactions: Add 1 μL of polyinosinic acid (Sigma, dissolved at 100 ng/μL) and then add 70 μL of RLT buffer (Qiagen) and 50 μL of 100% ethanol in sequence. Load samples onto Rneasy columns and treat according to the manufacturer's directions, except that the volume of RPE wash buffer is reduced to 150 μL per wash. Elute the cleaned aRNA in 30 μL of H$_2$O and dry down to 10 μL.

3.3.2. Second Round

10. Second first-strand cDNA reaction: Add 1 μg of random hexamers (Amersham Biosciences) to the aRNA and denature at 70°C for 10 min and cool on ice. Add 9 μL of first-strand cocktail (prepared as in **step 2**), and incubate the mix at room temperature for 10 min. Incubate at 37°C for 2 h. Heat-kill at 70°C for 10 min.

11. Optional: Remove 1 μL and dilute in 3 μL of water. Use 2 μL for real-time PCR to assess the efficiency of the first round of T7 amplification.

12. Add 1 μL RNase H (2U/μL, Invitrogen) and incubate at 37°C for 30 min.

13. Heat-denature at 95°C for 2 min. Spin briefly.

14. Add 0.5 μg T7dT$_{21}$ primer. Incubate at 70°C for 5 min, then at 42°C for 10 min. Cool on ice.

15. Second second-strand cDNA synthesis: Assemble second-strand cDNA synthesis master mix: 91 μL water, 30 μL second-strand buffer (Invitrogen), 3 μL 10 m*M*

dNTPs (Amersham Biosciences), 4 μL *E. coli* DNA pol. I (Invitrogen, 5 U/μL), and 1 μL Rnase H (Invitrogen, 2U/μL) per reaction. Add 129 μL mix per reaction. Incubate at 16°C for 2 h. Then add 2 μL T4 DNA pol. (Invitrogen, 5 U/μL). Incubate at 16°C for 15 min and then heat-kill at 70°C for 15 min.

16. Repeat **steps 6–9.** Addition of polyinosinic acid during the final purification of the transcription reactions is unnecessary. Elute final aRNA in 30 μL of water (*see* **Note 3**).

17. Add 5 μg of random hexamers to the eluted aRNA (which will be approx 28 μL after elution). Heat at 70°C for 10 min, and cool on ice. Add 10 μL first-strand buffer (Invitrogen); 5 μL 0.1 *M* DTT; 1.5 μL RNase Block (Stratagene); 1 μL 25 m*M* (each) dA-, dG-, dTTP; 2 μL 1 m*M* dCTP; 2 μL 1 m*M* Cy3-dCTP (Amersham Biosciences); and 2.5 μL Superscript II (Invitrogen, 200 U/μL) per reaction. Incubate at room temperature for 10 min, then at 37°C for 2 h.

18. Digest the RNA in the aRNA-cDNA hybrid by adding 0.1 U of RNase A (Sigma) per sample and incubating at 37°C for 20 min.

19. Purify using the Qiaquick Nucleotide Removal Kit (Qiagen).

20. Optional: Remove 1 μL and dilute in 299 μL of water. Use 2 μL for real-time PCR to assess the efficiency of the second round of T7 amplification.

The Cy3-labeled cDNA is ready to use as hybridization target on microarrays. We hybridize our targets to spotted cDNA microarrays in a conventional hybridization buffer containing 50% formamide. **Figure 3** shows a part of a microarray hybridized to a target generated from a single laser captured cell.

We strongly recommend testing the amplification protocol by starting with larger amounts of total RNA. Two ng of total RNA should give approx 50–70 μg of aRNA after two rounds of aRNA amplification. This way, the yield of aRNA can be measured by OD_{260} in a spectrophotometer. It is also important to judge the quality of the aRNA by running an aliquot on an agarose gel. We prefer running denaturing 1% agarose gels, containing 1 *M* urea. (Add three parts loading buffer and one part sample, denature at 90°C/1 min, cool on ice. Loading buffer: 8 M urea, 10 m*M* Tris-HCl, 1 m*M* ethylenediamine tetraacetic acid (EDTA), 1% Igepal CA-630 (Sigma), 0.05% Orange G). **Figure 4** shows an example of what the aRNA should look like after one and two rounds of aRNA amplification. After two rounds, the average length of the aRNA is approx 200–1000 bases.

4. Notes

1. Nissl staining of fresh frozen, cryo-sectioned tissue for LCM: Take out the slide from the freezer and put directly in 100% ethanol for 1 min. Proceed with the following steps: 95% ethanol/10 s, 70% ethanol/10 s, 50% ethanol/10 s, phosphate-buffered saline (PBS)/10 s, 0.8% Cresyl Violet/40 s, PBS/10 s ×3, 70% ethanol/10 s, 95% ethanol/10 s, 95% ethanol + 1.6% acetic acid/5–10 s, 95% ethanol/10 s, 100% ethanol/10 s, xylene/1 min, and finally left to air dry. For the Arcturus instrument, the final xylene step is critical. For the PALM instrument, it is not.

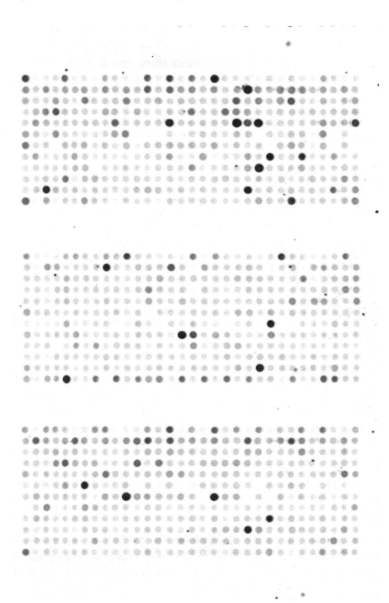

Fig. 3. Close-up of a microarray hybridized with the target from a single STT neuron, showing one-eighth of the total array. The microarray is a spotted-glass cDNA microarray, containing approx 9000 spots and printed using a Generation III spotter from Amersham Biosciences.

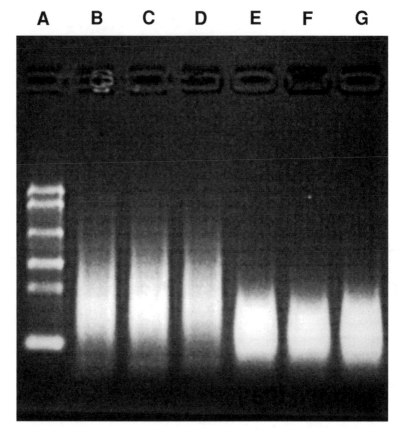

Fig. 4. Denaturing 1% agarose gel analysis of amplified aRNA. **(A)** 0.24–9.5 Kb RNA ladder (Invitrogen), **(B–D)** aRNA after one round of amplification. **(E–G)** aRNA after two rounds of amplification.

2. The importance of quantitative RT-PCR cannot be overstated. Quantitative RT-PCR (*see* **Chapter 18**) is used to assay the amount of RNA extracted from the laser captured tissue samples, even single cells, before T7 amplification. It is also used to monitor the T7 amplification and in the final validation of microarray data. As the amplified aRNA is biased towards the 3′-end of the mRNA sequence, it is advisable to choose a PCR amplicon that is close to the 3′-end. For neuronal tissue, we typically use neuron specific enolase as the PCR template.

3. For single-cell analysis, the final amount of aRNA will be less than a microgram. Hence, quantification of the aRNA by reading OD_{260} in a spectrophotometer or agarose gel analysis is not practical. Instead, the entire product is labeled and hybridized. For microarray analysis, there are different array platforms and several different options for labeling the hybridization target. The aRNA produced may be

labeled during transcription; alternatively, cDNA may be synthesized from the aRNA and labeled during synthesis. Labels may be radioactive, fluorescent, or tags (such as biotin) to which the reporter moiety is attached either prior or after hybridization. Our protocol synthesizes a Cy3-labeled cDNA from the final aRNA.

References

1. Luo, L., Salunga, R. C., Guo, H., et al. (1999) Gene expression profiles of laser-captured adjacent neuronal subtypes. *Nat. Med.* **5,** 117–122.
2. Eberwine, J., Yeh, H., Miyashiro, K., et al. (1992) Analysis of gene expression in single live neurons. *Proc. Natl. Acad. Sci. USA* **89,** 3010–3014.
3. Dell, D., Raghupathi, R., Crino, P. B., et al. (1998) Amplification of mRNAs from single, fixed, TUNEL-positive cells. *Biotechniques* **25,** 566–568, 570.
4. Nair, S. M., Werkman, T. R., Craig, J., et al. (1998) Corticosteroid regulation of ion channel conductances and mRNA levels in individual hippocampal CA1 neurons. *J. Neurosci.* **18,** 2685–2696.
5. Brooks-Kayal, A. R., Jin, H., Price, M., and Dichter, M. A. (1998) Developmental expression of GABA(A) receptor subunit mRNAs in individual hippocampal neurons in vitro and in vivo. *J. Neurochem.* **70,** 1017–1028.
6. Wang, E., Miller, L. D., Ohnmacht, G. A., et al. (2000) High-fidelity mRNA amplification for gene profiling. *Nat. Biotechnol.* **18,** 457–459.
7. Baugh, L. R., Hill, A. A., Brown, E. L., and Hunter, C. P. (2001) Quantitative analysis of mRNA amplification by in vitro transcription. *Nucleic Acids Res.* **29,** E29.
8. Van Gelder, R. N., von Zastrow, M. E., Yool, A., et al. (1990) Amplified RNA synthesized from limited quantities of heterogeneous cDNA. *Proc. Natl. Acad. Sci. USA* **87,** 1663–1667.

18

Semi-Quantitative Real-Time PCR for Pain Research

Hong Qing Guo and Sandra R. Chaplan

Summary

In this chapter we cover what we have found to be a "best practice" for real-time polymerase chain reaction (PCR) for relative mRNA quantification. We describe our techniques for tissue-sample collection and freezing, sample handling for quick and reproducible extraction of total RNA, first strand cDNA synthesis, real-time PCR amplification, and template dilution and storage for PCR. We offer our insights on intron-spanning primer design for genes (when applicable), effective primer selection vs reaction optimization, and relative quantification and sample normalization using housekeeping genes. Comments are also provided on the choice of PCR reagents including fluorescent probes, prevention of PCR "carry over," and on the practical aspects of real-time PCR theory and interpretation.

Key Words: RNA extraction; first-strand cDNA synthesis; polymerase chain reaction (PCR), semi-quantitative PCR; relative PCR; dorsal root ganglia; brain; spinal cord; SYBR® Green I; intron-spanning primers; cycle threshold; primer efficiency; housekeeping gene.

1. Introduction

The polymerase chain reaction (PCR) has dramatically changed the ability to study gene regulation in small tissue samples. Many different applications of PCR have been devised since the original description of the technique *(1–3)*. Real-time PCR in particular has developed into a popular research tool over the past decade since it was first pioneered by Higuchi and co-workers *(4)*. The advantage of real-time PCR over conventional "end-product" PCR is that it permits the analysis of the amount of product generated at each stage of progress of the reaction. The log-linear phase of the amplification can be identified readily. During this reaction phase, in a well-optimized reaction, the quantity of product is not subject to rate-limiting factors such as exhaustion of nucleotides or enzyme, and can be shown to bear a meaningful relationship to

From: *Methods in Molecular Medicine, Vol. 99: Pain Research: Methods and Protocols*
Edited by: Z. D. Luo © Humana Press Inc., Totowa, NJ

the amount of starting template. The efficiency of the reaction can be characterized as well. In end-point PCR, however, the amount of final product is likely to represent the plateau phase of the amplification reaction, the efficiency of the reaction cannot be judged without the use of additional special techniques, and the relationship between the starting quantity and the final amount of product is unknown.

In comparison studies, it is usually of greater interest to measure differences between treatments (relative quantification or semi-quantitative PCR) rather than to perform absolute quantitation of mRNA copy numbers (quantitative PCR). This chapter gives a simple approach to tissue collection, RNA extraction, and real-time semi-quantitative PCR comparisons of limited numbers of gene products using methodology we have successfully applied to several rodent preclinical neuroscience models *(5,6)*.

2. Materials

1. Dry ice.
2. Isopropanol 95%, sufficient quantity to make a dry ice slurry bath large enough to accommodate multiple cryomolds; add dry ice, let stand several minutes until fully chilled.
3. Suggested: vinyl specimen molds, e.g., Tissue-Tek® disposable cryomolds® (Cat. no. 4557, 25 × 20 × 5 mm, Sakura Finetek USA Inc., Torrance, CA) in which to place samples for freezing.
4. Water baths equilibrated at: 42°C, 37°C, 70°C (or 95°C).
5. Wet ice.
6. RNase-free microcentrifuge tubes; prefozen for tissue collection.
7. RNase-free filter (aerosol-resistant) pipet tips.
8. BioPulverizer (Cat. no. 59014H, BioSpec Products, Inc., Bartlesville, OK; or Cat. no. 141287, Research Products International, Corp., Mt. Prospect, IL); chilled on dry ice.
9. Small spatula; chilled on dry ice.
10. Ultrasonic processor (TEKMAR 130PB, Mason, OH or Cat. no. 15 338 53, Fisher Scientific. Pittsburgh, PA).
11. Vortexer.
12. Microcentrifuge.
13. (Optional) Vacuum manifold-QIAvac 24 (Cat. no. 19403, Qiagen, Valencia CA), and vacuum source.
14. Molecular biology grade RNase-free water.
15. WD-40.
16. Ethanol 95%.
17. β-Mercaptoethanol (Cat. no. M-3148, Sigma, St. Louis, MO); protect from light; store at room temperature.
18. Ethanol 70% (in molecular biology-grade RNase-free water).

19. RNeasy® mini-kit (Qiagen, Cat. no. 74104), containing the following buffers in addition to mini-spin columns and collection tubes; all may be stored at room temperature. Buffer RLT requires the addition of β-mercaptoethanol immediately prior to use (included in kit):

   a. Buffer RLT: contains guanidine isothiocyanate (GITC): harmful if ingested; incompatible with acids (contact releases very toxic gas); follow manufacturer's suggestions when handling.
   b. Buffer RW1: 95% ethanol must be added by user before use.
   c. Buffer RPE.

20. (Optional) Ultraviolet (UV) Spectrophotometer with microcuvette.
21. Oligo d(T)$_{12-18}$ 0.5 μg/μL (Cat. no. 277610-01, Amersham Biosciences, Piscataway, NJ) ; store at –20°C.
22. SuperScript™ II reverse transcriptase (Cat. no. 18064-014, Invitrogen, Carlsbad, CA); store at –20°C.
23. RNase Block Ribonuclease inhibitor (Cat. no. 300151, Stratagene, La Jolla, CA); store at –20°C.
24. dATP, dTTP, dCTP, dGTP at 100 mM (Cat. no. 27-2035-01, Amersham Biosciences, Piscataway, NJ); prepare as a 10 mM solution of dNTPs in RNase-free water; store at –20°C.
25. RNase H (Cat. no. 18021-071, Invitrogen); store at –20°C.
26. Poly-inosinic acid (Cat. no. P4154, Sigma, St. Louis, MO), 13.3 μg/mL solution in RNase-free water; store at –20°C
27. Genomic DNA (appropriate species); store at –20°C.
28. Gene-specific forward and reverse primers, diluted to 100 μM in RNase-free water; store at –20°C.
29. 2X *Taq* PCR Master Mix (Cat. no. 201445, Qiagen). Exact contents of the mix are proprietary, but include:

   a. *Taq* polymerase.
   b. dNTPs (200 μM final concentration of each dNTP).
   c. PCR buffer.
   d. MgCl$_2$ (1.5 mM final concentration).

30. TaqStart™ Antibody (Cat. no. 5400-1, Clontech, Palo Alto, CA); store at –20°C.
31. SYBR® Green I (Cat. no. S-7563, Molecular Probes, Eugene, OR), diluted 1:2000 in water (*see* **Note 1**); protect from light; store at –20°C.
32. Fluorescein (Cat. no. 170-8780, Bio-Rad, Hercules, CA); diluted to 500 nM in water (*see* **Note 1**); protect from light, store at room temperature.

3. Methods

3.1. General Considerations for RNA and PCR Work

RNA is highly vulnerable to degradation and must be handled with great care. Samples must be kept frozen at –80°C until use, and should be kept on ice after thawing. Gloves must be worn at all times, and changed frequently.

All labware that comes into contact with RNA must be RNase-free. Use only filter (aerosol-resistant) pipets, and keep samples securely capped whenever possible. Practice caution in the handling of any RNase used as a reagent. Designate a set of RNase-free laboratory equipment, including pipettors. In addition, it is critical to avoid contaminating RNA samples or laboratory equipment with amplified PCR products because this will lead to spurious results (false-positives); most laboratories designate one set of equipment for pre-PCR (RNA or template) work, and a separate set for post-PCR work.

3.2. RNA Extraction

Tissue specimens to be compared for pain work are generally very small and precious, and genes of interest may be quite rare. Techniques that maximize both the yield and the quality of the RNA are therefore extremely important.

3.2.1. Tissue Collection

The extraction protocol that follows is designed for samples up to 15 mg apiece (*see* below). Tissues should be harvested as quickly as possible, using clean instruments, and flash-frozen immediately. If removal of intravascular contents is desired, intracardiac perfusion with RNase-free buffer should be performed prior to tissue collection. Several options for flash-freezing exist. Liquid nitrogen, although the criterion standard, is not always convenient, and provided that samples are not very large, as an alternative we suggest floating them, e.g., in a small disposable mold, on a slurry of isopropanol and dry ice. For very small tissue samples, such as dorsal root ganglia (DRGs), freezing may be rapid enough if placed directly on dry ice alone. For these tiny samples, we recommend placing the fully frozen tissue in a labeled, prefrozen cryotube; otherwise, the tissue will freeze fast to the tube wall, and will be annoyingly hard to remove when needed. Tissues must be stored at $-80°$ until RNA extraction is performed.

3.2.2. Tissue Homogenization

We have found that complete solubilization of tissues in the extraction (lysis) buffer is critical to achieve maximal RNA recovery. Our routine practice is to extract total RNA using the RNeasy® kit because the procedure is convenient and fast, does not require phenol, does not call for nucleic acid precipitation (which may reduce yield), results in little DNA contamination, and gives reproducible recovery. This kit will handle samples up to 15 mg tissue with the buffer volumes described herein, or up to 30 mg tissue with increased buffer volumes; for further information or use with tissue cultures, the manufacturer's instructions should be consulted. For small tissues such as DRG and portions of spinal cord, we have found the most effective solubilization is achieved by first pulverizing the frozen tissue, then sonicating the fragments in the lysis buffer provided in the RNeasy® kit (Buffer RLT). Sonication is preferable to a micro-tissue grinder, which can retain small bits of tissue and lead to cross-contamination.

1. To pulverize these small samples, we recommend the BioPulverizer.
2. Apply a very light film of WD-40 (silicone lubricant) to the faces of the pulverizer to create a nonstick coating and wipe it off well.
3. Thoroughly prechill both pulverizer plates and a small clean spatula on dry ice. Keep samples on dry ice while assembling for processing.
4. Pre-aliquot 300 µL of the Buffer RLT (containing 10 µL/mL β-mercaptoethanol) into each labeled tube destined to receive pulverized sample.
5. Working quickly, place each deeply frozen sample on the pulverizer, smash one or more times until the tissue is reduced to a pancake of fine granules, use the spatula to scrape the tissue particles immediately into the Buffer RLT, and vortex vigorously. Once tissues are dispersed in this solution, or in any comparable lysis buffer that contains GITC, RNA is substantially protected from degradation. Clean the pulverizer between samples disposable, lint-free with a wipe. Place pulverizer on dry ice between samples to keep metal plates fully chilled.
6. To sonicate, we use an ultrasonic processor with a micro-probe tip, which works well with both 1.5-mL and 15-mL tubes. Adjust to a pulse level that does not cause heating, splashing, or foaming of the sample, and pulse intermittently until the sample is fully dispersed, usually about 5–6 s.

When fully sonicated, the sample should appear to be a turbid solution that does not contain visible particles. Wipe the sonicator tip and rinse generously in between samples with RNase-free water. Equipment may be definitively cleaned after use (once at room temperature) with a 10% solution of household bleach followed by copious rinsing in RNase-free water.

3.2.3. RNA Extraction

To date, no extraction technique gives complete freedom from contaminating genomic DNA. If isolation of mRNA is necessary, a number of kits are available that enable extraction of poly-A tailed mRNA using, e.g., magnetized beads. The PolyATract® mRNA isolation system (Promega, Cat. no. Z5300) is one that we have used successfully, combined with the aforementioned tissue homogenization technique; mRNA extraction will not be described in this chapter, but the manufacturers' instructions with these kits are very simple to follow.

As mentioned earlier, our routine practice is to extract total RNA using the RNeasy® kit, and genomic DNA contamination is generally not problematic. Although DNase treatment of samples is often recommended elsewhere in the literature, in our hands this has not sufficiently improved sample purity to warrant the additional steps. We follow the manufacturer's instructions for the RNeasy® extraction procedure using either the spin or vacuum column protocol; the vacuum protocol is briefly summarized below.

1. Add 1 volume 70% ethanol (300 µL) to lysate, mix well, do not centrifuge.
2. Apply the sample to an RNeasy® minicolumn; aspirate.
3. Add 700 µL Buffer RW1 to the column, aspirate.
4. Add 500 µL Buffer RPE to the column; aspirate.
5. Repeat addition of 500 µL Buffer RPE; aspirate thoroughly to dry column.
6. Place RNeasy® column in a clean collection tube; pipet 50 µL RNase-free water directly onto membrane; let stand 1 min, then spin in microcentrifuge 1 min at full speed to elute RNA into collection tube.

Upon completion of the manufacturer's protocol for the RNeasy kit, we aliquot the RNA as desired, then store at –80°C until use. The protocol usually yields about 3 µg of total RNA per rat DRG in a volume of about 50 µL, or approx 1 µg/mg tissue. Yields are ordinarily somewhat lower for whole spinal cord tissue, and somewhat higher for total brain.

3.2.4. RNA Quantification

If sample sizes permit, RNA recovery can be measured by spectrophotometry; however, a microcuvette or specially designed device is usually necessary to measure the small amounts in question. We use either the Beckman DU 530 spectrophotometer with a 50 µL microcell accessory (accurate down to an OD of .05 corresponding to 100 µg/mL undiluted total RNA with a dilution factor of 50) or the RNA 6000 Nano Lab Chip® kit (Agilent Technologies, 5065-4476), which can measure down to 20 ng total RNA in a 5 µL volume with accuracy, and in addition allows inspection of total RNA quality.

3.3. First-Strand cDNA Synthesis

We perform first-strand cDNA synthesis with a 10 µL aliquot (about 0.5 µg RNA for rat DRG) of the total RNA generated above, according to the following recipe.

1. Add 0.5 µg oligo d(T)$_{12–18}$ (1 µL) primer to 10 µL of total RNA.
2. Incubate at 70°C for 10 min.
3. While the above reaction is incubating, prepare a 10 mM mixture of dNTPs in RNase free water and keep on ice. May be frozen and re-used (*see* **Note 2**).
4. Prepare the following master mix (allow extra for pipetting losses).

   Per reaction:

   a. 4 µL 5X First-strand buffer (Invitrogen).
   b. 2 µL 0.1 mM dithiothreitol (DTT) (Invitrogen).
   c. 1 µL 10 mM dNTPs.
   d. 40 U RNase block.
   e. 1 µL SuperScript™ II reverse transcriptase.
5. Chill the total RNA/oligod(T) reaction on ice for 1 min.

6. Spin the tubes briefly.
7. Add 9 µL of the above master mix to each reaction.
8. Incubate at 42°C for at least 30 min and up to 2 h.
9. Add 1 µL of RNase H to each reaction.
10. Incubate at 37°C for 30 min.
11. Inactivate the enzymes at 95°C for 2 min, or 70°C for 10 min.
12. Spin tubes briefly.
13. Keep reaction on ice.

While this standard recipe calls for oligo d(T) primer, which permits subsequent amplification of any polyadenylated mRNA, specific sequences of interest can be more robustly amplified using gene-specific primers designed to hybridize at 42°C. If the mRNA of interest is rare, gene-specific primers are likely to boost its detection. One or more gene-specific primers may be used in combination with the oligo d(T) primer.

3.4. Real-Time PCR (see Note 3)

3.4.1. Template Pre-Treatment

The cDNA samples generated above can be stored at –20°C. For use in real-time PCR reactions, we recommend diluting them 4× with water containing poly-inosinic acid [poly(I)] to a final concentration of 10 ng poly(I)/µL, i.e., to a 20 µL cDNA reaction, add 60 µL water containing 13.3 ng/µL of poly(I). The poly(I) serves as a carrier and prevents losses of rare genes owing to sticking to plasticware. Dilution of the cDNA improves the chemistry of subsequent PCR reactions in real-time thermal cyclers, and usually provides sufficient dilution of common housekeeping genes to bring them into a good working range for real-time PCR detection.

3.4.2. Designing Intron-Spanning Primers

Whenever possible, we design PCR primers to hybridize with sequences that lie on different exons, separated in the genomic sequence by one or more large introns, or to lie across a splice junction such that they will only hybridize with the uninterrupted cDNA sequence. Contaminating genomic DNA sequences will thus be too long to amplify under the reaction conditions, and the signal will be specifically from cDNA. If genes do not contain an intron but are abundant, such as housekeeping genes, the amount of genomic contamination is usually slight enough to disregard (several orders of magnitude below cDNA amount). The amount of genomic contamination can be estimated by using a mock cDNA synthesis reaction, i.e., all reagents included in the reaction except reverse transcriptase. Genomic DNA contamination is more likely to be problematic for rare, intronless genes, and one of two possible strategies is suggested to address this scenario: either correction for genomic contamination using parallel non-RT samples, or purification of mRNA.

The online availability of the human genome sequence has made designing intron-spanning primers much easier. The genomic structure of most genes is not specifically published. However, the sites of intron splicing can usually be quickly deduced by comparison of the human cDNA sequence to the human genome. This simply involves BLAST searching the cDNA sequence of interest against either the draft or the curated genome sequence, and noting the size and location of the discontinuities in the genomic alignment compared to the cDNA. Most of these discontinuities represent areas where introns are excised. In some cases, the length of the gaps in the cDNA and the genomic sequence will match; these gaps do not represent introns but areas of repetitive sequence that were not aligned. Occasionally a large gap will indicate the end of one genomic contig and the start of another. Conservation of sequences between humans and, e.g., rodents is such that it is usually possible to deduce the location of introns in the rodent sequence based on the intron-splicing sites in the human ortholog simply by performing an alignment of the two genes. In all cases we have examined so far, the introns correspond. High-sequence homology between gene family members on one or both sides of the intron-splicing junction may be observed; however, we have had little trouble designing primers that distinguish between closely related genes. Standard considerations for primer design (e.g., primer length, G + C content, etc.) should be respected.

3.4.3. Primer Optimization

For each new gene to be assayed, we recommend ordering at least three forward and three reverse primers to be tested in all possible combinations. Primers that may have worked well in conventional end-point PCR may not be the most efficient for the chemistry of real-time PCR and should be re-evaluated. Primer efficiency varies greatly, and cannot be predicted "in silico." Bad primers will either fail to amplify, give nonspecific products (affectionately known as "ampli-schmutz" [7] or "primer dimer"), amplify more slowly, or give broad melting curves/gel bands indicating multiple products. It is much more practical to select a selective, highly efficient pair of primers that work well under standard reaction conditions than to attempt to optimize a substandard primer pair by varying reaction conditions. Primers should be tested in all combinations against cDNA, genomic DNA (if intron-spanning), and no-template control. Keep looking for a primer pair that gives a clean melting curve with a single sharp peak, and no product in the genomic DNA or control reactions. Do not despair if the first three primer pairs fail to provide an optimal result; do consider whether the stretch of sequence to be amplified might have strong secondary structure, and whether a higher annealing temperature (and higher primer melting temperature [T_m]) might help. During primer assessment, run the product on a gel at least once to verify that the size is as expected; size cannot be deduced from a melting curve. In rare cases, double peaks in the melting curve can be seen despite single bands when run on a gel; this may reflect strong secondary structure in the amplicon. Choose the primer pair that gives the most efficient reaction, exemplified by both lower cycle threshold and optimal amplification (*see* **Note 6**). Efficiency can be improved by varying the annealing temperature and Mg^{2+} concentrations. It is not usually necessary to experiment widely with reaction conditions. Always dilute primers in water.

3.4.4. Standard Curve and Internal Control

For relative quantification, it suffices to use a cDNA source to generate the standard curve, as long as the gene of interest is sufficiently abundant to amplify from serially diluted samples. To calculate copy numbers, however, the amplicon must be cloned into a vector in order to generate a standard curve based on amplification of a dilution series (six to eight dilutions are recommended) of known copy numbers of the plasmid. A more detailed discussion of absolute copy number detection is beyond the scope of this essay, and can be found in the Applied Biosystems "User's Bulletin no. 2" at the following url: http://docs.appliedbiosystems.com/pebiodocs/04303859.pdf

For relative quantitation, because sample extraction, reverse transcription efficiency, and loading all introduce error, it is necessary to choose a housekeeping gene as an internal control against which to normalize the gene of interest. We use cyclophilin A (peptidylprolyl isomerase A) for this purpose. Cyclophilin A, although it has introns, does have the disadvantage of possessing multiple pseudogenes; therefore, genomic DNA contamination amplifies as well. However, the mRNA is sufficiently abundant that the contaminant amplification, following the aforementioned extraction procedure, is three orders of magnitude below the specific signal, which is acceptable. Regulation of cyclophilin A appears not to occur in brain, DRG, or spinal cord after a variety of interventions (*8–10*). Other putative housekeeping genes may, however, be regulated; if this is not known prior to your preparation, assessment is advised.

3.4.5. Setting Up the PCR Reaction (see **Note 4**)

The following is a recipe for an fairly inexpensive home brew for a 50 µL reaction in the iCycler IQ™ (Bio-Rad Laboratories Inc.)

Prepare enough of the following two master mixes to allow for the number of reactions you plan to do, plus sufficient extra to cover for pipetting losses.

Per reaction:

1. 25 μL 2X *Taq* PCR Master Mix.
2. Add 0.2 μL TaqStart™ Antibody.
3. Let this first mixture stand for 5 min to allow *Taq* antibody to bind to and inactivate *Taq* polymerase until released by the first heating cycle during PCR (hot-start technique).
4. In the meantime, prepare the second master mix in a separate tube as follows:

    Per reaction:

    a. 18.55 μL water (*see* **Note 1**).
    b. 0.125 μL forward primer, 100 μ*M*
    c. 0.125 μL reverse primer, 100 μ*M*
    d. 2 μL 1:2000 diluted SYBR® Green (*see* **Note 5**). (Suggested: 2 μL 500 n*M* fluorescein for final concentration of 20 n*M;* if used, reduce water to 16.55 μL.)
    e. 2 μL 50 m*M* MgCl$_2$.
    f. 2 μL cDNA template (may be increased to 5 μL if desired, reducing water accordingly, to allow for more convenient aliquotting using a repeating pipetor). (Note that templates may be omitted from the master mix and individually aliquoted into reactions as appropriate.)
5. Add 24.8 μL of the second master mix to each PCR master mix/Taq antibody well (or tube).
6. Spin the reaction plate (or tubes) briefly.
7. Program the thermal cycler according to the manufacturer's instructions to include a 2-min initial denaturation step to activate the hot-start, followed by a standard protocol consisting of 40 cycles of PCR, with collection of real-time data during the extension phase (*see* **Note 6**). We use a three-step protocol (denaturation/annealing/extension), but good results should be obtainable using the faster two-step protocol as well.
8. Program a melting curve procedure to follow the completion of the PCR (*see* **Note 7**).
9. Begin thermal cycling protocol.

If fluorescein is omitted, initialization of the iCycler is sometimes unsuccessful using this recipe (without fluorescein) owing to the presence of insufficient background fluorescence to collect baseline "well factors." This problem is easily circumvented by adding 20 n*M* final concentration of fluorescein to the reaction as suggested; we use this routinely without interference with the amplification or signal detection. Commercially available SYBR® Green I premixes in general similarly include an additional fluorophore for this purpose.

3.4.6. A Simple Method for Normalizing Samples

At the completion of the amplification, data may be exported to an Excel spreadsheet for further analysis. In order to perform statistical analysis, or for graphic display, results will need to be normalized to the housekeeping gene. Many methods of normalization of results can be devised. One simple approach is to assume that the sample showing the largest yield of housekeeping gene represents optimum recovery of RNA from the experimental tissue, and arbitrarily designate this "calibrator" sample as corresponding to 100% recovery, or a fractional recovery of 1. The relative recovery of other housekeeping gene samples is then compared to the calibrator by dividing all housekeeping gene sample starting copy number values by the copy number of the calibrator. Use this fractional recovery value (between 0 and 1) to normalize the copy numbers of the respective paired samples of the gene of interest, by dividing each test sample by the fractional recovery of the housekeeping gene.

More detailed discussion of the mathematics of sample analysis can be found in user bulletin no. 2 courtesy of Applied Biosystems, at the following url: http://docs.appliedbiosystems.com/pebiodocs/04303859.pdf

4. Notes

1. The water used for PCR reactions does not have to be RNase-free. However, the quality of the water is very important.
2. dNTPs are among the more labile components of the RT-PCR cocktails, and if reactions that were previously successful suddenly start to fail, often the cause is degraded dNTPs.
3. In general, we have found it desirable to assay six to eight different samples per treatment per run in order to achieve statistical significance. A minimum experiment (testing one target gene and a housekeeping gene) thus requires at least six test samples on each for control and experimental conditions, serial dilutions for a standard curve for each gene, and suitable negative controls. Many investigators prefer to run duplicates for each sample. It can therefore easily be seen that the convenience of 96-well format is appreciated. Among models offering plate formats, we have used the BioRad iCycler IQ™ with satisfaction, and the ABI Prism® is also suitable for this purpose. Other real-time PCR machines based on the individual tube format do offer accelerated amplification times such as the LightCycler® (Roche) and the Smart Cycler® (Cepheid). In addition, the Smart Cycler® offers the flexibility of being able to vary amplification protocols for each well. The Smart Cycler® and the LightCycler® are particularly useful for speed of turnaround, selection of primer pairs, and optimization of cycling conditions. The ergonomic drawbacks of handling large numbers of small tubes are factors to consider, however.
4. We have had success with a variety of PCR master mix kits, as well as home recipes. Be advised however that not all commercial PCR master mix kits will work in all real-time PCR machines (owing to different reaction tubes and varying additives in each mix.). Using the Bio-Rad iCycler IQ, we recommend the Applied Biosystems SYBR Green PCR master mix (Cat. no. 4309155), the IQ™ SYBR Green Supermix (Bio-Rad, Cat. no. 170-8880), Qiagen 2X Taq PCR Master mix (requires the addition of SYBR Green). The varying denaturation times required to activate these

mixes must be taken into consideration when programming the initial thermal cycle. Many commercial premixes use the "UNG" technique to prevent carry-over from previous PCR reactions. With this approach, dUTP is used in the nucleotide mix (dNTPs) instead of dTTP. The addition of uracil *N*-glycosylase (UNG) excises uracil residues, resulting in fragmentation of the product. However, this adds expense to the reaction kits, and may be unnecessary if the lab is careful to separate pre- and post-PCR areas as conventionally advised. Substitution of uracil for thymidine residues also prevents the convenient use of real-time PCR products for cloning.

5. Real-time PCR technology is based on the generation and detection of increasing sample fluorescence as amplification progresses. There are two basic reporter chemistries in all real-time PCR systems in which signal of the reporter increases in direct proportion to the amount of PCR product in the reaction. The more specific system uses a fluorescence-labeled hybridization probe for quantitation. The alternative system employs a DNA binding dye such as SYBR Green I.

   Probe-based systems are more specific, because probes are designed to hybridized fluoresce only when with the desired product; nonspecific products generate no signal. Probes are also suitable for multiplexing PCR reactions, because fluorescent dyes with different emission spectra may be attached to different probes. A probe-based system is advantageous in the case where an assay will be conducted repeatedly and the amount of available RNA is very small, because it enables simultaneous assaying of a housekeeping gene as a control for each test sample. The number of samples is also halved if the necessity of running duplicate preparations with housekeeping genes is eliminated, permitting, e.g., running duplicates for each test preparation for tighter quality control. Popular types of probes include TaqMan® and Molecular Beacons®, which both rely on Förster (fluorescence) resonance energy transfer (FRET). We have not opted for this approach because obtaining effective fluorescence-tagged probes can be very costly and time-consuming, and calls for the design of an additional high-efficiency oligonucleotide sequence over and above the forward and reverse primers.

   We rely exclusively on SYBR Green I, which fluoresces only when it binds to double-stranded DNA. The advantages of the SYBR Green system are that it is simple to use, less expensive, versatile, and enables rapid assay design for new targets. In addition, because multiple SYBR® Green molecules bind to each product molecule, this system provides more sensitive detection capability than a probe-based system, in which the stoichiometry of hybridization is only 1:1. We have had good results with amplicons around 100 bp and up to 400 bp using this system. The disadvantage is that SYBR Green will bind to any double-stranded DNA, which may result in an overestimation of the target concentration if the reaction conditions are not optimized. We have not found this to be a significant drawback, because we routinely select primers that give only specific product. Brightness of the signal also depends on the size of the amplicon; the longer the sequence, the more SYBR Green will bind.

6. Reaction progress is displayed as the graph of cycle number vs fluorescence. The cycle threshold (or crossing threshold) (C_T) is the cycle number at which the fluo-

rescence exceeds a designated threshold. The higher the starting template copy number, the earlier the reaction will enter the log-linear phase of amplification and result in fluorescence distinguishable from background. The threshold may be automatically chosen by current real-time cycler software, or may be manually selected. To permit background subtraction, samples should be run at a template concentration that results in a cycle threshold greater than 10.

When comparing genes, primers should be chosen that are of similar and satisfactory efficiency, as judged by their amplification reaction slopes, or the slopes of standard curves generated by amplification of a template dilution series. A perfectly efficient PCR amplification would in theory result in doubling of the product with every cycle. Efficiency of the actual reaction can be evaluated by comparing the slope of the amplification of a single standard sample (or of a standard curve) generated by a given primer pair to the slope of a perfectly efficient PCR reaction. A perfect reaction would be described by the function, $y = 2^x$, where y = copy number and x = number of cycles.[1] When represented on a semilog scale, with copy number on the y-axis and cycle number on the x-axis, the formula for this hypothetical reaction is thus $\log_{10} y = 0.301x + b$. If represented as a standard curve, with log (starting quantity) on the y-axis and cycle threshold on the x-axis, the relationship between template quantity and cycle threshold is inverse (the higher the initial quantity, the lower the cycle threshold), so the slope takes on a negative value $(-.301)$. Any reaction with less than perfect efficiency will have a slope less than the absolute value of this hypothetical perfect slope. If the axes are inverted, as they are in the representation on some real-time thermal cycler software, with cycle increments on the y-axis and log (quantity) on the x-axis, the slopes are the reciprocal of the foregoing (3.322 or -3.322), and larger absolute values indicate declining reaction efficiency.

7. The specificity of the product is evaluated at the end of the reaction by a melting curve. Temperature is ramped up or down past the melting point of the product, detected as the rate of change of fluorescence. Uniform products melt rapidly over a narrow temperature range, giving "sharp" melting peaks. The T_m of the product will depend on both the length and the base content, and is not well-predicted by readily available tools, but will be reproducible using the same reaction chemistry; however, it will vary if different PCR mixes are used. Once the T_m of a product is verified by comparing the product band size on a gel with the expected amplicon size, a particular T_m may be considered characteristic of the correct product.

References

1. Mullis, K. B. and Faloona, F. A. (1987) Specific synthesis of DNA in vitro via a polymerase-catalyzed chain reaction. *Methods Enzymol* **155**, 335–350.

---

[1] In actuality, the efficiency has some inherent limitations, and, due to the linear amplification of long products, is better described by $y = 2^x - 2x$; this is beyond the scope of this discussion, however.

2. Mullis, K., Faloona, F., Scharf, S., et al. (1986) Specific enzymatic amplification of DNA in vitro: the polymerase chain reaction. *Cold Spring Harb. Symp. Quant. Biol.* **51 Pt 1,** 263–273.
3. Saiki, R. K., Gelfand, D. H., Stoffel, S., et al. (1988) Primer-directed enzymatic amplification of DNA with a thermostable DNA polymerase. *Science* **239,** 487–491.
4. Higuchi, R., Dollinger, G., Walsh, P. S., and Griffith, R. (1992) Simultaneous amplification and detection of specific DNA sequences. *Biotechnology (NY)* **10,** 413–417.
5. Chaplan, S. R., Guo, H. Q., Lee, D. H., et al. (2003) Neuronal hyperpolarization-activated pacemaker channels drive neuropathic pain. *J. Neurosci.* **23,** 1169–1178.
6. Bonaventure, P., Guo, H., Tian, B., et al. (2002) Nuclei and subnuclei gene expression profiling in mammalian brain. *Brain Res.* **943,** 38–47.
7. Mullis, K. B., Ferre, F., and Gibbs, R. A. (eds.) (1994) *The Polymerase Chain Reaction.* Birkhauser, Boston.
8. Schmid, H., Cohen, C. D., Henger, A., et al. (2003) Validation of endogenous controls for gene expression analysis in microdissected human renal biopsies. *Kidney Int.* **64,** 356–360.
9. Semple-Rowland, S. L., Mahatme, A., Popovich, P. G., et al. (1995) Analysis of TGF-beta 1 gene expression in contused rat spinal cord using quantitative RT-PCR. *J. Neurotrauma* **12,** 1003–1014.
10. Harrison, D. C., Medhurst, A. D., Bond, B. C., et al. (2000) The use of quantitative RT-PCR to measure mRNA expression in a rat model of focal ischemia: caspase-3 as a case study. *Brain Res. Mol. Brain Res.* **75,** 143–149.

19

Functional Genomic Analysis in Pain Research Using Hybridization Arrays

Stephen J. Walker, Travis J. Worst, Willard M. Freeman, and Kent E. Vrana

Summary

Hybridization array technology makes it possible to compare global gene-expression patterns in any experimental context for which good-quality RNA can be generated. To date, DNA arrays have been used as a tool to compare functional genomic changes (differences in wholesale gene expression) in studies that cover an impressive variety of research disciplines including cancer, yeast genomics, and, more recently, neuroscience and behavior. The basic premise of the array experiment is that one interrogates a panel of probes (gene-specific cDNA fragments or gene-specific oligonucleotides that have been immobilized on a solid support) with RNAs (targets) from control and treated experimental samples that have been either radioactively or fluorescently labeled. Signal derived from either competitive (both samples on a single chip) or differential (one sample/one chip) hybridization is used to calculate relative gene expression. There are three widely used platforms available to perform array experiments (Affymetrix GeneChips, oligonucleotide arrays, and membrane-based cDNA arrays) and each platform offers advantages and limitations. The experimental description in this chapter explains, in detail, how to perform a hybridization array using the macroarray platform.

Key Words: Microarray; macroarray; hybridization; deoxyribonucleic acid (DNA); ribonucleic acid (RNA); oligonucleotides; gene expression; functional genomics; normalization.

1. Introduction

With the advent of hybridization array technology, it is now possible to compare global gene-expression patterns in any experimental context for which RNA can be generated. The basic premise of the array experiment is that one queries a panel of targets (gene-specific cDNA fragments or gene-specific oligonucleotides) that have been immobilized on a solid support (e.g., glass, nylon, or plastic; *see* **Fig. 1**). The arrays are hybridized with RNAs (targets) from

From: *Methods in Molecular Medicine, Vol. 99: Pain Research: Methods and Protocols*
Edited by: Z. D. Luo © Humana Press Inc., Totowa, NJ

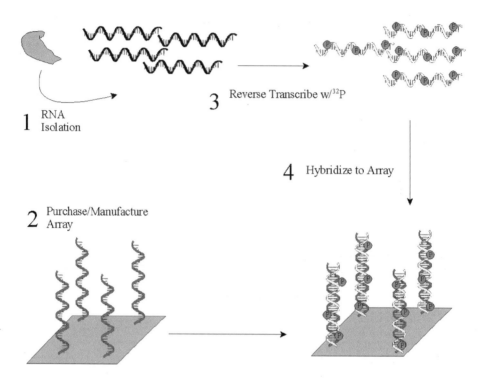

Fig. 1. Basic experimental design from tissue isolation to hybridization.

"control" and "treated" experimental samples that have been either radioactively or fluorescently labeled. The RNAs are labeled as complementary DNAs (cDNAs) or amplified antisense RNAs (aRNAs). The labeled probes either competitively hybridize to each particular target location *(spot)* on a single array (fluorescence-based assay; detection based on labeling the two RNA samples with different color fluorescent dyes), or the signal intensities from two distinct but identical arrays (radioactivity-based and fluorescence-based labeling) are compared at each spot to assess which genes are up- or downregulated.

Hybridization array technology has been used as a tool to compare functional genomic changes (differences in "wholesale" gene expression) under an impressive variety of experimental paradigms including cancer research, yeast genomics studies, and, more recently, neuroscience and behavior. A current review of the use of this technology *(1)*, specifically in the field of neuroscience, reports an exponential growth within the last decade in the number of articles published that contain the word "microarray" in the title (from less than 10 in 1994 to more than 750 in 2001). This is testament to the widespread applicability of this technology and to the growing popularity of arrays as a means to screen genes in a high-throughput fashion. This will certainly apply to the field of pain research as well, where techniques such as ribonuclease protection analysis (RPA) *(2)*, *in situ* hybridization *(2,3)*, and differential display *(4)* are already being employed to assess the expression of many genes. There are three major array platforms available for wide-spread use—the GeneChip®, the microarray, and the macroarray—and we offer a brief description of each.

The undisputed leader in the field of hybridization array technology is Affymetrix. In the mid-1990s they introduced the *GeneChip,* a glass wafer onto which thousands of gene-specific oligonucleotides are synthesized by a patented process known as photolithography. Experiments that involve the use of the Affymetix platform rely on labeling of two RNAs (one control and one treated) with subsequent hybridization to two distinct chips. The Affymetrix technology continues to be used widely and provides an excellent platform for high-throughput functional genomic analysis. It is now becoming more affordable to the standard academic laboratory, especially in light of the growing number of University Core Facilities that are set up to offer this platform.

A second platform that offers slightly less throughput per experiment is the microarray. Microarray, for the purposes here, will refer to glass slides onto which either gene-specific cDNAs or gene-specific oligonucleotides are deposited manually or by robot. Microarrays rely on labeling of two sets of RNAs (one control and one treated) with two different color fluorescent dyes, followed by hybridization of the resulting cDNAs on the same chip. Generally, the RNAs are labeled by converting to cDNAs by reverse transcription in the presence of fluorescent precursor nucleotides (tagged with Cy3 and Cy5 dyes). The microarray industry grew out of a need to provide an alternative platform to the (initially) cost-prohibitive Affymetrix product, at a level of quality and price that academic labs could justify. There are currently dozens of companies offering microarrays, representing large gene sets from numerous species.

Finally, there is the macroarray, which for our purposes here, refers to any nylon membrane or plastic surface onto which is spotted hundreds to thousands of gene-specific cDNAs or oligonucleotides. The macroarray experiment requires that the two populations of RNA be radioactivity-labeled and then used to query two identical, but separate, membranes. This is an obvious disadvantage of the macroarray platform because the use of two different membranes has great potential to introduce error. Macroarrays do, however, afford a robust fold-change sensitivity detection (we can detect as low as 50% change in gene expression in repeat experiments), a feature that can be very advantageous, especially when looking for differential gene expression in brain tissue where the changes are often quite modest. The experimental description that follows explains, in detail, how to perform a hybridization array using the macroarray platform. For a more complete review of these platforms, *see* Freeman et al. *(5)*.

2. Materials

2.1. Reagents

1. Source of RNA (tissue, cell culture, etc.).
2. Liquid nitrogen.
3. RNA extraction reagent (e.g., TRI Reagent; Molecular Research Center, Inc., Cincinnati, OH; Trizol, Gibco, Carlsbad, CA).
4. Chloroform.
5. Isopropanol.
6. 75% ethanol.
7. Nuclease-free water or diethlypyrocarbonate (DEPC)-treated water.
8. Agarose (for denaturing nucleic acid gels).
9. MOPS buffer.
10. TE buffer: 10 mM Tris-HCl, pH 8.0, 1 mM ethylenediamine tetraacetic acid (EDTA), pH 8.0.
11. Ethidium bromide.
12. Formamide.
13. Formaldehyde.
14. cDNA labeling kit (Clontech Laboratories; Palo Alto, CA).
15. α-^{32}P-dATP (3,000 Ci/mmol, 10 µCi/µL; ICN).
16. Prehybridization and hybridization solutions (Express Hyb; Clontech).
17. Salmon sperm DNA.
18. 20X SSC (standard saline citrate) stock solution.
19. Denaturation buffer: 1.0 M NaOH, 10.0 mM EDTA.
20. Neutralization buffer: 1.0 M NaOH, pH 7.0; 27.6 g NaH$_2$PO$_4$ + 180 mL H$_2$O, pH to 7.0 using 10 N NaOH and the qs to 200 mL with H$_2$O.
21. Wash buffer 1: 2X SSC with 1% SDS.
22. Wash buffer 2: 0.1X SSC with 0.5% SDS.
23. Wash buffer 3: 2X SSC.

2.2. Equipment and Supplies

1. Stainless-steel mortar and pestle.
2. Cryovials.
3. Sonicator.
4. Agarose gel apparatus and power supply.
5. Light box (with UV lamp).
6. Spectrophotometer (with UV lamp).
7. Gel documentation/image capture camera (UVP ImageStore 7500, UVP, Upland, CA).
8. Arrays (nylon-based cDNA macroarrays; Atlas Arrays, Clontech Laboratories, Palo Alto, CA).

9. Thermocycler.
10. Size-exclusion columns (Chroma Spin-200 DEPC-water column; Clontech).
11. Sigmacote (Sigma Chemical Co.).
12. Hybridization bottles.
13. Hybridization oven.
14. Water bath(s).
15. Saran wrap.
16. Laminate plastic.
17. Bag sealer.
18. Phosphorimaging cassette.
19. Phosphorimager.

2.3. Software

1. RNA quantification (e.g., TINA, Raytest, Wilmington, NC; for providing analysis and quantification of RNA. The Agilent Bioanalyzer 2100 performs a similar function with less material).
2. Array image capture (Photoshop, Adobe, San Jose, CA).
3. Array analysis (AtlasImage 2.01).

3. Methods

The methods outlined in this section describe a typical experiment using the macroarray format and include a brief discussion of post-hoc analysis following the generation of results from the array experiment. This format is chosen for discussion because the authors have extensive experience with these methods, and because the equipment, supplies, and expertise needed to perform this type of array experiment are readily available to most laboratories that do molecular biology work (especially, e.g., Northern blots). With this platform, an array consists of hundreds to thousands of unique cDNAs (200–500 base pairs in length) spotted onto nylon; or, alternatively, thousands of oligonucleotides, representing a nonredundant unique gene set, spotted onto plastic. Because radioactivity is used for the labeling step, each array "experiment" consists of two separate, but identical, membranes. This unitary ($n = 1$) array experiment is then replicated twice in order to assess variability and then followed by an appropriate *post hoc* experimental series such a quantitative reverse transcription polymerase chain reaction (RT-PCR) and/or quantitative Western-blot analysis to confirm changes.

3.1. Tissue Selection

Sample collection is a basic element of experimental design for many molecular biological experiments, but it is worth reiterating. In the field of neuroscience, it is often imperative to use dissected tissue from treated and control animals. Therefore, it is often unavoidable that the samples will contain multiple cell types. In complex samples such as brain tissue, there is routinely a heterogeneous cell population. Therefore, observed changes may represent a change in one cell type or multiple cell types. Similarly, smaller changes occurring in only one type of cell may be hidden if the expression of this gene in other cell types is unchanged. Thus, researchers must be mindful of this heterogeneous population when drawing conclusions. A promising technological solution is laser-capture microdissection, which allows very small and identified cellular populations to be dissected.

3.2. RNA Isolation

The single most important factor in the ability to generate quality results from an array experiment is the preparation and use of high-quality RNA (*see* **Note 1**). Total RNA (or mRNA) can be reliably and repeatedly generated from any number of biological samples including whole blood, other tissues (e.g., brain, liver), and from cells in culture. In this section we discuss the isolation and assay of total RNA from brain tissue.

3.2.1. Tissue Dissection and Storage

The most reliable preparations of RNA come from tissue samples that have been rapidly dissected and "flash-frozen" in liquid nitrogen. For retrieving tissue, because brain regions are not absolutely discrete, it is best to have the same individual perform the dissections on all samples for a given experiment (and any subsequent repeat experiments) to ensure relative uniformity in sample collection. Once the whole brain has been removed from an animal's skull, and working as rapidly as possible, individual brain regions are dissected, immediately put into prelabeled and weighed tubes, tissue weights are determined, and the samples dropped into liquid nitrogen or buried in crushed dry ice. Tissue collected and frozen in this fashion can then be stored at –80°C for long periods of time.

3.2.2. Creating a Tissue Powder

Tissue that has been previously dissected and stored frozen at –80°C can be readied for array and post-hoc analysis by the creation of a frozen tissue powder. This procedure is especially useful in that a homogenous powder is formed that can be aliquoted for subsequent RNA or protein purification. First, a stainless-steel mortar and pestle is chilled on dry ice. Frozen tissue is transferred, without thawing, into the mortar and covered with liquid nitrogen. The sample is then ground to a fine powder (keeping it covered with liquid nitrogen at all times). The frozen powder at the bottom of the bowl is then retrieved with a (prechilled) stainless-steel spatula and quickly deposited into prechilled, preweighed cryovials. We routinely place half of the tissue into each of two tubes, one to be used for RNA extraction, the other for protein preparation. The tubes, containing tissue, are quickly reweighed (without thawing), returned to liquid nitrogen or dry ice, and stored at −80°C until further processing can be performed.

3.2.3. RNA Isolation

RNA is extracted from frozen tissue powder using a modification of the single-step method originally developed by Chomczynski and Sacchi *(6,7)*. There are a number of commercially available reagents; this laboratory routinely uses TriReagent®.

1. Sonicate tissue in TriReagent using 10 μL/mg tissue (40–80% sonicator power; 3 × 5 s with 20-s rest intervals).
2. Leave at room temperature for 5 min, then centrifuge at 12,000*g* for 15 min at 4°C.
3. Remove and use the aqueous layer (top portion).
4. Add 1/5 original TriReagent volume of chloroform ($CHCl_3$) and vortex.
5. Leave at room temperature for 5 min, then centrifuge at 12,000*g* for 15 min at 4°C.
6. Remove and use the aqueous layer (use organic layer for protein).
7. Add $^1/_2$ original TriReagent volume of isopropanol and vortex.
8. Let sit 5 min or more at room temperature.
9. Centrifuge at 12,000*g* for 15 min at 4°C.
10. Remove supernatant and save pellet.
11. Wash pellet with 1 volume (1 μL/μL TriReagent) of 75% EtOH.
12. Centrifuge at 12,000*g* for 15 min at 4°C.
13. Remove supernatant and dry pellet by inverting tube on a kimwipe for 5–10 min.
14. Resuspend pellet in DEPC H_2O.
15. Place in 55–60°C water bath for 10 min.
16. Store RNA at −80°C.

3.2.4. RNA Quality Assessment and Quantification

Quantity and relative quality of RNA can be determined spectrophotometrically by diluting an aliquot into TE buffered water (pH 8.0; unbuffered water can produce spurious results) and measuring the UV absorbance at 260 nm and 280 nm.

1. Thaw RNA samples on wet ice.
2. Analyze the samples at 260 nm and 280 nm and determine the ratio; ratio of 1.9–2.0 is ideal.
3. RNA concentration is determined by multiplying the absorbance at 260 nm by 40 μg/mL/OD_{260} and the dilution factor.
4. Resolve one μg of each RNA sample on a denaturing gel using denaturing solution.
5. Assess RNA quality; there must be minimal/no evidence of RNA degradation **(Fig. 2)**.

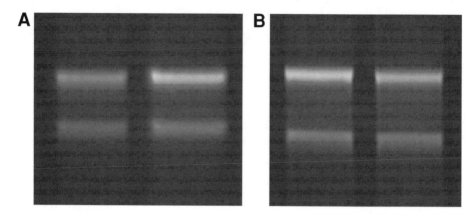

Fig. 2. RNA qualification. (**A**) Poor-quality RNA on the left, showing little difference in 18S and 28S band intensities, and broad bands, and smearing between bands.
Compare this with the lane on the right, noticing that the 28S intensity is approximately twice that of the 18S. It should be noted that many laboratories might consider
the RNA on the left to be acceptable, whereas this laboratory has had the greatest success using RNA of the quality on the right. (**B**) Good-quality total RNA showing the
18S band at half the intensity of the 28S band and sharp bands. In addition, these two
samples were loaded at approximately equal concentrations, which has been confirmed by the gel electrophoresis.

Although this laboratory routinely employs denaturing agarose gel electrophoresis for determining quality, a new platform from Agilent Technologies
(Palo Alto, CA) provides a workstation that will quantify RNA and produce
information on degradation and quality from as little as 5 ng of total RNA.

3.3. RNA Equilibration: Creating Pools

Once the quantity and quality have been determined, RNA pools of individual treatment and control groups can be made. The intent, at this stage, is to
create a population mean of individual samples. In this manner, genes illuminated by an array experiment will more likely represent the biological phenomenon rather than animal-to-animal variability. An equal amount of RNA should
be added from each sample to create pooled RNA. The pools may be composed
of different volumes and should be adjusted to 1 μg RNA/μL with DEPC-
treated water. This may require vacuum concentration of the sample pools. The
Clontech macroarrays require 4 μg total RNA to be hybridized to the membranes. Therefore, pools of 6 μg of total RNA are generally prepared. This permits an excess of 2 μg of RNA to run on a denaturing gel (1 μg at a time) to

ensure an equal quantity of RNA is being loaded on each membrane. The 28S bands should be with within 10% of each other as determined by a densitometry program, such as TINA. The pooled RNA is now and ready for use in the experiment.

3.4. Reverse Transcription

Note: Use radioactive safety procedures.

1. Prepare the Master Mix (per labeling reaction: 5X Reaction Buffer, 2 µL; 10X dNTP Mix 1 µL; DTT at 100 m*M*, 0.5 µL) except for α-^{32}P dATP and MMLV.
2. Create RNA and primer mixture using 4 µL (4 µg) pooled RNA and 2 µL primer mixture (supplied with the array).
3. Incubate RNA/primer mixture in a thermocycler at 70°C for 2 min, then 50°C for 2 min.
4. Add α-^{32}P-dATP (3.5 µL/rxn.) and MMLV (1 µL/rxn.) to the Master Mix **(step 1)** and vortex.
5. Add 14 µL complete Master Mix to each sample.
6. Incubate for 25 min at 50°C.
7. Meanwhile, prepare the size exclusion columns and label tubes for probe purification (*see* **Subheading 3.5.**).
8. Add 2µL Termination Solution at the end of the 25-min incubation.

3.5. Probe Purification and Equilibration

The RNA has now been reverse transcribed to create radioactive cDNA targets. The next step is to remove the unincorporated ^{32}P-dATP using size-exclusion columns. To accomplish this, we use gravity-fed Chroma Spin-200 columns.

1. Suspend Chromaspin resin by inverting column several times and tapping. Shake resin down from cap and allow it to settle. If the resin is much below the 1.0-mL mark, add some resin from another column. Be sure there are no air bubbles.
2. Snap off the bottom of the column, then remove the top. Allow the column to drain into a 2.0-mL screw-cap tube. Discard the tube and water and place column into a fresh screw-cap tube. Carefully apply the sample to the center of the column and allow the liquid to enter the column completely.
3. Chase with 100 µL of sterile DEPC water, adding carefully to the center of column in a drop by drop manner. Repeat this step once.
4. Label seven 2.0-mL screw cap tubes (Fraction 1–7) per column and open tops. Place column in the first tube and add 100 µL of sterile water. Let the column drain completely and knock off any "drips." Remove column and place in "Fraction 2" tube. Add 100 µL of sterile water and collect as before. Continue for a total of 7 fractions.
5. Cap fractions tightly and place into 20-mL glass scintillation vials. Count in scintillation counter (Cerenkov counting of ^{32}P). Plot counts profile and identify void fraction (or fractions). Experiment will require at least 1×10^6 cpm per filter.
6. Store fractions at –80°C until ready to use.

Poor Experiment   **Good Experiment**

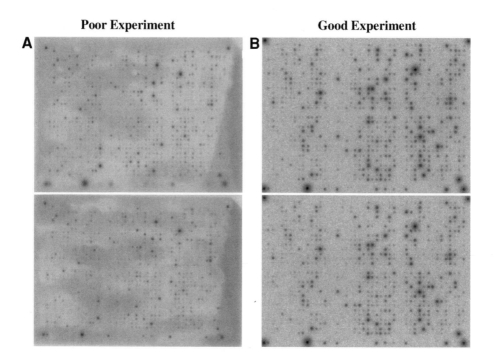

Fig. 3. Hybridization arrays showing normal and clouded backgrounds. (**A**) An example of poor array experiment in which the two arrays had inconsistent and prominent background problems. This clearly results from nonspecific binding and poor membrane washing. Frequent "shaking" of the prehybridization and hybridization steps minimizes this problem. Note that high background decreases the specific signal and produces diffuse images. (**B**) An example of two arrays showing low background and high-intensity binding.

3.6. Prehybridization

Prior to the actual hybridization, the membranes are prehybridized (to block subsequent nonspecific interaction with radiolabeled target). The importance of effective prehybridization is illustrated in **Fig. 3.**

1. On the day of labeling, place hybridization solution stock bottle into 68°C water bath.
2. Once target preparation is successful, then remove array membranes from freezer.
3. Clean hybridization bottles using Alconox and rinse thoroughly. Treat bottles with Sigmacote (or Rain-X). Allow to dry. Clean excess Sigmacote using Kim-wipe.
4. Once dry, fill bottles with DEPC-treated water.
5. Wet membranes in DEPC-treated water and insert into bottles, probe side away from glass.

6. Pour off water and briefly allow to drain.
7. Add 25 mL of hybridization buffer and 250 µL denatured Salmon Sperm DNA (10 mg/mL) in 50 mL conical and mix well: this is the prehybridization solution.
8. Add 12.5 mL of prehybridization solution into each bottle and shake in circular fashion.
9. Prehybridize at 68°C in oven at least 4 h (or, for best results, overnight).
10. Shake often to improve distribution of buffer and therefore reduce background (*see* **Note 2**).

3.7. Hybridization

After prehybridizing to the arrays, the radiolabeled targets must be prepared before hybridization.

1. Remove samples from freezer and allow to thaw.
2. Add one-tenth total volume of Denaturing solution and incubate at 68°C for 20 min.
3. Add an equal volume of Neutralizing solution and 5 µL Cot-DNA (supplied with arrays), incubate at 68°C for 10 min.
4. Add labeled cDNAs to appropriate labeled bottles (treated, control) and hybridize overnight in incubation oven.
5. Shake often to improve distribution of probe and therefore decrease background inconsistencies.

3.8. Washing and Phosphorimaging

Note: Prewarm Wash Solutions 1 and 2 to 68°C before starting.

1. Pour radioactive target solution into radioactive waste container.
2. Rinse each array with 50 mL Wash Solution 1 quickly and pour into same waste container.
3. Wash with 50 mL Wash Solution 1 for 30 min, shaking at 15-min intervals.
4. Repeat **Step 3** for three washes, pouring first and second washes into radioactive waste and the third and subsequent washes down the drain.
5. Wash with 50 mL Wash Solution 2 for a total of two washes with shaking.
6. Wash with 50 mL Wash Solution 3 for 15 min at room temperature on shaker.
7. Prepare laminate mounting surfaces.
8. Remove excess wash solution and lay on mounting surface, probe side up.
9. Cover in plastic wrap and carefully remove bubbles.
10. Enclose membrane using bag sealer and mount in phosphorimaging cassette.
11. Expose for 3–5 d.
12. Plate can then be read and analyzed using an imaging program such as Clontech's Atlas Image 2.01.

3.9. Data Analysis

Data analysis is a critical component of hybridization array experiments and poses a number of challenges owing to the large amount of data generated even in a single experiment. The most basic goal of array data analysis is to identify genes that are differentially regulated. Hybridization arrays are prone to false-positives and therefore analysis strategies attempt to decrease this error rate without increasing false-negatives. The analysis method described here is a simple, empirical approach. There are now more advanced statistical approaches to data analysis *(8)*.

3.9.1. Background Subtraction

The first steps in data analysis are background subtraction and normalization. The principals of both are similar to the techniques used with conventional nucleic acid or protein blotting. Background subtraction corrects for nonspecific background noise and permits comparison of specific signals. For illustration, if the signal intensities for the control and experimental spots are 4 and 6, respectively, it would appear that the experimental is 50% higher. However, if a background of 2 is subtracted from both signal intensities, the experimental value is actually 100% higher than control (2 vs 4). Background is often taken from the blank areas on the array. A complication to background subtraction is that differences in background across the array can affect some spots more than others. An alternative is to use either a local background for the area around each spot or designate spots with the lowest signal intensities for background determination. The latter may be a more accurate determination of nonspecific background because it represents the nonspecific binding of targets to probe. Background intensities from blank areas (no nucleic acids) do not contain probe, and therefore are arguably a different form of background.

3.9.2. Normalization

Normalization is the process by which differences between separate arrays are accounted for. All macroarray experiments require the use of normalization for accurate comparisons. For example, when a pair of macroarrays representing control and treated samples show a difference in overall or total signal intensity, such differences can arise from unequal starting amounts of RNA or cDNAs, from labeling reactions of different efficiencies, or from differences in hybridization. Any of these factors can skew the results. One common method of normalization is to use a housekeeping gene(s)—a gene thought to be invariant under experimental conditions—for comparison. If the signal for this gene is higher on one array than the other, it can be used to normalize the data. Housekeeping genes may be problematic because they themselves vary under some experimental conditions. To overcome the variability of these genes, some researchers have turned to a "basket" or "sum" approach for normalization. This strategy is based on the precept that the global radiolabeled target synthesis should be constant. That is, even though the compared samples will have selected increases and decreases, on balance the total hybridization signal should be constant. Therefore, arrays can be normalized by equilibrating the sum of the intensities for all control and experimental spots. In a similar vein, the median value of signal intensities can be used. This value is less susceptible to distortions caused by outliers.

3.9.3. Gene Calling and Differential Expression

The next step is to determine which genes were detected by the array analysis. When using large-scale arrays, there will be probes for genes that are not expressed in the tissue sample or are expressed below the level of detection. In fact, arrays are inherently much less sensitive than RT-PCR for example. This means that there must be some method for "calling" a gene as being detected by the array. The simplest method for use with macroarrays is to set a threshold, expressed as a percentage above background, that a signal must exceed for the gene to be called as present. In our experience, a 50% above background threshold has worked well. This threshold can be increased or decreased. Genes with low signal intensities are more variable, so decreasing the gene-calling threshold will increase the number of genes analyzed (as well as increasing the attendant variability). The converse is true when increasing the gene-calling threshold.

Once genes have been called as being detected by the array, the next step is to determine which genes are changed in their expression by the experimental condition. Differential expression calls are more problematic and there are no commonly accepted standards. We will describe the most basic method. The normalized signal for each gene is converted into a ratio of the treated signal intensity over the control signal intensities. Previous work by our laboratory has shown that macroarrays can reliably detect a 50% increase and greater or a 33% decrease and greater *(9)*. These amounts are equivalent on a natural log scale (+0.4 and –0.4, respectively). Genes whose expression ratios exceed these cut-offs are potential differentially regulated genes. Relying on only one array experiment is likely to result in a number of false-positives. Therefore, it is highly recommended that array experiments be repeated one or two times **(Fig. 4)**. Genes that consistently exceed the differential expression ratio across multiple experiments are less likely to be the result of random error and more likely to represent real changes in mRNA abundance.

4. Notes

1. RNA quality is the number one predictor of a successful hybridization array experiment. Make sure that the tissue is kept on dry ice or in the presence of liquid nitrogen while extracting the RNA to ensure minimal tissue thawing. Thawing will compromise the RNase protection provided by the extreme temperatures and cause RNA degradation. When removing extracted RNA from the –80°C freezers for use in an experiment, always thaw the RNA on wet ice and not at room temperature for the

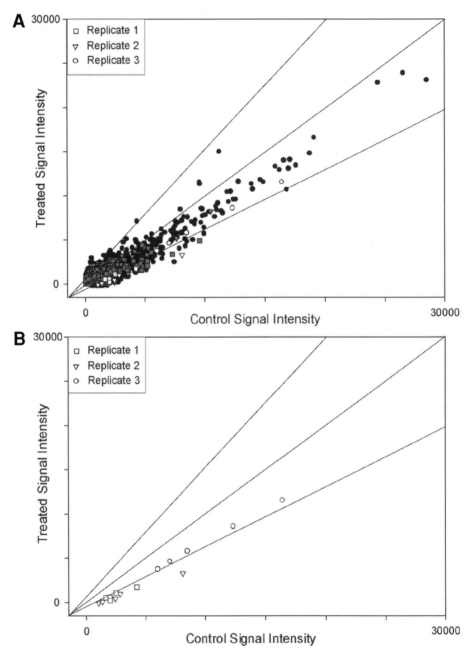

Fig. 4. Macroarray analysis of treated Cerebellar Granule Neuron cultures. (**A**) Scatterplot representing the ratio determined by comparing treated signal intensity to control signal intensity from three independent hybridization experiments. (**B**) Restricted scatterplot generated by removing the nonreplicating data points.

same reason. Additionally, repeated freeze-thawing will ultimately lead to degradation of the RNA, so this must be kept to a minimum. Finally, never perform an experiment with RNA that has not been carefully and fully characterized.

2. Shaking is such an important step in the process that it bears mentioning again. During both prehybridization and hybridization, shaking ensures that "clouds" do not appear at corners of edges of the membranes, which can complicate analysis. Examples of this problem are illustrated in **Fig. 3**.

References

1. Nisenbaum, L. K. (2002) The ultimate chip shot: can microarray technology deliver for neuroscience? *Genes Brain Behav.* **1**, 27–34.
2. Xie, J., Lee Y. H., Wang, C., et al. (2001) Differential expression of alpha1-adrenoceptor subtype mRNAs in the dorsal root ganglion after spinal nerve ligation. *Mol. Brain Res.* **93**, 164–172.
3. Boom, A., Mollereau, C., Meunier, J.-C., et al. (1999) Distribution of the nociceptin and nocistatin precursor transcript in the mouse central nervous system. *Neuroscience* **91**, 991–1007.
4. Berthele, A., Schadrack, J., Castro-Lopes, J. M., et al. (2000) Neuroplasticity in the spinal cord of monoarthritic rats: from metabolic changes to the detection of interleukin-6 using mRNA differential display. *Prog. Brain Res.* **129**, 191–203.
5. Freeman, W. M., Robertson, D. J., and Vrana K. E. (2000) Fundamentals of DNA hybridization arrays for gene expression analysis. *Biotechniques* **29**, 1042–1046. (Review.)
6. Chomczynski, P. and Sacchi, N. (1987) Single step method of RNA isolation by acid quanidinium thiocyanate-phenol-chloroform extraction. *Anal. Biochem.* **162**, 156–159.
7. Chomczynski., P. (1993) A reagent for the single-step simultaneous isolation of RNA, DNA and proteins from cell and tissue samples. *BioTechniques* **15**, 532–537.
8. Tusher, V. G., Tibshirani, R., and Chu, G. (2001) Significance analysis of microarrays applied to the ionizing radiation response. *Proc. Natl. Acad. Sci. USA* **98**, 5116–5121.
9. Freeman, W. M., Nader, M. A., Nader, S. H., et al. (2001) Chronic cocaine-mediated changes in non-human primate nucleus accumbens gene expression. *J. Neurochem.* **77**, 542–549.

20

Generation of Transgenic Mice

Guoping Feng, Jing Lu, and Jimmy Gross

Summary

In this post-genomic era, emphasis has shifted from identifying genes to understanding the physiological functions of gene products and their implications in human diseases. The use of transgenic mice is one of the key approaches in elucidating gene function and regulation. Transgenic mice have wide applications in biomedical research. These include (1) gain-of-function studies by overexpressing a protein in a tissue-specific manner; (2) loss-of-function studies by overexpressing a dominant-negative construct; (3) mapping functional domains by expressing various mutated constructs in a null (knockout mice) background; (4) mapping regulatory elements using a reporter gene; and (5) labeling subsets of cells with fluorescent proteins for live in vivo imaging of cell structure and function. In this chapter, we provide overviews as well as detailed protocols for each step involved in the generation of transgenic mice, including the selection of regulatory elements, purification of DNA, obtaining fertilized eggs, pronuclear injection, and genotyping of transgenic mice.

Key Words: Transgenic mice; pronuclear injection; promoter; regulatory elements; overexpression; superovulation; genotyping.

1. Introduction

Transgenic animals have been widely used in both the biotech/pharmaceutical industry and the biomedical research community. It is now possible to generate transgenic animals in a wide range of mammalian species, such as mice, rats, pigs, sheep, and cows. The larger transgenic mammals are mainly used to produce pharmaceutical reagents *(1)*, whereas mice are the most common choice for laboratory research. In this chapter, we will focus on the techniques that are involved in producing transgenic mice. The potential uses of transgenic mice in biomedical research are numerous. These include: (1) gain-of-function studies by overexpressing a protein in a tissue-specific manner; (2) loss-of-function studies by overexpressing a dominant- negative construct; (3) mapping

From: *Methods in Molecular Medicine, Vol. 99: Pain Research: Methods and Protocols*
Edited by: Z. D. Luo © Humana Press Inc., Totowa, NJ

functional domains by expressing various mutated constructs in a null (knockout mice) background; (4) mapping regulatory elements using a reporter gene; and (5) labeling subsets of cells with fluorescent proteins for live in vivo imaging of cell structure and function.

There are several different ways to generate transgenic mice. The most common way is to directly inject the DNA into the pronuclei of a fertilized oocyte *(2)*. A second approach is to introduce the DNA into mouse embryonic stem (ES) cells and select for ES cell colonies that have the transgene randomly integrated into their genomes. Transgenic mice can then be produced by injecting these ES cells into blastocysts *(3)*. Transgenic mice can also be produced by infecting embryos with viral vectors *(4,5)*. The pronuclear injection approach will be the main topic of this chapter because this is still the most commonly used and least reagent-dependent way to generate transgenic mice.

General steps involved in generating transgenic mice are:

1. Constructing a transgene.
2. Superovulating and obtaining fertilized eggs.
3. Injecting DNA into the pronuclei of the fertilized eggs.
4. Implanting injected eggs into the ovary ducts of pseudo-pregnant mice.
5. Genotyping transgenic mice.
6. Establishing lines of transgenic mice.

2. Materials

2.1. Purification of DNA for Pronuclear Injection

1. SeaPlaque low-melting agarose (FMC).
2. Tris-ethylenediamine tetraacetic acid (TE) buffer: 1 m*M* EDTA, 10 m*M* Tris-HCL, pH 8.0.
3. Tris-buffered phenol, phenol/chloroform/isoamyl alcohol (25:24:1), chloroform/isoamyl alchohol (24:1).
4. 3 *M* sodium acetate, pH 5.2.
5. 70% and 100% ethanol.
6. Rapid polymerase chain reaction (PCR) Purification System (Marligen Bioscience, Cat. no. 11458-015).
7. MF-Millipore membrane filter (Millipore Cat. no. VCWP02500).
8. Injection buffer: 10 m*M* NaCl, 0.25 m*M* ethylenediamine tetraacetic acid (EDTA), 10 m*M* Tris-HCl, pH 7.4. It is important to adjust pH accurately to 7.4. Sterilize by filtration.

2.2. Superovulation

1. Dulbecco's phosphate-buffered saline (PBS).
2. Gonadotropin from pregnant mare serum (PMSG), 2000 IU (Sigma Cat. no. G4877).
3. Human chorionic gonadotropin, 10,000 IU (Sigma Cat. no. CG-10).

2.3. Isolation of Fertilized Eggs

1. M2 and M16 medium (Specialty Media).
2. Hyaluronidase (Sigma Cat. no. H3884) solution in M2 medium (300 μg/mL). Make 10 mg/mL stock solution in M2 media. Filter-sterilize, aliquot, and store at –20°C. Dilute to 300 μg/mL with M2 media on the day of use.
3. Mineral oil (Sigma Cat. no. M8410).
4. 35-mm tissue-culture Petri dishes; 10-cm Petri dishes.
5. Fine forceps and scissors.
6. Glass capillaries for making egg-transfer pipets (Fisher Cat. no. 12-141-1) (*see* **Note 1**).
7. Latex tubing for mouth pipetting (VWR Cat. no. 62996-350).
8. Small Bunsen burner (VWR Cat. no. 62379-523).
9. Dissecting microscope with 20× and 40× magnification.
10. CO_2 incubator.

2.4. Pronuclear Injection

1. Glass capillaries for making holding pipet (VWR Cat. no. 53432-7289) (*see* **Note 2**).
2. Glass capillaries with an internal glass filament for making injection pipet (Sutter Instrument Cat. no. BF100-78-10) (*see* **Note 3**).
3. Mechanical pipet puller (Sutter P-87, P-97).
4. Microforge.
5. Injection chamber (*see* **Note 4**).
6. Microinjection setup, including stereomicroscope with a 40× objective; micromanipulators, vibration-free table (*see* **Note 5**).

2.5. Implantation of Injected Eggs

1. Avertin: To make a 100% stock solution, dissolve 10 g of 2,2,2-tribromoethanol (Aldrich Cat. no. T48402) in 10 mL of tert-amyl alcohol. Dilute to 2.5% with PBS for daily use. Wrap with aluminum foil and store at 4°C.
2. Fine forceps, scissors, suture, and animal clippers.
3. Egg-transfer pipet and latex tubing.
4. Dissecting microscope with 20× and 40× magnification.

2.6. Genotyping Transgenic Mice

1. Tail digestion buffer: 1 mM $CaCl_2$, 1% Tween-20, 50 mM Tris-HCl, pH 8.0.
2. Proteinase K solution: 10 mg/mL proteinase K in 50% glycerol, 20 mM $CaCl_2$, 10 mM Tris-HCl, pH 7.5. Keep at –20°C.

3. Methods

3.1. Construction of Transgenes

A transgene construct generally includes four components: 5′ regulatory sequences (a promoter region), a coding sequence, 3′ regulatory sequences (a polyadenylation signal sequence), and a vector for propagation in *Escherichia coli.* Promoter sequences determine the spatial and temporal pattern and level of transgene expression. A polyadenylation signal sequence is required for the polyadenylation of mRNA, and thus the stability of mRNA.

3.1.1. Select a 5′ Regulatory Element

5′ Regulatory sequences from a large number of genes showing tissue-specific expression have been characterized in transgenic mice. These in vivo characterized regulatory sequences are usually the best choices because many 5′ regulatory elements characterized in cultured cells may not convey the same specificity when used in transgenic mice. It is also important to point out that if a 5′ regulatory element is characterized as a whole gene (a whole genomic fragment contains 5′ regulatory sequences, coding regions, and 3′ regulatory sequences), then this 5′ regulatory element may not show the same degree of specificity when used to express another gene (for example, a reporter gene). This may be due to tissue-specific regulatory elements residing in the introns of the coding region *(6,7)*. Sometimes it may be critical that the expression pattern of a transgene matches precisely that of an endogenous gene and no such a promoter has been characterized. In such case, use of a large fragment (100–200 kb) of the 5′ regulatory region of the endogenous gene to drive the transgene expression is highly recommended. This can be accomplished by using BAC (bacterial artificial chromosome) clones, which have an insert of genomic DNA that can be up to the size of 300 kb. Both human and mouse genomes are sequenced and overlapping BAC clones are mapped in the genome databases of Genbank. BAC clones containing the gene of interest (and its 5′ regulatory sequences) are available for free (only shipping and handling charges) and suppliers are listed with each BAC clone. Several efficient methods have been developed to manipulate BAC clones (such as insertion of a reporter gene in the first coding exon) and reagents and protocols are readily available from these investigators *(8–10)*.

3.1.2. Coding Sequences

Coding sequences can be in the form of either a genomic fragment, which contains the complete intron and exon structure, or a cDNA. Owing to the existence of large-sized introns in mammalian genes, cDNA is the more commonly used form. It should be noted that several studies have shown that the expression levels of some transgenes are significantly lower in cDNA-based constructs than those of intron-containing genomic constructs *(11)*. It also has been shown that including an endogenous intron or addition of an exogenous intron in cDNA constructs increases the level expression of cDNA constructs *(12–14)*. This approach should be considered when high levels of transgene expression are important.

To improve transgene expression at the translational level, it is important that there is no in-frame or out-of-frame ATG before the true translation initiation ATG codon. Furthermore, a consensus sequence for translation initiation (Kozak sequence, ACCATGG where ATG is the translation initiation codon) can be introduced to ensure a strong translational start signal *(15)*.

3.1.3. 3′ Regulatory Sequences

A 3′ regulatory sequence containing a polyadenylation signal is critical for the stability of mRNA. The polyadenylation signal can be from the endogenous gene by using either the 3′ untranslated region of the gene or by using the full-length cDNA. More often, an exogenous polyadenylation signal is added to the 3′ end of the transgene. This is because: (1) the 3′ untranslated region of some genes may contain signals for increasing mRNA turnover; and (2) many of the isolated cDNA clones are not full-length and thus do not contain the polyadenylation signal. Many exogenous polyadenylation signals have been successfully used in transgenic mice. The most commonly used ones include the polyadenylation signal sequences from the SV40 T-antigen *(16)* and from the human or bovine growth hormone gene *(18,19)*.

3.2. Purification of DNA for Pronuclear Injection

DNA of standard plasmid clones can be propagated in *E. coli,* and isolated with commercial plasmid DNA purification kits. For large constructs, such as BAC clones, we recommend using special kits designed for large constructs (e.g., NucleoBond BAC maxi kit from BD Biosciences). For standard plasmid constructs, it is important to remove all vector sequences before pronuclear injection. It has been shown that inclusion of prokaryotic sequences in the injected construct can severely inhibit the expression of the transgene in mice *(17)*.

3.2.1. Phenol Extraction of DNA From Agarose Gel

1. To separate vector backbone from the insert, digest 6–10 μg DNA using appropriate enzymes. Make sure the digestion is complete.
2. Separate insert and vector by electrophoresis using 1% low-melting agarose.
3. Cut out the band with a razor blade, taking care to minimize gel volume.
4. Estimate volume by weighing and add equal volume of TE buffer.
5. Heat at 65–70°C for 20 min. Aliquot melted gel (500–600 μL/tube) into microcentrifuge tubes.
6. Add 1 volume of Tris-buffered phenol and vortex. Centrifuge for 10 min at maximum speed in a microcentrifuge and transfer the aqueous phase (top) to new tubes.
7. Add 150 μL TE to the phenol phase of each tube, vortex, and centrifuge as above. Combine the aqueous phase with previous tubes.

8. Add equal volume of phenol/chloroform/isoamyl alchohol to the aqueous phase, vortex, and centrifuge for 3 min.
9. Transfer the aqueous phase to new tubes.
10. Add equal volume of chloroform/isoamyl alchohol to the aqueous phase, vortex, and centrifuge for 3 min.
11. Transfer the aqueous phase to new tubes.
12. Add 1/10 volume of 3 M sodium acetate, pH 5.2, and 2 volumes of 100% ethanol to precipitate the DNA. Keep at –20° or –80°C for 15 min and centrifuge for 10 min.
13. Very carefully remove all the supernatant. Air-dry pellets for a few minutes. Dissolve all pellets in a total of 100 µL of TE.

3.2.2. Purification on Spin Column

1. Use the Rapid PCR Purification System (Marligen Bioscience). Prepare all the solutions according to manufacturer's instruction. Warm a tube of dH$_2$O at 65°C for later use.
2. To the DNA tube, add 400 µL Binding Solution (H1) and mix well.
3. Place a cartridge into a 2-mL wash tube. Load the sample from **step 2** into the cartridge. Centrifuge at 1,000g for 2 min, then at 12,000g for 1 min. Discard the flow-through.
4. Place the cartridge back into the 2-mL wash tube. Add 700 µL Wash Buffer (H2, containing ethanol) to the cartridge. Centrifuge at 12,000g for 1 min. Discard the flow-through. Centrifuge again at 12,000g for 1 min to remove all residual wash buffer.
5. Place the cartridge into a 1.5-mL recovery tube (supplied). Add 100 µL warm dH$_2$O to the cartridge. Incubate at room temperature for 2 min, then centrifuge at 12,000g for 2 min.
6. Precipitate DNA by adding 20 µL of 5 M NaCl and 200 µL of 100% ethanol. Keep at –20° or –80°C for 15 min and centrifuge for 10 min.
7. Very carefully remove all the supernatant and rinse the pellet with 150 µL 70% ethanol, then air-dry the pellet for a few minutes. Dissolve the pellet in 100 µL of injection buffer.

3.2.3. Dialysis

1. Add 5 mL injection buffer to a sterile 6-cm dish.
2. Float a 0.1-µm Millipore filter on buffer (Cat. no. VCWP02500). Be very careful not to wet the top of the filter (or you will lose all the DNA!).
3. Gently pipet DNA solution onto the center of the filter and leave for 3 h.
4. Transfer DNA solution to a sterile tube, recovering as much as possible.
5. Add 50 µL injection buffer to the filter and leave a few minutes. Recover this sample and combine with the previous sample.
6. Centrifuge at maximum speed for 15 min and transfer the top 90% of the solution to a sterile tube.
7. Estimate DNA concentration accurately by comparison with known standards on an agarose gel.

3.3. Preparation of Mice for Pronuclear Injection

To generate transgenic mice by pronuclear injection, it is necessary to routinely obtain a large number of preimplantation embryos and an adequate supply of pseudopregnant recipients. This requires a standard mouse facility equipped with proper ventilation, temperature, humidity, and light controls in addition to the proper personnel for cage washing, husbandry, and veterinary care.

3.3.1. Mouse Strain Selection

Mice for the production and breeding of transgenic mice can be divided into five categories:

1. Female mice for matings to produce fertilized eggs for DNA injection.
2. Fertile stud male mice.
3. Female mice to serve as pseudopregnant recipients.
4. Sterile stud male mice for the production of pseudopregnant females.
5. Desired inbred mice to be crossed to founder transgenic mice for establishing and maintaining transgenic lines

The mouse strain to be used as donor of the eggs for microinjection will depend on the nature of the research project. If genetic background is not critical to the experiment, injections are often performed with F2 hybrid zygotes from matings of F1 hybrid mice. This is mainly because hybrid mice can produce fertilized eggs more efficiently than inbred mice. Furthermore, fertilized eggs from hybrid matings are generally healthier, and thus survive in vitro manipulations better. Some of the most commonly used F1 hybrids are C57BL/6J × SJL, C57BL/6J × CBA/J, C57BL/6J × DBA/2J, C3H/HeJ × C57BL/6J, C3H/HeJ × DBA/2J.

If a defined genetic background is important, such as for immunological studies, then an appropriate inbred strain should be used. Many inbred strains have been successfully used to produce transgenic mice (e.g., FVB/N, C57BL/J6, BALB/cJ, and C3H). When using inbred strains, it will be necessary to set up more matings than with F1 hybrid mice to collect the same amount of healthy, fertilized eggs for microinjection.

Outbred (e.g., ICR) mice can be used as pseudopregnant recipients. They cost less and are generally better caretakers of pups.

To maximize the production of fertilized eggs, superovulated female mice are used. On average, 20–30 eggs can be collected from a 4- to 5-wk-old super-ovulated hybrid female mouse. Generally, twelve 4-wk-old females are super-ovulated and mated, and 6–10 of them will have vaginal plugs. This will yield a total of 150–250 viable eggs for a session of microinjection. 90% of these eggs will usually be fertilized. Approximately 60–80% of the injected eggs will survive and be reimplanted into the oviducts of pseudopregnant foster mothers, approx 25–30 embryos per mouse. Typically, two to five oviduct transfers can be performed after each session of microinjection.

The same numbers of fertile stud males as egg-donor females are required. Stud males must be placed in individual cages to avoid fighting and injury. Separate them 1 wk before mating with a superovulated female. Most F1 hybrid males can be used as studs for up to 1 yr.

For producing pseudopregnant females, any strain with a good breeding performance can be used. Twelve vasectomized males of at least 2 mo of age will be needed and can be repeatedly used for more than a year. Pseudopregnant females should be at least 6 wk of age and weigh at least 20 g, but obese mice make egg transfer difficult because of the large fat pads surrounding the ovaries. In general, 20–24 females will be needed and those in estrus will be placed with vasectomized males to obtain pseudopregnant females.

3.3.2. Superovulation

Gonadotropins are often administered to females prior to mating to increase the number of eggs that are ovulated. Gonadotropin from pregnant mare's serum (PMSG) and human chorionic gonadotropin (hCG) are used to mimic the follicle-stimulating hormone (FSH) and luteinizing hormone (LH), respectively.

1. Add 4 mL of Dulbecco's PBS to a 2,000 IU bottle of PMSG, and add 20 mL of distilled water to a 10,000 IU bottle of hCG. Aliquot 100 µL per tube of both hormones. Keep the hormones at –20°C.
2. Three days before microinjection, thaw one tube of PMSG. Add 0.9 mL of PBS to the tube and mix well. Draw hormone into a 1-mL syringe. Give i.p. injection of 0.1 mL per mouse at 1:30 PM. Label cage with time and date of injections.
3. 46–48 hours following PMSG injection, thaw a tube of hCG. Add 0.9 mL of PBS to the tube mix well. Draw hormone into a 1-mL syringe. Give i.p. injection of 0.1 mL per mouse. After injections, place each mouse into a cage overnight with a breeder male.
4. The next morning, check females for vaginal plugs. Mice with plugs are suitable to use for isolation of fertilized eggs.

3.3.3. Pseudopregnant Recipient Females

Selection of females for pseudopregnant recipient matings is most efficiently done by visual appearance of the external genitalia. Females go through a series of estrous cycling through which natural ovulation occurs. The easiest way to identify the correct estrus cycle is to examine the vaginal opening, which should be of a light pink color, slightly moist and swollen with pronounced striations. To set up matings, females are usually set up with sterile males in the afternoon (two females in each cage with one male). These matings are set up on the same day as the matings for fertilized eggs. The females are allowed to breed overnight and are examined for a vaginal plug the following morning. It is important to check for vaginal plugs early in the morning because they could fall out as early as 10–12 h after copulation.

3.4. Isolation of Fertilized Eggs

Fertilized eggs may be collected several hours before they are to be injected.

1. Preparing microdrop culture: Use a micropipet to dispense 20–40 µL drops of M16 or M2 medium on the bottom of a 35-mm Petri dish, then flood the dish with mineral oil.
2. Sacrifice the mouse by cervical dislocation. Lay the animal on its back and wipe abdomen with 70% ethanol.
3. Cut and pull the skin until the abdomen is completely exposed. Open the abdominal cavity by cutting and pull the coils of gut out of the cavity.
4. Cut between the oviduct and ovary with a pair of fine scissors and collect the oviducts, put them in a 35-mm Petri dish containing 0.2 mL M2 medium.
5. Release the eggs surrounded by cumulus cells by tearing the ampulla with fine forceps in hyaluronidase solution under 20× magnification using a dissecting microscope. The eggs will be released as the digestion removes the sticky cumulus cells.
6. Wash the separated eggs with transfer pipets by pipetting the eggs up and down several times in M16 medium drops.
7. Transfer the separated eggs with transfer pipets to new M16 medium drops in a 35-mm Petri dish.
8. Incubate all the eggs in a CO_2 incubator until ready to inject.

3.5. Pronuclear Injection

The time of administration of the hCG will determine the exact time of pronuclear injection. Typically, hCG is administered at 12–1 PM and the eggs can be injected between 12 noon and 6 PM on the following day.

1. Just before injection, 50 one-cell eggs are washed by pipetting up and down several times in M2 medium droplets, and then transferred into the M2 droplet of the injection chamber. The injection should be finished within 20–30 min each time.
2. Fill the tip of an injection pipet with DNA solution (1–2 ng/µL) by dipping the blunt end into the DNA solution.
3. Place holding pipet and injection needle into position.
4. Place the tip of the holding pipet close to an egg and then suck it onto the end of the pipet. If the position of the pronucleus is not convenient enough for injection, reorient the egg by releasing and sucking it again with the help of the injection pipet. The male pronucleus is usually larger then the female pronucleus and nearer the surface and therefore easier to hit.
5. Refocus on the pronucleus to be injected using microscope focusing control. Move the tip of the injection pipet next to the egg and bring it into the same focal plane using the vertical control on the micromanipulator.

6. Push the injection tip forward carefully into one of the pronuclei. Take care not to touch the nucleoli.

7. Squeeze on the syringe connected to the injection pipet. If the pronucleus visibly swells, it has been successfully injected.

8. Withdraw the injection needle out of the egg quickly but gently. If any cytoplasmic granules are accidentally pulled out of the egg after removing the needle, the egg may be starting to lyse. If this happens in succession, the injection needle needs to be replaced. On average, one injection needle can be used to inject 20–25 eggs.

9. Place the correctly injected cell on one side of the M2 microdroplet. Inappropriately injected eggs, including eggs that are going to lyse after injection, are placed on the opposite side.

10. After all the eggs have been injected, the healthy-looking eggs are transferred to a M16 microdroplet in a 35-mm Petri dish. Wash the eggs by pipetting up and down several times in M16, and then transfer to a M16 microdroplet marked with "post" in the same 100-mm Petri dish. Incubate in a CO_2 incubator until transplantation.

3.6. Implantation of Injected Eggs

Injected one-cell stage eggs can be transferred into the ampullae of 0.5-d p.c. pseudopregnant recipients. But if the eggs are kept in the incubator until they grow into 3.5-d blastocysts, they can also be transferred into the uterine horns of a 2.5-d p.c. pseudopregnant recipients. We will only discuss the former procedure.

1. Anesthetize the pseudopregnant recipient mouse by injecting it i.p. with 0.015 mL of 2.5% avertin per gram of body weight.

2. Wash the injected eggs with transfer pipets by pipetting the eggs up and down several times in M2 medium droplets, and then load the transfer pipet with eggs as follows: fill the transfer pipet with mineral oil to just past the shoulder. Take up a small air bubble into the pipet followed by M2 medium, and then a second air bubble. Draw up the eggs in a minimal volume of M2 medium. Take up a third air bubble followed by a short column of M2 medium.

3. Soak and wipe the lower back of the recipient mouse with 70% ethanol.

4. Cut a small transverse incision (less then 1 cm) on the lower back. Through the body wall, the fat pad on the ovary is visible. Pick up the body wall and make a small incision just over the white fat pad. Pick up the fat pad and pull out the ovary and oviduct with a pair of blunt forceps. Clip a serrefine clamp onto the fat pad and keep the oviduct outside the body wall.

5. Put the mouse on a 10-cm Petri dish on the stage of a stereomicroscope with its head to the left. Find the infundibulum under 20–40× magnification. Carefully make a hole in the bursa over the infundibulum with two pairs of fine forceps.

6. With the help of a pair of blunt fine forceps, insert the egg-loaded transfer pipet into the infundibulum. Blow on the transfer pipet until air bubbles 2 and 3 have entered the ampulla.

7. Release the fat pad and place the uterus, oviduct, and ovary back inside the body wall. Sew up the body wall with one stitch and close the skin with wound clips.
8. If necessary, implant more eggs to the other oviduct.
9. Put the mouse back in the cage on top of a 37°C warm plate. The mouse should be kept warm until it recovers from anesthetics.

3.7. Genotyping Transgenic Mice

Typically 10–40% of the mice born from the foster females contain the transgene. These are called transgenic "founder" mice. These mice are identified by either Southern-blot analysis or PCR of genomic DNA from the tail clips. We routinely use the PCR method to genotype transgenic mice and have found it very reliable. We recommend amplifying a fragment of about 300–600 base pairs if using the following crude tail DNA preparation method.

1. At postnatal d 7–10, cut 0.3–0.5 cm tail, put into a 1.5-mL microcentrifuge tube.
2. To each tube, add 100 µL tail buffer and 10 µL proteinase K solution (10 mg/mL). Incubate at 55°C overnight.
3. Centrifuge briefly. Boil samples for 10 min to inactivate proteinase K. Samples are ready for PCR.
4. PCR reactions: Assemble PCR reactions on ice. For a 25 µL reaction, add 18.9 µL distilled H_2O, 2.5 µL 10X PCR buffer with proper concentration of Mg^{2+}, 0.5 µL dNTPs (10 mM dATP, dGTP, and dTTP), 0.5 µL of each primer (10 µM), 0.1 µL Taq polymerase (5U/µL), 2 µL tail DNA.
5. Heat the PCR block to 96°C, then put tubes in. This will minimize nonspecific amplification.
6. Cycles: **Step 1,** 96°C for 3 min; **step 2,** 96°C for 1 min; **step 3,** 62°C for 1 min; **step 4,** 68°C for 3 min; repeat **steps 2–4** for 34 more times; **step 5,** 68°C for 10 min; **step 6,** keep at 4°C.
7. Run 10 µL on a 2% agarose gel.

4. Notes

1. Making transfer pipets: soften the glass tubing by rotating it in a fine flame of a small Bunsen burner. Pull both ends to produce a tube with an internal diameter of approx 200 µm. Score the tubing with a diamond-point pencil to obtain a neat break.
2. Making holding pipets: Soften the glass capillary tubing by rotating it in a fine flame of a small Bunsen burner. Pull both ends to produce a tube with an outside diameter of approx 80–120 µm, score the tubing with a diamond-point pencil to obtain a neat break. Clamp the pipet into the microforge, position the drawn tip of the pipet directly above the heating filament of the microforge, and heat the tip of the pipet until the inside diameter shrinks to approx 15 µm.
3. Making injection pipets: Use a mechanical pipet puller to pull a piece of 10–15 cm long glass capillary tubing. Design an optimal program setting of the puller by trying various settings. A good injection pipet should have a tip with a diameter of less than 1 µm. Pipets should be pulled the same day they are to be used.

4. Making injection chamber: Fix two small rubber bars on a siliconized microscopic slide with Vaseline® as cover glass holder, add a droplet of 10 µL of M2 medium, put a cover glass on the rubber bar, and make sure the M2 medium reaches the cover glass. Add enough mineral oil to surround the medium drop. The chamber should be made just before use.
5. For a detailed description of how to set up a microinjection station, please refer to ref. *(20)*.

References

1. Houdebine, L. M. (2000) Transgenic animal bioreactors. *Transgenic Res.* **9,** 305–320.
2. Gordon, J. W., Scangos, G. A., Plotkin, D. J., et al. (1980) Genetic transformation of mouse embryos by microinjection of purified DNA. *Proc. Natl. Acad. Sci. USA* **77,** 7380–7384.
3. Gossler, A., Joyner, A. L., Rossant, J., and Skarnes, W. C.. (1989) Mouse embryonic stem cells and reporter constructs to detect developmentally regulated genes. *Science* **244,** 463–465.
4. Jaenisch, R. (1976) Germ line integration and Mendelian transmission of the exogenous Moloney leukemia virus. *Proc. Natl. Acad. Sci. USA* **73,** 1260–1264.
5. Lois, C., Hong, E. J., Pease, S., et al. (2002) Germline transmission and tissue-specific expression of transgenes delivered by lentiviral vectors. *Science* **295,** 868–872.
6. Vidal, M., Morris, R., Grosveld, F., and Spanopoulou, E. (1990) Tissue-specific control elements of the Thy-1 gene. *EMBO J.* **9,** 833–840.
7. Mckeon, C. (1993) Transcriptional regulation of the insulin receptor gene promoter. *Adv. Exp. Med. Biol.* **343,** 79–89.
8. Lee, E. C., Yu, D., Martinez de Velasco, J., et al. (2001) A highly efficient *Escherichia coli*-based chromosome engineering system adapted for recombinogenic targeting and subcloning of BAC DNA. *Genomics* **73,** 56–65.
9. Gong, S., Yang, X. W., Li, C., and Heintz, N. (2002) Highly efficient modification of bacterial artificial chromosomes (BACs) using novel shuttle vectors containing the R6Kgamma origin of replication. *Genome Res.* **12,** 1992–1998.
10. Misulovin, Z., Yang, X. W., Yu, W., et al. (2001) A rapid method for targeted modification and screening of recombinant bacterial artificial chromosome. *J. Immunol. Methods* **257,** 99–105.
11. Brinster, R. L., Allen, J. M., Behringer, R. R., et al. (1988) Introns increase transcriptional efficiency in transgenic mice. *Proc. Natl. Acad. Sci. USA* **85,** 836–840.
12. Hammer, R. E., Krumlauf, R., Camper, S. A., et al. (1987) Diversity of alpha-fetoprotein gene expression in mice is generated by a combination of separate enhancer elements. *Science* **235,** 53–58.
13. Choi, T., Huang, M., Gorman, C., and Jaenisch, R. (1991) A generic intron increases gene expression in transgenic mice. *Mol. Cell. Biol.* **11,** 3070–3074.
14. Palmiter, R. D., Sandgren, E. P., Avarbock, M. R., et al. (1991) Heterologous introns can enhance expression of transgenes in mice. *Proc. Natl. Acad. Sci. USA* **88,** 478–482.

15. Kozak, M. (1986) Point mutations define a sequence flanking the AUG initiator codon that modulates translation by eukaryotic ribosomes. *Cell* **44,** 283–292.

16. Weis, J., Fine, S. M., David, C., et al. (1991) Integration site- dependent expression of a transgene reveals specialized features of cells associated with neuromuscular junctions. *J. Cell Biol.* **113,** 1385–1397.

17. Bamber, B. A., Masters, B. A., Hoyle, G. W., et al. (1994) Leukemia inhibitory factor induces neurotransmitter switching in transgenic mice. *Proc. Natl. Acad. Sci. USA* **91,** 7839–7843.

18. Townes, T. M., Lingrel, J. B., Chen, H. Y., et al. (1985) Erythroid-specific expression of human beta-globin genes in transgenic mice. *EMBO J.* **4,** 1715–1723.

19. Chada, K., Magram, J., Raphael, K., et al. (1985) Specific expression of a foreign beta-globin gene in erythroid cells of transgenic mice. *Nature* **314,** 377–380.

20. Hogan, B., Beddington, R., Constantini, F., and Lacy, E. (1994) *Manipulating the Mouse Embryo: A Laboratory Manual,* 2nd ed. Cold Spring Harbor Laboratory Press, Cold Spring Harbor, New York.

21

Knockout Mouse Models in Pain Research

Andrée Dierich and Brigitte L. Kieffer

Summary

Gene targeting in mice by homologous recombination is a powerful approach to study the role of specific genes in vivo. This technology is now applied to pain-related genes to understand molecular mechanisms of nociceptive behaviors. In this chapter, we provide detailed methodological information for the construction of knockout animals, exemplified by the generation of mice lacking opioid receptor genes. We report our protocols for the production, maintenance, transfection, and selection of embryonic stem (ES) cells, as well as for blastocyst injection, which are generally applicable to any gene-targeting project. We also describe strategies for the construction of targeting vectors, as well as for ES cell and animal genotyping, in the context of μ, δ, and κ opioid receptor genes. We finally provide a few examples of mouse phenotyping in pain behavioral assays.

Key Words: Pain; opioids; μ; δ; and κ receptor; knockout mice; targeting vector; embryonic stem (ES) cells; homologous recombination; blastocyst; genotype; phenotype; behavior.

1. Introduction

Gene targeting in mice was established in the laboratory of M. Capecchi *(1)*, as the successful combination of two discoveries. One was the demonstration that DNA recombination can occur in mammalian cells between a chromosomal locus and an homologous, but modified, cloned DNA sequence leading to a mutant locus *(2)*. The other was the isolation of totipotent embryonic stem (ES) cells, which can contribute to any mouse tissue, including the germ-line, and can be genetically modified *(3,4)*. Gene targeting by homologous recombination is now widely used to modify specific genes in the mouse genome. Initial and most current manipulations are insertions of a foreign gene into an essential exon of the targeted gene, thus leading to a nonfunctional gene. The resulting animals—so-called knockout mice—are then examined anatomically, biochemically, and behaviorally, and modifications

From: *Methods in Molecular Medicine, Vol. 99: Pain Research: Methods and Protocols*
Edited by: Z. D. Luo © Humana Press Inc., Totowa, NJ

observed in the mutant animal—referred as to "the phenotype"—provide unique insights into in vivo functions of the gene of interest.

Among the several genetic approaches currently available in pain research (*see* ref. *5*), knockout mice have proved exquisite tools to assess the molecular basis of pain responses in vivo. Mutant strains lacking pain-related genes have been generated and significant alterations of pain sensitivities in the knockout animals have been reviewed recently for more than 20 genes *(6,7)*. Examples are the genetic inactivation of neurotrophins and their receptors, which have identified nerve growth factor (NGF) *(8)* and TrkA *(9)* as developmental players of pain sensitivity, or null mutations in cytokine genes that show a role for interleukin (IL)-6 *(10)* and interferon (IFN)-α *(11)* in the development of inflammation and neuropathic pain, respectively. Analyses of mice lacking receptors for algogene substances or pain mediators have implicated the prostacyclin receptor PGI_2 as a target for nonsteroidal anti-inflammatory drugs *(12)*, demonstrated low receptor selectivity for clinically relevant adrenergic and serotoninergic drugs (*see* **ref. *6***), showed limited implication of B_2 compared to B_1 bradykinin receptors in inflammatory responses *(13)*, and revealed a role for vanilloid VR1 receptors in the perception painful heat and thermal hypersensitivity during inflammation *(14)*. Also from knockout mice studies, the preprotackykinin gene product was suggested to modulate the perception of various noxious stimuli in an intensity-related mode *(15)* and to play a role in supraspinal nociception *(16)*. The absence of one tackykinin receptor (NK1) produced a different phenotype, with no incidence on acute pain thresholds and limited consequences on inflammatory and stress-induced responses *(17)*. Null mutations in intracellular signaling molecule genes have demonstrated a role for the regulatory subunit RIβ of protein kinase A (PKA) in neurogenic inflammation but not neuropathic pain *(18)*, whereas protein kinase C (PKC) γ is critically involved in neuropathic pain *(19)*. Although by far not exhaustive, these few examples clearly illustrate the usefulness of gene targeting in the exploration of pain-related molecules.

Another system involved in pain is the opioid system. Opiate drugs are most powerful analgesics and the endogenous opioid system is critical in regulating nociception (*see* **refs. *20,21***). Mice lacking each of the three opioid receptor genes as well as each of the three opioid peptide genes have been generated by us and others (reviewed in **refs. *22–24***). The analysis of opioid receptor knockout mice has allowed identifying the molecular targets of several prototypic opiates in vivo, including morphine *(22)*. Also, first data indicate a tonic implication of opioid receptors in response to some painful stimuli, which differ across opioid receptor subtypes and suggest the existence of a mu receptor/enkephalin tone in supraspinal responses to thermal pain (*see* ref. *24*). Although persistent pain has been little investigated in knockout mice of the opioid system so far, one report demonstrates the pronociceptice activity of dynorphin in the development and maintenance of neuropathic pain *(25)*. Mice lacking opioid receptors that have been generated in our laboratory *(26–28)* will be used as examples here.

The purpose of this chapter is to provide basic methodological information on the construction of knockout animals. We will first describe the general strategy used to inactivate a gene of interest in mice and then focus on the methodological approach. We have chosen to particularly develop materials and methods that are specific to the generation of any knockout animal and involve the manipulation of ES cells. These are the protocols that we have successfully used in the past years (*see* also **refs. *29–31***). For other steps, which are specific for each targeted gene (targeting construct and genotyping), our description will stand at the level of rationales for cloning and analysis and our mice lacking opioid receptors will serve as illustrations. In those steps, protocols for gene cloning, DNA modification, and genomic DNA analysis will be briefly described and the reader is referred to classical molecular biology handbooks.

1.1. The Knockout Strategy

Steps involved are summarized in **Fig. 1.**

Step 1. Creation of a targeting construct by gene cloning and modification. A portion of the gene of interest, including coding exons, is cloned from a mouse genomic library. The gene fragment is mapped or fully sequenced to localize unique restriction sites necessary to create the construct. A foreign gene encoding antibiotic resistance (neomycin or hygromycin resistance) is then inserted into, or in place of, a coding exon using suitable restriction sites. Because of lack of translation initiation codon and/or frame shift, the resulting gene fragment is nonfunctional. This modified portion of the gene is called the targeting construct.

Step 2. Gene transfer into ES cells. The targeting construct is transfected into totipotent ES cells, classically prepared from the mouse strain 129 (most of which are agouti-colored). Cells are then submitted to antibiotic treatment in order to select cells that have irreversibly integrated the DNA construct in their genome.

Step 3. ES cell genotyping. Most ES cell clones have integrated the transgene randomly. Homologous recombination, i.e., replacement of the endogenous locus by the homologous targeting construct, is a rare event and has eventually occurred in some clones. To detect the latter clones ("positive clones"), several hundred ES cell clones are amplified separately. Their genomic DNA is prepared and analyzed at the level of the gene locus. Because homologous recombination is unlikely to occur simultaneously at both alleles, the positive clone will contain a mutant and a wild-type allele at the locus of interest and will therefore be heterozygous for the mutation.

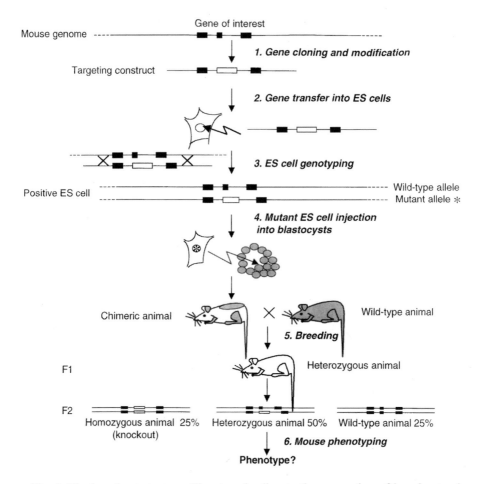

Fig. 1. The knockout strategy. The steps leading to the generation of knockout animals are numbered and explained in the Introduction. Each step is detailed in the Methods section. The gene of interest is represented by a solid line (introns) and black boxes (exons). The transgene—classically a gene encoding neomycin resistance—used to perturbate gene expression is represented by a white box. The targeting construct is transfected into pluripotent ES cells and a mutant ES clone, where the construct has replaced the homologous wild-type region, is identified. This ES clone is injected into blastocysts and participates to produce chimeric animals, which in turn are bred to generate F1 heterozygous mutant mice. F1 interbreeding leads to animals homozygous for the inactivated allele (knockout mice).

Step 4. Production of chimeric animals by injection of mutant ES cells into blastocysts. The positive ES clone is amplified and cells are injected into blastocysts from a different mouse strain, usually C57BL/6 (dark-colored). Blastocysts are then implanted into the uterus of a pseudopregnant foster mother for further development. The pluripotent mutant 129 ES cells colonize C57BL/6 embryos and both cell types participate in generating the novel mouse. This animal, also named the chimeric mouse, will display coat color patches indicating that parts of the tissues derive from mutant ES cells.

Step 5. Breeding and production of knockout animals. Chimeric males are bred with C57Bl/6 females in order to search for germ-line transmission. Genomic DNA from the offspring is analyzed at the level of the gene locus (mouse genotyping), as previously done for ES cells in step 3. If mutant ES cells have produced germ cells, chimeras should be able to pass the mutant allele onto the next generation. In this case, some of the F1 animals show the targeted mutation. These animals, which are heterozygous for the mutation, are interbred to obtain F2 homozygous, heterozygous, and wild-type littermates at a Mendelian frequency. Animals homozygous for the mutation are currently referred as to the knockout mice.

Step 6. Mouse phenotyping. The absence of gene function should then be verified, either at the RNA or protein level, to determine whether the targeting strategy was successful. Animals from each genotype (wild-type, heterozygous, and homozygous) can now be compared to assess the role of the targeted gene in vivo.

The reader should be aware that a year, at least, is required to achieve steps 1–5. Further, our description here is limited to the basic method for obtaining knockout mice. More sophisticated approached have now derived from initial homologous recombination protocols either to subtly modify the targeted gene by site-directed mutagenesis (knockin) or to inactivate the gene of interest in a temporally and regionally controlled manner (conditional knockout). For these approaches, the construction of targeting constructs slightly differs and involves the introduction of Lox*P* sites flanking the targeting exon and the selection gene (step 1). Also an additional step is required where either ES cells (step 3) or the mutant animal (step 5) are exposed to the enzyme Cre recombinase. Rationales and appropriate references are reviewed in Metzger et al. *(32)*.

2. Materials

A key step in the generation of knockout animals is the preparation of ES cells that are used to modify the mouse genome. Preparation of these cells is therefore the subject of the Materials section.

2.1. Mouse ES Cell Preparation

Mouse embryonic stem cells, also named ES cells, are isolated from the inner cell mass (ICM) from a mouse blastocyst. Most ES cell lines available up to now have been isolated from blastocysts originating from different 129 mouse substrains. From these strains the yield (number of blastocysts actually producing ES cells/total number of blastocysts) is 10–30% *(33–37)*. For some reason, not yet solved, only few ES cell lines have been isolated from other mouse strains, such as C57BL/6, BALB/c, or DBA/1, but yields are often below 1% *(38–41)*.

Blastocysts are isolated from mated females at 3.5 d postcoitum (p.c). Females are killed by CO_2 inhalation. The uteri are isolated in one piece by cutting at the uterus–ovary junction on both sides and at the vulva level where they join. Uteri are kept in a Petri dish in DMEM + 10% FCS + 40 μg/mL gentamicin, refered as to blastocyst medium. Using a dissection microscope, blastocysts are flushed in a Petri dish from each uterus horn (at the uterus–ovary junction) by injection of 0.5 mL blastocyst medium with a syringe attached to a 25-G hypodermic needle. Uterus and needle are firmly clamped with fine forceps. After 5–10 min, blastocysts have settled down in the Petri dish and are collected using a mouth controlled glass pipet. Glass pipets (haematocrit capillaries, internal diameter 1 mm) are prepared by rotating the center of the capillary over a small gas flame and stretching both ends at the melting point to reach the desired internal diameter for collecting the blastocysts. After collection, the blastocysts are washed once in fresh blastocyst medium, then transferred to a 6-mm Petri dish precoated with feeder cells (*see* **Note 2**) and supplemented with ES culture medium (*see* **Subheading 2.2.**) + 1X nonessential AA (MEM 100X, GIBCO BRL, Cat no: 11140–035; also called embryo-ES culture medium). Dishes are placed in an incubator at 37°C and 5%CO_2. Generally 10–15 blastocysts are transferred to one Petri dish.

After 2 d in culture, and self-disruption of the zona pellucida, trophoblast cells spread over the feeder layer. ICMs begin to proliferate and form cell clusters 2–3 d later, which can be picked for disagregation. The time chosen for disagregation of ICMs is critical for establishment of a new ES cell line. There is variability in the size of the growing ICMs, so it is crucial that cells are watched and disagregation is done before an endoderm layer develops around the core of the growing ICM.

ICM can be disagregated either mechanically or after trypsination. For mechanic disruption the ICM is picked, transferred into a 5 μL drop of ES medium (*see* **Subheading 2.2.**) and passed gently several times (controlled by mouth pipetting) through a glass capillary (diameter $^1/_2$ of the ICM mass) to get clumps of 10–15 ES cells. These clumps are transferred to a single well of a 4-well culture dish (Nunc 4 × 16 mm) precoated with feeder cells in 1 mL of embryo-ES medium and reincubated. Alternatively, each ICM can be transferred in a drop of PBS first, then to a 5 μL drop of trypsin solution (For 1000 mL: NaCl 8 g, KCl 0.4 g, Glucose 1 g, $NaHCO_3$ 0.589 g, ethylenediaminotetraacetic acid (EDTA) 0.29 g, trypsin 0.5 g from Sigma type XI; T-1005). After few minutes when the cells began to lose contact with each other, 3 μL FCS are added to inactivate the trypsin and the ICM is processed as above. Both methods of disagregation were used successfully in our hands.

Cultures have to be watched every day to locate potential growing ES-like colonies. ES-like colonies can first be distinguished from non-ES colonies by their typical morphology. ES cells grow in tight colonies with clear edges, which can be recognized by their large nuclei containing one or two dark nucleoli. ES colonies also proliferate actively without differentiation compared to contaminating differentiated cells. After about 1 wk in culture, all ES-like colonies from one well are picked and treated as the ICMs. Cell suspensions from 1–5 colonies are expanded into a new well (16 mm) coated with new feeders in embryo-ES medium. This step is considered passage 1. ES cell colonies are shown in **Fig. 2A.**

Isolation of new ES cell lines (especially from mouse strains other than 129SV) needs some practice with ES cell handling, but success is also largely dependent on the quality of the serum (*see* **Note 1**) and feeder cells. Putative ES cell lines are then further characterized by genotyping, karyotyping, and by testing their capability to colonize the germ-line after microinjection into mouse blastocysts (*see* below).

2.2. Culture Conditions

ES cell culture requires the cytokine Leukemia Inhibitory Factor (LIF) to maintain their proliferating undifferentiated state *(42,43)*. LIF can be provided by culturing ES cells on feeder cells. Alternatively, some ES cell lines have been adapted to feeder-free conditions, providing the addition of exogenous recombinant LIF to the culture medium *(44)*. It seems, however, that ES cells derived from mouse blastocysts cultured in absence of feeder cells contain higher number of cells with aneuploïd karyotypes *(44)*. Also, in our laboratory, we have observed that the contribution of ES cell lines to the germ line is considerably impaired in feeder-free culture of ES cells. Accordingly, we grow our ES cell lines on feeders and, in addition, we add recombinant LIF to our ES culture medium to minimize variations in the quality of the different feeder preparations.

Therefore, to establish new ES cell lines and to run standard ES culture, we typically grow cells on feeder cells-coated dishes using the following medium (ES culture medium):

1. Dulbecco's Modified Eagle's Medium (DMEM) high glucose (Invitrogen Cat no. 31966-021).
2. 10% Fetal calf serum (FCS tested batch; *see* **Note 1**)
3. 40 µg/mL gentamicin (sulphate)
4. 0.1 mM β-mercaptoethanol (Sigma, Cat. no. M 7522)
5. 500–1000 U/mL LIF (recombinant LIF prepared from transfected COS cells)

The preparation of feeder cells and LIF are detailed in **Notes 2** and **3.** In our hands, optimal growth is obtained on Falcon plastic dishes, and particularly on 6-cm dishes.

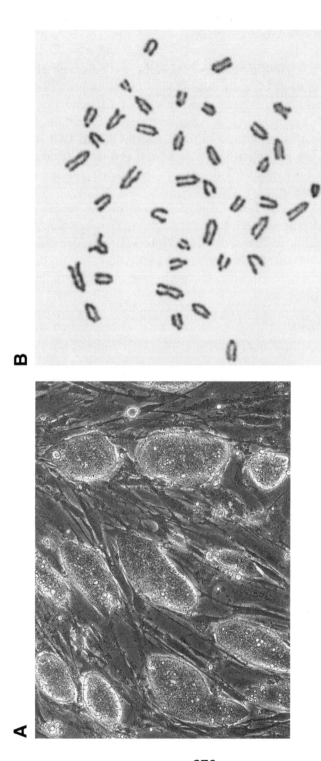

Fig. 2. Preparation of ES cells. (A) Embryonic stem cells in optimal culture conditions. The ES clumps are growing on a feeder layer of inactivated mouse fibroblasts. (B) Chromosome spread of 40 chromosomes from a male ES cell line after Giemsa staining. Magnification 100X. Bar = 100 μm.

2.3. Freezing and Thawing ES Cells

For freezing, ES cultures should be at about 70% confluency. Medium is changed 2–3 h before freezing. ES cells are washed and trypsinised as described above. Freezing medium (90% FCS + 10% dimethyl sulfoxide [DMSO]) is added to the cell pellet, which is gently resuspended and transferred in cryovials. ES cells are frozen at 1–5 × 10^6 cells/mL freezing medium. Cryovials are placed into a styrofoam box at –80°C. Next day, cryovials are transferred into a liquid nitrogen container for long-term storage.

For thawing, the content of the cryotube is quickly thawed in a water-bath at 37°C, cells resuspended in ES cell medium to dilute DMSO, and centrifuged. Pellet is resuspended in ES culture medium and plated on feeder-coated dishes or plates, at a density corresponding to the freezing density.

2.4. Characterization of the ES Cell Lines

Karyotype is done according to Robertson (45) for newly established ES cell lines to identify cells that have an euploid karyotype and are preferably male. Karyotype is also done later for each targeted ES clone before microinjection (*see* **Subheadig 3.4.**), because long manipulations of ES cells in vitro are favorable to mutations. Routinely we count the modal number of chromosomes (40 chromosomes in mice), a method that seems sufficient to detect loss or gain of chromosomes and any translocations. Briefly, ES cells are grown on a 6-cm Petri dish without feeders in ES medium and used at an exponentially growing state (24 h after subculture on average). Culture medium is changed 3 h before processing. Colcemid (Sigma D-1925, 10 µg/mL) is added to each dish at a final concentration of 2 µL/mL of culture medium and the cells incubated for 2–3 h. Cells are harvested as for standard culture and collected in a 15-mL conical tube. After centrifugation 3 min at 200*g,* the pellet is resuspended by adding dropwise 2 mL of hypotonic KCl (0.56% w/v), completed to 6 mL with hypotonic KCl and mixed by inverting the tube. Cells are kept 20 min at room temperature for swelling. Six drops of freshly prepared fixative (3 vol absolute methanol/1 vol glacial acetic acid) are added with a Pasteur pipet and cells are pelleted 5 min at 200g. The pellet is resuspended by adding again the fixative dropwise (6 mL) under gentle stirring to avoid clump formation and let stand 10 min at room temperature. This treatment is repeated three times. The final pellet is resuspended as a single-cell population into 0.5–1 mL of freshly prepared fixative solution depending on the pellet size. Pellets of cells can be kept at –20°C and spread later on.

Spreading of the cells is done on microscope slides, cleaned by 70% ethanol or also in fixative before use. Slides are put onto a grid over a water bath at 55°C, and 3 drops of cell suspension are deposited on the slide using a Pasteur pipet.

The drops spread over the slide and the fixative evaporates. We verify the quality of the chromosomes spreads under microscope and prepare an average of six to eight slides for one karyotype. The mitotic spreads are then stained by immersing (10–15 min) the slides in a 3% (vol/vol) Giemsa stain solution in phosphate-buffered saline (PBS) and then rinsed several times in distillate water and dried. Analysis and counting of the chromosomes of the mitotic spreads are processed using a computer program (IKAROS, Meta System). **Figure 2B** shows result from a typical ES cell karyotype. Normal karyotype is a good indication, although not a guarantee, for successful germ-line transmission.

The Y chromosome is characterized by its size (one of the three smallest chromosome in mouse). It can also be confirmed by polymerase chain reaction (PCR) analysis and we generally genotype our new established ES cell lines by a Y-chromosome-specific PCR reaction *(46)*. Genomic DNA prepared from ES cells cultured in feeder-free conditions is isolated. A 102 bp region of the Y chromosome is amplified using the following PCR conditions: DNA (100 ng) is incubated with a forward primer (5′ GAATTCATATATATGACAGAGGCA 3′), a reverse primer (5′ CCATTCCCTTCAAATATCATACT 3′) 100 pM each in 50 mM KCl, 10 mM Tris-HCl, pH 8.3, 1.5 mM MgCl$_2$, 0.2 mM dNTPs, and 1 U of Taq polymerase for 1 min at 94°C (denaturing), 2 min at 50°C (annealing), 3 min at 72°C (extension). After 35 cycles, samples are held 10 min at 72°C and cooled. PCR products are separated on a 2% agarose gel prestained with ethidium bromide to verify the presence of the 102 bp band.

3. Methods

3.1. Step 1: Gene Cloning and Modification

3.1.1. General Methods

Different types of vectors for gene targeting have been developed, essentially replacement and insertion vectors, which differ by the mechanism of integration and targeting efficiencies. The design of such targeting vectors has been exhaustively described (*see* **refs.** [*47–52*]). Here we report targeting constructs that we have used to generate mice lacking opioid receptors, as examples. Gene cloning techniques used to produce the constructs are classical molecular biology methods and will not be detailed here (e.g., *see* **ref.** *53*).

3.1.2. Opioid Receptor Gene Targeting Constructs

The targeting construct should first present a strong perturbation of the coding region to render the gene nonfunctional. This is achieved by insertion of the neomycin resistance gene (Neo) at a critical location (targeted region). Second, the construct should contain long portions of chromosomal homologous DNA (ideally a minimum of 3000 base pairs) upstream and downstream the site of

Neo insertion to favor homologous recombination. Targeting constructs that we have used to inactivate μ (MOR), κ (KOR), and δ (DOR) opioid receptor genes are schematized on **Fig. 3.**

Opioid receptors are G protein-coupled receptors with a seven-transmembrane topology. MOR, KOR, and DOR genes display a highly similar genomic organization, with coding regions spanning three (DOR and KOR) or four (MOR) exons, and splice junctions located at conserved positions downstream the encoded transmembrane domains I and IV *(54)*. To create the MOR targeting construct, we first cloned a 6.8 kb SalI/SpeI genomic fragment containing exon 2 and 3 from a SvPas 129 mouse genomic library. It is important that genomic DNA isolated to create the targeted construct is isogenic (i.e., same mouse substrain) to the ES cell genome *(55,56)*. Similarly, for the KOR construct, we have isolated a large BamHI genomic fragment containing exon 1, and to target the DOR gene we have cloned a 8.5 kb SacI/EcoRI genomic fragment harboring exon 1.

Perturbation of the coding region is achieved by insertion of an antibiotic-resistance gene. We routinely use either Neo *(57)* or Hygro *(58)* cassettes, i.e., transgenes encoding resistance to neomycin or hygromycine, respectively, under the control of the phosphoglycerate kinase (Pgk-1) promoter. For MOR, we inserted the Neo cassette into a unique BamHI restriction site located in exon 2 of the cloned DNA fragment. This mutation introduces a STOP codon into the encoded first intracellular loop of the μ receptor, leading to a truncated and presumably inactive protein. For both KOR and DOR constructs, exon 1 was excised by a SmaI digestion and replaced by Neo. The correct production of receptor proteins is presumed impossible from these mutated DNA portions, because both exon 1 contain the START translation codon necessary for receptor expression.

In the final constructs, 5′ homologous regions were 5.1 kb, 1.3 kb, and 1.2 kb in size and 3′ homologous regions were 1.7 kb, 5.2 kb, and 6.4 kb, for MOR, KOR, and DOR, respectively. Although at least one homologous arm was shorter than 3 kb for each of the constructs, homologous recombination occurred and positive ES cells were isolated. Targeting frequencies using these constructs varied largely. About 10% of neomycin-resistant ES clones showed the mutated locus in the case of MOR targeting *(26,56)*, whereas only 1 over 50 neomycin-resistant ES clones was positive for KOR *(27)* and 1 over 350 for DOR (28). Homologous recombination frequencies not only depend on the length of homologous sequences *(59)*, but also rely on specific DNA sequences of targeted loci and the occurrence of numerous DNA repeats at the exon 1 DOR locus seemed unfavorable. For all three constructs, the targeting strategy was successful because a complete absence of μ *(26,60)*, κ *(27,61)*, and δ *(28,62)* opioid receptors was demonstrated in the brain of resulting homozygous mutant mice.

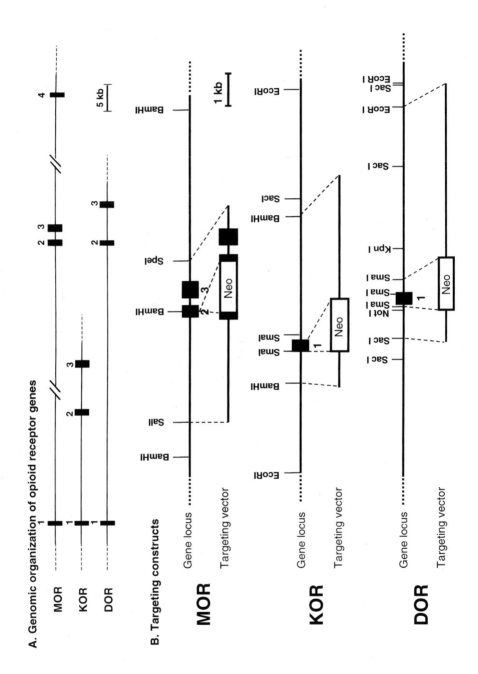

A. Genomic organization of opioid receptor genes

B. Targeting constructs

←

Fig. 3. Examples of targeting constructs used to inactivate opioid receptor genes. (**A**) The coding regions of opioid receptor genes are distributed over three (KOR and DOR) or four (MOR) exons. Splicing between exon 1 and 2, as well as 2 and 3 occurs at conserved positions corresponding to the first intracellular and second extracellular loops of the seven-transmembrane spanning proteins. The KOR gene is the smallest, whereas the MOR gene is over 53 kb in length. (**B**) Strategies for gene inactivation. Targeting constructs (bottom) are represented with their corresponding wild-type loci (top), with dashed lines indicating homologous regions. Introns are shown as solid lines, exons are numbered and represented by black boxes. The Neo cassette is shown as a white box. For MOR the Neo gene was inserted into exon 2 leading to a frame shift (MOR). For KOR and DOR genes, exon 1 was deleted and replaced by the Neo gene, preventing correct initiation of protein translation.

Once cloning steps to construct the targeting vector are completed, the plasmidic DNA is amplified using the XL1-Blue *Escherichia Coli* strain and purified using a Qiagen Plasmid Maxikit (Cat no. 12163). DNA (about 20 µg) is linearized using a unique restriction site located in the plasmidic part of the construct and complete linearization is verified by agarose electrophoresis. The digestion mixture is phenol/chloroform extracted and the DNA purified by EtOH precipitation. The DNA pellet is resuspended in sterile water at a 1 mg/mL concentration for gene transfer.

3.2. Step 2: Gene Transfer into ES Cells

The pluripotent stem cells are prepared as described in the Materials section. The targeting construct is transferred into the cells and cellular clones that have integrated the transgene either randomly (heterologous recombination) or at the locus (homologous recombination) are selected in the presence of antibiotic. It is critical that ES cells remain undifferentiated along DNA transfer, antibiotic selection, amplification, and genotyping, for successful colonization of the germ line.

3.2.1. Transfection

ES cells are electroporated at an exponentially growing phase. Maximal homologous recombination is obtained in the S phase of the cell cycle. The ES cells (low passage number: 10–13) are plated onto 6-cm dishes and subcultured 24 h to 48 h (depending of the division rate of the ES cell line) before electroporation. Medium is changed 3 h before harvesting the cells. ES cells are trypsinised (1 mL/dish) and after trypsin inactivation with 1 mL of ES culture medium, gently dissociated with a pipet to get a single-cell suspension. The cells are centrifuged 2 min at 200*g* and the pellet is resuspended in ES culture medium as a single-cell suspension at a density of 10^7 cells/0.5 mL. Cells are distributed in Bio-Rad cuvets (0.5 mL suspension/cuvet). For each cuvet, 10 μg of linearized targeting vector (1 mg/mL) is added to the cell suspension and a single pulse 400 V/250 μF at room temperature is delivered with a Bio-Rad gene pulser. Approximately 50% cell death is expected for optimal electroporation efficiency. After electroporation, each cuvet is maintained 10 min at room temperature and then cells are resuspended in 50 mL ES medium and plated onto five dishes (10 cm)/cuvet, coated with feeders. Importantly neomycine- or hygromycine-resistant feeder cells need to be used, depending on selectable gene cloned in the targeting vector. These are prepared from Neo+ or Hygro+ genetically modified embryos available in the laboratory. Culture medium is changed the next day. Selection against the selectable marker gene is performed using ES medium complemented with 150 μg/mL antibiotic. Selection is started 48 h after electroporation and maintained for 8–10 d, until resistant clones have reached a suitable size for being picked. Selection culture medium is daily changed in order to remove dead ES cells.

3.2.2. Picking and Amplification of Resistant Clones

Before picking, culture dishes are rinsed once with PBS and then overlaid with PBS to prevent from drying out. The resistant colonies are picked using a stereomicroscope and transferred individually into separate wells from V-shaped 96-well plates containing 50 μL of trypsin solution. The colonies are pipetted up and down several times for dissociation. Ten min later, 150 μL of ES medium is added to stop trypsin action and the cell suspensions are transferred again individually into 48-well plates coated with feeders. Plates are incubated at 37°C. We usually pick 384 colonies for one targeting experiment (eight 48-well plates).

The culture medium is changed every day. When cells reach 80% confluence, they are split into two new 48-well plates, one coated with feeders to make frozen stocks and one coated with gelatine (0.1%) for DNA preparation and genotyping.

To successfully freeze ES cells directly in the plates, most cell clones should be at a 80–90% confluency. The culture medium of each well is aspirated and cells are rinsed with PBS followed by treatment with 100 μL trypsin solution for 5 min. Freezing solution A (DMEM 70% + FCS 30%) is added to the cells (100 μL), to dilute the trypsin, and cells are resuspended several times. Freezing solution B (DMEM 50% + FCS 30% + DMSO 20%) is then added (200 μL) and the suspension is homogenized again. The culture plate is wrapped with tape and placed into a sealed plastic bag. Plates are then placed into a styrofoam box and stored at –80°C until the clones have been genotyped.

For genomic DNA preparations, the ES colonies are transferred into 24-well plates until near confluence, washed once with PBS, and 500 μL lysis buffer (Tris-HCl, pH 7.5, 50 m*M,* EDTA 5 m*M,* SDS 1%, NaCl 200 m*M*) is directly added into each well. At this stage, plates can be stored at –20°C until DNA analysis is completed, or immediately processed.

3.3. Step 3: ES Cell Genotyping for the MOR Gene Null Mutation

Genotyping aims at screening antibiotic-resistant ES clones to search for cellular clones where homologous recombination has occurred. Genomic DNA is prepared from each ES clone and the analysis of the gene locus is performed either by PCR or Southern blotting according to classical techniques, as described in molecular biology handbooks (see for example **ref. 53**.)

3.3.1. DNA Preparation

Proteinase K (20 mg/mL stock solution) is added to each well (5 μL/well) containing ES cells in lysis buffer (*see* above) and incubation of the 24-well plates is performed overnight at 37°C with gentle agitation. DNA is precipitated by adding 500 μL isopropanol/well and shaking the plate for 15 min. The DNA precipitate is then transferred into 500 μL EtOH 70% and spun for 5 min at 10,000*g* and 4°C. The DNA pellet is air-dried, resuspended in 50 μL 10 m*M,* Tris-HCl, pH 8.0, 1 m*M* EDTA, and heated at 65°C for 5 h for complete dissolution. Typically 5 μg to 20 μg genomic DNA is obtained from each well, and half of the DNA preparation (25 μL) is used for Southern-blot analysis.

3.3.2. Screening by Southern Blot

Southern blotting is the most currently used method to screen for and then confirm the targeting event. The strategy designed to detect homologous recombination at the MOR locus is schematized on **Fig. 4A.** First, unique restriction sites flanking the targeted MOR genomic region have been identified previously by mapping (**step** 1) and the size-specific restriction fragments obtained from wild-type or mutant genome can be predicted. Second, to ensure that the targeting construct is accurately inserted into the locus, i.e., exactly replaces the wild-type region, detection of restriction fragments should be performed using DNA probes located outside the targeting construct portion itself ("external probes"). Using an upstream probe (5′ probe) will confirm correct insertion of the targeting vector at its 5′ end, whereas a downstream probe (3′ probe) will do so at the 3′ end of the vector.

In **Fig. 4A** we show a typical genotyping experiment using a 5′ probe. The genomic DNA (about 10 μg) is digested using the enzyme BamHI, DNA fragments are size-resolved by electrophoresis on a 0.7% agarose gel and transferred

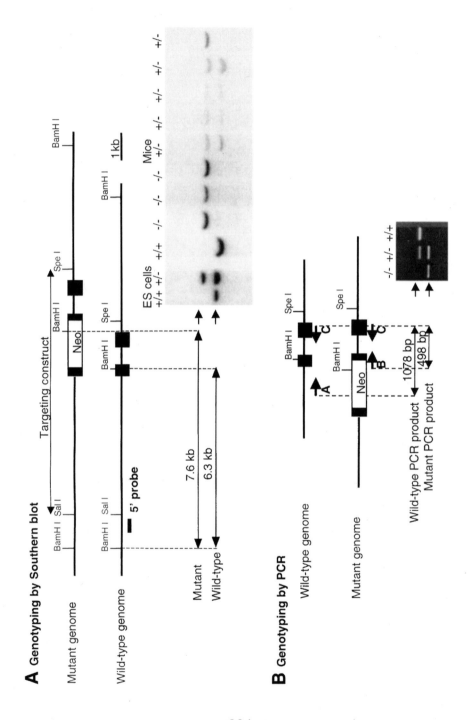

A Genotyping by Southern blot

Targeting construct

Mutant genome

BamH I   Sal I   BamH I   Spe I   BamH I   BamH I
                                   Neo

Wild-type genome

BamH I   Sal I   Spe I   BamH I   BamH I

5' probe

1kb

            ES cells   Mice
+/+ +/- +/+ -/- -/- -/- +/- +/- +/- +/- +/- +/- +/-

Mutant   7.6 kb
Wild-type 6.3 kb

B Genotyping by PCR

Wild-type genome

BamH I   Spe I
                A   B   C

Mutant genome

BamH I   Spe I
          Neo   C

Wild-type PCR product   1078 bp
Mutant PCR product   498 bp

-/- +/- +/+

284

Fig. 4. Examples of genotyping experiments following MOR gene targeting. (**A**) In the Southern-blot procedure, genomic DNA is digested using BamHI, DNA is size-resolved by electrophoresis on agarose gel, blotted onto a nylon membrane and probed with the 5′ P^{32}-labeled probe to reveal wild-type and mutant alleles. Representative experiments are shown for ES cell genotyping (*see* **Subheading 3.3.**) and F1 inter-breeding offspring (*see* **Subheading 3.5.**). Similar experiments are performed using a 3′ and a Neo probe to fully confirm homologous recombination. (**B**) A simpler PCR procedure is used for mouse genotyping when mutant mice colonies are established. Primer pairs specifically amplify a 1078 bp fragment from the wild-type allele (A and C) and a 498 bp fragment from the mutant allele (B and C).

onto a nylon membrane. A 5′ DNA probe (classically 500 bp in size) is generated by PCR from the BamHI-SalI region, which is located upstream the SalI-SpEI region corresponding to the targeting construct (*see* **Fig. 4A**).

The probe is radiolabeled using ^{32}P-labeled dCTP in a random priming procedure, and hybridized to the nylon membrane. After washing under stringent conditions, the membrane is exposed to a X-ray film to reveal BamHI fragments hybridized to the probe. In our example, a 6.3 kb band is expected from a wild-type allele, whereas a 7.6 kb band should be labeled on the mutant allele. Most ES clones show the 6.3 kb band only (random integration), whereas a positive ES clone shows both 6.3 kb and 7.6 kb bands (integration at the targeted locus, heterozygous genotype). The same genotyping protocol is later applied to mouse tail biopsies (*see* **Subheading 3.5.**). The genotyping profile for a negative (+/+) and a positive (+/−) ES cell clone is shown on **Fig. 4A,** together with a representative genotyping experiment of an offspring obtained from F1 heterozygous mice interbreeding (*see* **Subheading 3.5.**).

Screening several hundred ES cell clones is performed using one external probe. When positive ES cells are identified, it is important that a similar strategy is applied using the other external probe (3′ in our example) on the ES candidate clones, to confirm correct insertion of the construct at both ends (not shown). Finally, Southern blotting should also be performed using a fragment of the antibiotic-resistance gene as a probe, as a second confirmation of accurate vector integration, and to verify that no other construct has been inserted randomly elsewhere in the genome (not shown). Using the Neo probe, negative ES clones typically show one or several bands of variable size (random integration(s)). In contrast, a genuine positive clone should display one band only and at the predicted size (7.6 kb in our example for BamHI digested genomic DNA hybridized with probe consisting of a 5′ portion of the Neo gene; *see* **Fig. 4A**).

After the screening step, therefore, positive mutant ES cell clones are re-amplified for complete genomic analysis.

3.3.3. Positive ES Cell Amplification

The plate with positive-targeted ES colonies is placed in an incubator at 37°C, and the cell suspension of one well is transferred into a sterile tube containing 5 mL ES medium and centrifuged 3 min at 200*g*. The pellet is resuspended in 0.5 mL ES culture medium and plated onto a new well of the same size coated with new feeders. The ES cells are then subcultured and expanded in 6-cm dishes. The amplified cells are also karyotyped to verify correct number of chromosomes (*see* **Subheading 2.4.**), and frozen for storage in liquid nitrogen. Finally some of the cells are injected into mouse blastocysts for germ-line transmission (*see* **Subheading 3.4.**).

3.4. Step 4: Mutant ES Cell Injection into Blastocysts

The genetically modified ES cells are now introduced into embryos and participate in creating a novel mouse. There are several methods to transfer ES cells into embryos and general guidelines are provided to the reader, with appropriate references.

3.4.1. The Mutant ES Cell

Most ES cell lines used for gene targeting are derived from 129 substrains (agouti or light-colored mice). After in vitro manipulation (*see* above), these cell lines are injected into blastocysts of mice from another strain and pigmentation, giving rise to chimeric mice. Coat color of live-born pups is our eyewitness for the contribution of mutant ES cells to development of the animal. The presence of light-colored regions is a good indication that mutant ES cells indeed have contributed to forming the animal. It is hoped that some of the ES cells have produced germ cells. When more than 75% of injected blastocysts produce chimeric animals, the majority of them are later found able to transmit the mutation to their offspring (germ-line chimera). In our laboratory, all ES cell lines were derived from the 129 SvPas mouse substrain. When prepared as described in **Subheading 2.**, these cells were found to contribute to the germ-line even after 30–40 passages in vitro.

ES cells for microinjection are prepared as follows: cells are plated 1 d before microinjection onto Petri dishes coated with gelatine without feeders. The next day cells are trypsinized as usual. After centrifugation, the pellet is washed once in PBS and centrifuged again. The final pellet is suspended in a small volume (20 µL for a 3-cm dish) of blastocyst injection medium (DMEM HEPES modified Sigma D 6171 + 10% FCS + 40 µg/mL gentamicin). After appropriate dilution, 10–15 ES cells are injected per recipient blastocyst.

3.4.2. The Recipient Blastocysts

Chimeric mice can be obtained either by injection of ES cells into blastocyst or by morula aggregation with ES cell clumps.

Different mouse strains—BALB/c, CD1, MF1, NMRI, C57BL/6—were tested as recipient blastocysts. Injection of ES cells into C57BL/6 blastocysts gave highest frequencies of germ-line chimeras both in our laboratory and others *(63–66)*.

For blastocyst injection, recipient blastocysts are isolated as for establishment of a new ES cell line (*see* **Subheading 2.1.**). We favor natural mating with the C57BL/6 females because superovulation in our hands does not increase the yield of blastocyst collection. Natural mating is under the control of the light cycles in the animal facility: 12 h light and 12 h dark. We obtain 4–5 blastocyst/female on average. Before microinjection, blastocysts are maintained in ES cell-culture medium without LIF.

3.4.3. Microinjection

Microinjection conditions and transfer of the manipulated embryos in recipient foster mothers have been exhaustively described *(67,68)* and will not be detailed here. Chimeras can also be obtained by injection into morula *(69)*. The procedure of injection is identical to that of blastocyst injection. In our hand, assays using this technique does not increase the yield of obtention of germ-line chimeras. Finally, ES cells can be aggregated with 8-cell stage embryos in vitro *(70,71)*. This methods does not need any sophisticated injection apparatus and is relatively easy to be applied, but has been successful for only few ES cell lines in our hands.

Chimeric mice have an agouti (129 Sv)/black (C57BL/6) coat color. The chimerism becomes apparent 1 wk after birth. Extent of chimerism can be extremely variable, from some agouti patches to nearly an entire agouti coat.

3.5. Step 5: Breeding

3.5.1. The F1 Generation

Germ-line transmission is tested by mating the chimeric mice (129 Sv-C57BL/6) with C57BL/6 mice. Preferably chimeric males are used because mating with several wild-type C57BL/6 females allows generating numerous F1 animals. Agouti is dominant to black. Black F1 pups are not tested for genotype, because this color indicates that only C57Bl/6 (i.e., nonmutant) cells contributed to mouse development, suggesting that both male and female germ cells are wild-type. Agouti F1 animals are analyzed and, typically, 50% animals on average harvest the targeted mutation. Breeding is performed in a standard animal facility with 12 h dark-light cycles and food at libitum.

3.5.2. F1 and Mouse Genotyping

Agouti chimera offsprings are analyzed for germ-line transmission. Genomic DNA is prepared from mouse tail biopsies about 3 wk after birth. Typically, a small portion of mouse tail (1 cm) is cut and transferred into 500 μL lysis buffer (Tris-HCl, pH 8.5, 100 mM, EDTA 5 mM, sodium dodecylsulfate (SDS) 0.2%, NaCl 200 mM, with proteinase K 300 μg/mL) and incubated at 55°C for 3–4 h. After vigourous shaking, the mixture is spun down for 10 min at 10,000g. The supernatant is transferred into 500 μL isopropanol and let stand for 5 min at 4°C until genomic DNA precipitation is completed. The DNA precipitate is manually picked, transferred into 500 μL EtOH 70%, pelleted by centrifugation for 10 min at 10,000g, and air-dried. The pellet is resuspended in 100 μL 10 mM, Tris-HCl, pH 8.0, 1 mM EDTA, for 2 h at 65°C.

DNA is first analyzed by Southern blot, using a protocol identical to that used for ES cell genotyping (*see* **Subheading 3.3.** and **Fig. 4A**). Once heterozygous animals have been identified and confirmed using both 3′ and 5′ external probes, further routine genotyping of F2 mice is performed using the PCR. This simpler and faster procedure (about 4 h total) allows analysis of a limited portion of the genome, and usually does not extend beyond the targeted region owing to limitations in the size of PCR products. For this reason, we use PCR genotyping only when correct targeting has been established by Southern analysis for F1 and F2 animals. Sets of specific oligonucleotide primers framing the targeted locus are synthesized, based on known genomic sequences, and designed to amplify regions that differ in size in wild-type and mutant alleles.

The PCR strategy for routine genotyping of our established MOR mutant colonies is shown in **Fig. 4B.** In our example, a common reverse primer (primer C) hybridizes to both wild-type and mutant alleles. Two forward primers are used. Primer A hybridizes to both alleles, whereas primer B (Neo sequence) hybridizes to the mutant allele only. When the three primers are mixed to genomic DNA, the PCR reaction typically yields a 1078 bp fragment from the wild-type genome (primers A and C) and a 498 bp fragment from the mutant genome (primers B and C). A typical genotyping profile from wild-type, heterozygous, and homozygous mutant DNA is shown. A 2700 bp band is also generated from the hybridization of A and C on the mutant allele, but the yield of this PCR product is lower than that of the 498 bp product and this fragment is rarely visible under our standard experimental conditions.

Each PCR reaction needs to be optimized, depending on the gene sequence and primers. As an example, for genotyping our MOR mutant animals we proceed as follows: 1 μL of genomic DNA solution (as prepared above) is incubated with primer A (5′ GGA CAT GGA TGT GCC TAT GAT GTG 3′, 0.25 μM), primer B (5′ ACC GCT TCC TCG TGC TTT ACG GTA 3′, 0.25 μM), primer C (5′ GTG GTC AAG TCT GAC ATT CAT GG 3′, 0.5 μM), dNTPs

(0.2 mM each), MgCl$_2$ 1.5 mM, standard PCR buffer (provided by the Enzyme supplier) and 1 U Taq Polymerase in a total volume of 50 μL. PCR is performed for 30 cycles, 1 min at 94°C, 1 min at 62°C, 1 min at 72°C. The PCR product is analyzed by electrophoresis on 1% agarose gel. Results are shown in **Fig. 4B.**

3.6. Step 6: Mouse Phenotyping in Pain Models

As for most behavioral models, paradigms to assess pain responses have been historically developed in rats. Behavioral nociceptive assays are now progressively applied to mice owing to the rapidly growing number of transgenic and knockout mouse models and availability of inbred mouse strains for quantitative trait loci mapping, associated with practical considerations such as fast and less expensive breeding. The diversity of pain tests validated in mice is expanding rapidly. Because behavioral models of pain are largely described in other chapters of this book, we will simply overview here phenotyping procedures that have been successful in assessing pain responses in knockout mice.

Experimental conditions to apply thermal, mechanical, and electrical stimulations have been set and several tests to assess pain sensitivity have been validated in mice *(7,72)*. Along general phenotyping screens, the tail-flick and the hot-plate tests (noxious heat) or measurements of responses to mild electric footshocks, are currently incorporated into sensory-ability testing sessions to evaluate pain sensitivity in large numbers of mutant mice *(72)*. When modifications of pain responses are detected, or expected from knowledge of the targeted gene, the battery of pain tests is broadened. The Hargreaves test (thermal pain; *see* Chapter 2), the formalin test (chemical pain; *see* Chapter 3), the tail pressure or the application of von Frey hairs (mechanical) can also be used (*see* description in **ref. 7**). Advantages/disadvantages of each applied noxious stimulus, as well as considerations such as handling, habituation, stimulus intensity, repeated testing, or end-point choice in mice have been discussed by Wilson and Mogil *(73)*.

Pain thresholds first evaluate responses to acute noxious stimulation. Modifications of pain thresholds in knockout mice suggest a possible role of targeted genes in "physiological" pain or normal pain perception. Pain thresholds are also used as end-point measurements to evaluate hyperalgesia and allodynia, which may develop in pathological pain states. Several behavioral models for inflammatory and neuropathic pain have been successfully applied to knockout mice. These include the Seltzer partial sciatic nerve ligation *(74)*; the Chung spinal nerve ligation (*see* **ref. 25** and Chapter 4); formalin, capsaicin, or PGE$_2$-evoked inflammation (*see* **ref. 18** and Chapter 3); and bladder inflammation *(75)*. Other models of inflammation have used Complete Freund Adjuvant (CFA) *(76)* or carrageenan *(77)*. A number of examples now exist in the literature and we believe that many more will follow.

Finally, in pain models as for other behaviors, issues related to the background genotype of mutant mice should be considered. F2 mutant mice generated from chimeras are most often 50% 129 and 50% C57BL/6 hybrids whose parental strains differ largely in nociceptive and analgesic responses *(78)*. It is therefore recommended to backcross F2 animals for at least 10 generations on a specific background to obtain mutant animals with a so-called "pure" genetic background *(79)* and reduce interindividual variability. Also, differences in experimental conditions and laboratory environments can significantly influence the phenotype *(80)* and efforts should be made to standardize experimental conditions to allow cross-laboratory and cross-mutant strain comparisons. Only under those conditions will the knockout approach be fully exploitable to identify genes and their interactions in pain research.

To illustrate phenotyping of knockout animals using pain models, **Fig. 5** shows the complete lack of morphine analgesia in the MOR-deficient mice that we generated using the construct presented in **Fig. 3.** These experiments used the tail-immersion test and the hot-plate test and demonstrated that mu receptors represent the molecular target for morphine analgesia in vivo *(26)*. Similarly, U-50488H, a prototypical kappa agonist did not produce analgesia in KOR-deficient mice, indicating high kappa selectivity of this compound in vivo *(27)*. Finally, DOR- and KOR-deficient mice were exposed to a number of distinct acute noxious stimuli. All tested thresholds were unchanged in the DOR mutant, suggesting that delta receptors are not important in the perception of acute pain, or that the absence of delta receptors in the knockout animals has been compensated by unknown mechanisms *(28)*. In contrast, enhanced number of abdominal contractions in response to peritoneal acetic-acid injections in KOR mutant mice showed a clear tonic implication of kappa systems in the perception of chemical visceral pain *(27)*. Together, mice lacking opioid receptors have been and will be instrumental in revisiting the molecular targets of clinically relevant opiates, as well as opiates to be developed in the future. These mice will also allow researchers to examine involvement of the endogenous system in pain and other opioid-controlled behaviors.

4. Notes

Here we describe key features that have greatly contributed to our success in the manipulation of ES cells and production of mutated animals. These are the serum quality for ES cell preparation and culture, as well as feeder cells and LIF that we use to maintain ES cell undifferentiated.

1. Serum Tests for ES Cultures. A critical point in the establishment of ES cell lines, as well as in ES cell culture, is the quality of the fetal calf serum (FCS) used. It is absolutely necessary to test different batches, to select the best one, and then to use

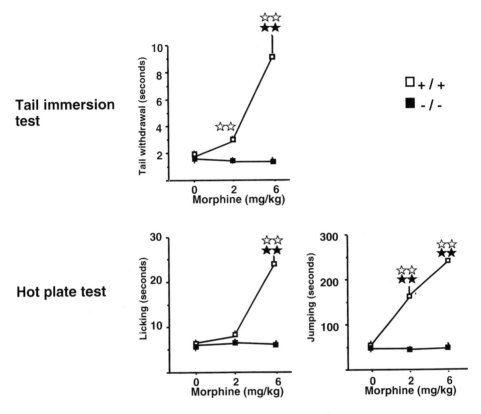

Tail immersion test

Hot plate test

Fig. 5. Morphine analgesia in mice lacking the MOR gene. Antinociceptive responses to thermal pain are shown using two models. In the tail-immersion test, tail withdrawal latencies are indicated. In the hot-plate test, both of licking and jumping latencies are measured. Subcutaneous injections of morphine dose-dependently increase tail withdrawal, licking, and jumping latencies in wild-type animals, but not in MOR homozygous mutants. Black stars indicate significant treatment effect (morphine analgesia) and white stars show a significant difference between wild-type and mutant mice ($p > 0.01$). Data adapted with permission from **ref. 26**.

the selected one for 1–2 yr without changing culture conditions. Sera can be stored frozen at –20°C for 2–3 yr.

To select the best batch of FCS, we first perform a colony-forming assay to determine the number of ES colonies growing in each batch following plating as a single-cell suspension. Two to three hundred ES cells are plated onto squared 6-cm dishes coated with feeders. Each assay is duplicated for each batch under test, the current FCS batch used as a control. After 1 wk in culture, medium being changed every other day, the ES cell colonies formed are counted under a stereomicroscope. For easier counting, the ES colonies can be stained for 5 min with a 2% methylene blue solution, washed several times with distillate water, and air-dried. A serum is considered good if 40% of the plated cells form colonies (i.e., plating efficiency is 40%). FCS batches are tested at three different concentrations 10 or 15% (usual concentrations where the ES cells are cultured), as well as 30% to test toxicity. This latter concentration permits also to select one batch among several batches giving similar results at the 10 or 15% concentrations. The plating efficiency has to be the same at 10 or 15% and 30% FCS.

To further test the selected sera after this first screen, ES cells are further cultured both with or without feeders in parallel, for two to three passages using standard ES cell culture conditions (medium and density; *see* **Subheading 2.2.**). The typical morphology of the undifferentiated ES cells should be maintained for at least two passages even in the absence of feeder cells.

The ultimate test in our laboratory before definitive choice of FCS batch is an assay of differentiation of the ES cells to cardiomyocytes *(81)*. In short, ES cells are cultured for one passage without feeders, and then approx 10^6 ES cells are grown in a 10-cm (hydrophobic) Petri dish in ES medium supplemented with 20% FCS and without LIF. Under these conditions, the ES cells aggregate and give rise to floating embryonic bodies of different sizes. Medium is changed every other day (be careful: do not aspirate the embryonic bodies). After 8 d using these culture conditions, contractile areas of cardiomyocytes should appear in the embryonic bodies. This last test is not time-consuming and reflects the good quality of a FCS batch.

2. Feeder cell preparation. Feeders are mitotically arrested primary mouse embryonic fibroblasts (MEFs). Inactivation of division can be done either by mitomycin-C treatment or X-ray irradiation. In our laboratory, we use mitomycin treatment, because no source for irradiation is available. Genetic background of the embryo does not seem important for the feeder effect.

Mouse embryos are isolated from uteri of females at 13.5 or 14.5 d.p.c. With fine forceps, the placenta, amnion, and yolk sac are removed. Embryos are washed two times in PBS to eliminate as much blood as possible. Head, liver, heart, and intestine are discarded and the carcasses washed one time in PBS. Embryos (10–12) are minced into small pieces in 1–2 mL of PBS, and incubated in 50 mL of trypsin solution in an Erlenmeyer flask containing sterile small glass beads for 30 min at 37°C under gentle agitation on a magnet stirrer. During this time, if the solution becomes viscous, add 100 µL of concentrated crude DNAase solution 10 mg/mL (sterile-filtered). After adding 50 mL of trypsin solution a second time for 30 min at 37°C, trypsin action is stopped by adding 5 mL of FCS and the cell suspension is poured over a sieve (48 µm Falcon: 352340) into 50-mL tubes (Falcon) and centrifuged 5 min at 200g. Viable cells are resuspended in fibroblast medium (DMEM + 5% FCS + 40 µg/mL gentamicin), counted and plated onto 15-cm Petri dishes at 5×10^6 cells/plate. From 10 embryos, we expect 5×10^7–10^8 cells. Fibroblasts are then expanded for 5 d. At this state, the cells can be either frozen (1P15/cryovial) and stored in liquid nitrogen until further use, or used as feeder cells immediately.

To be used as feeder cells, primary fibroblasts are further cultured, split at no more than 1 to 5. After two or three passages, fibroblasts are treated for 2 h 45 min with 10 μg/mL mitomycin-C (Sigma M-0503). After mitomycin treatment, feeder cells are washed twice with PBS, collected after trypsination, and counted. At this state, as for fibroblasts, feeders can be frozen until further use or expanded on gelatinized (0.1%) culture dishes or plates for ES cell culture. Fibroblasts are only good as feeders for three to four passages. Feeders have to be distributed at an adequate number of cells to form a monolayer of cells (on average 5×10^4 cells/cm^2) and preferentially at least 1 d before adding ES cells. Feeders can be kept for up to 2 wk before they should be discarded. Fibroblast medium has to be changed to ES medium prior to use for ES cell culture. Quality of feeders may vary from different fibroblast preparations, so it is important to verify the feeder effect on test ES cells.

3. LIF Preparation and Titration. LIF is a member of the IL-6 cytokine family that exhibits pleiotropic effects on different cell types. LIF not only maintains pluripotency of ES cells *(42,43)*, but has a broad range of biological actions on early embryos *(82,83)*, primordial germ cells *(84)*, myocytes *(85,86)*, neurons *(87,88)*, and adipocytes *(89)*. LIF exists under two isoforms, a diffusible and an extracellular matrix-bound isoform *(90)*. LIF acts by binding to a specific receptor and a signal transducer (gp130), which mediate LIF signaling through JAK/STAT and MAP kinase pathways *(91)*.

Recombinant human LIF is prepared by electroporating the LIF expression plasmid pC10-6R DIA/LIF (generous gift from Dr. Austin Smith) into COS-7 cells *(44)*. Briefly, cells are diluted at 5×10^7 cells/0.5 mL and electroporated with 100 μg LIF plasmid at 960 μF and 200 V (5×10^7 cells/cuvet). After 10 min at room temperature for recovery, cells from one cuvet are diluted into 450 mL culture medium and distributed into 15 culture flasks (175 cm^2). The next day, culture medium is replaced by 40 mL fresh medium/flask. Medium is collected 48 h, as well as 96 h later and filtrated on 22 μm. Both harvested media are pooled, aliquoted (20 mL), and stored at –80°C until use.

LIF preparations are titrated at 1/250, 1/500, and 1/1000 dilutions using several ES cell preparations, cultured under standard conditions either on feeders or only on gelatinized plates during 1–2 wk. ES cells are examined each day for their typical morphology. ES colonies should stay round and tightly packed. The best titer of LIF corresponds to the dilution where ES cells show lowest rate of differentiation in the feeder-free series. In our hands, the different LIF preparations were highly reproducible and a 1/750 dilution has been routinely used over the past several years.

References

1. Capecchi, M. R. (1989) Altering the genome by homologous recombination. *Science* **244**, 1288–1293.
2. Thomas, K. R., Folger, K. R., and Capecchi, M. R. (1986) High frequency targeting of genes to specific sites in the mammalian genome. *Cell* **44**, 419–428.
3. Evans, M. J. and Kaufman, M. H. (1981) Establishment in culture of pluripotential cells from mouse embryos. *Nature* **292**, 154–156.

4. Martin, G. R. (1981) Isolation of a pluripotent cell line from early mouse embryos cultured in medium conditioned by teratocarcinoma stem cells. *Proc. Natl. Acad. Sci. USA* **78,** 7634–7638.

5. Mogil, J. S., Yu, L., and Basbaum, A. I. (2000) Pain genes?: natural variation and transgenic mutants. *Ann. Rev. Neurosci.* **23,** 777–811.

6. Mogil, J. S. and Grisel, J. E. (1998) Transgenic studies of pain. *Pain* **77,** 107–128.

7. Crawley, J. N. (2000) *What's Wrong with My Mouse.* Wiley-Liss, New York.

8. Crowley, C., Spencer, C. D., Nishimurai, M. C., et al. (1994) Mice lacking nerve growth factor display perinatal loss of sensory and sympathetic neurons yet develop basal forebrain cholinergic neurons. *Cell* **76,** 1001–1011.

9. Smeyne, R. J., Klein, R., Schnapp, A., et al. (1994) Severe sensory and sympathetic neuropathies in mice carrying a disrupted Trk/NGF receptor gene. *Nature* **368,** 246–249.

10. Xu, X. J., Hao, J. X., Andell-Jonsson, S., et al. (1997) Nociceptive responses in interleukin-6-deficient mice to peripheral inflammation and peripheral nerve section. *Cytokine* **9,** 1028–1033.

11. Robertson, B., Xu, X. J., Hao, J. X., et al. (1997) Interferon-gamma receptors in nociceptive pathways: role in neuropathic pain-related behaviour. *Neuroreport* **8,** 1311–1316.

12. Murata, T., Ushikubi, F., Matsuoka, T., et al. (1997) Altered pain perception and inflammatory response in mice lacking prostacyclin receptor. *Nature* **388,** 678–682.

13. Rupniak, N. M., Boyce, S., Webb, J. K., et al. (1997) Effects of the bradykinin B1 receptor antagonist desArg9[Leu8]bradykinin and genetic disruption of the B2 receptor on nociception in rats and mice. *Pain* **71,** 89–97.

14. Caterina, M. J., Leffter, A., Malmberg, A. B., et al. (2000) Impaired nociception and pain sensation in mice lacking the capsaicin receptor. *Science* **288,** 306–313.

15. Cao, Y. Q., Mantyh, P. W., Carlson, E. J., et al. (1998) Primary afferent tackykinins are required to experience moderate to intense pain. *Nature* **392,** 390–394.

16. Zimmer, A., Zimmer, A. M., Baff, J., et al. (1998) Hypoalgesia in mice with a targeted deletion of the tackykinin 1 gene. *Proc. Natl. Acad. Sci. USA* **95,** 2630–2635.

17. De Felipe, C., Herrero, J. F., O'Brien, J. A., et al. (1998) Altered nociception, analgesia and aggression in mice lacking the receptor for substance P. *Nature* **392,** 394–397.

18. Malmberg, A. B., Brandon, E. P., Idzerda, R. L., et al. (1997) Diminished inflammation and nociceptive pain with preservation of neuropathic pain in mice with a targeted mutation of the Type I regulatory subunit of cAMP-dependent protein kinase. *J. Neurosci.* **17,** 7462–7470.

19. Malmberg, A. B., Chen, C., Tonegawa, S., and Basbaum, A. I. (1997) Preserved acute pain and reduced neuropathic pain in mice lacking PKCgamma. *Science* **278,** 279–283.

20. Dickenson, A. H. (1991) Mechanisms of the analgesic action of opiates and opioids. *Br. Med. Bull.* **47,** 690–702.

21. Ossipov, M. H., Malan, T. P., Jr., and Lai, J. (1997) Opioid pharmacology of acute and chronic pain, in *Handbook of Experimental Pharmacology* (Dickenson, A. and Besson, J. M., eds.), Springer Verlag, Berlin, vol. 130, pp. 305–327.

22. Kieffer, B. L. (1999) Opioids: first lessons from knock-out mice. *Trends Pharmacol. Sci.* **20,** 537–544.

23. Hayward, M. D. and Low, M. J. (1999) Targeted mutagenesis of the murine opioid system. *Results Probl. Cell Differ.* **26,** 169–191.

24. Kieffer, B. L. and Gavériaux-Ruff, C. (2002) Exploring the opioid system by gene knockout. *Prog. Neurobiol.* **66,** 285–306.

25. Wang, Z., Gardell, L. R., Ossipov, M. H., et al. (2001) Pronociceptive actions of dynorphin maintain chronic neuropathic pain. *J. Neurosci.* **21,** 1779–1786.

26. Matthes, H. W. D., Maldonado, R., Simonin, F., et al. (1996) Loss of morphine-induced analgesia, reward effect and withdrawal symptoms in mice lacking the μ-opioid receptor gene. *Nature* **383,** 819–823.

27. Simonin, F., Valverde, O., Smadja, C., et al. (1998) Disruption of the κ-opioid receptor gene in mice enhances sensitivity to chemical visceral pain, impairs pharmacological actions of the selective κ-agonist U-50,488H and attenuates morphine withdrawal. *EMBO J.* **17,** 886–897.

28. Filliol, D., Ghozland, S., and Chluba, J. (2000) δ- and μ-opioid receptor-deficient mice exhibit opposing alterations of emotional responses. *Nature Genet.* **25,** 195–200.

29. Dolle, P., Dierich, A., Le Meur, M., et al. (1993) Disruption of the Hoxd-13 gene induces localized heterochrony leading to mice with neotenic limbs. *Cell* **75,** 431–441.

30. Saudou, F., Amara, D. A., Dierich, A., et al. (1994) Enhanced aggressive behavior in mice lacking 5-HT1B receptor. *Science* **265,** 1875–1878.

31. Dierich, A., Sairam, M. R., Monaco, L., et al. (1998) Impairing follicle-stimulating hormone (FSH) signaling in vivo: targeted disruption of the FSH receptor leads to aberrant gametogenesis and hormonal imbalance. *Proc. Natl. Acad. Sci. USA* **95,** 13612–13617.

32. Metzger, D. and Feil, R. (1999) Engineering the mouse genome by site-specific recombination. *Curr. Opin. Biotech.* **10,** 470–476.

33. Doetschman, T. C., Eistetter, H., Katz, M., et al. (1985) The in vitro development of blastocyst-derived embryonic stem cell lines: formation of visceral yolk sac, blood islands and myocardium. *J. Embryol. Exp. Morphol.* **87,** 27–45.

34. Robertson, E., Bradley, A., Kulhn, M., Evans, M. (1986) Germ-line transmission of genes introduced into cultured pluripotential cells by retroviral vector. *Nature* **323,** 445–448.

35. Hooper, M., Hardy, K., Handyside, A., et al. (1987) HPRT-deficient (Lesch-Nyhan) mouse embryos derived from germ-line colonization by cultured cells. *Nature* **326,** 292–295.

36. McMahon, A. P. and Bradley, A. (1990) The Wnt-1 (int-1) proto-oncogene is required for development of a large region of the mouse brain. *Cell* **62,** 1073–1085.

37. Nagy, A., Rossant, J., Nagy, R., et al. (1993) Derivation of completely cell culture-derived mice from early-passage embryonic stem cells. *Proc. Natl. Acad. Sci. USA* **90,** 8424–8428.

38. Ledermann, B. and Burki, K. (1991) Establishment of a germ-line competent C57BL/6 embryonic stem cell line. *Exp. Cell. Res.* **197,** 254–258.
39. Kontgen, F., Suss, G., Stewart, C., et al. (1993) Targeted disruption of the MHC class II Aa gene in C57BL/6 mice. *Int. Immunol.* **5,** 957–964.
40. Roach, M. L., Stock, J. L., Byrum, R., et al. (1995) A new embryonic stem cell line from DBA/1lacJ mice allows genetic modification in a murine model of human inflammation. *Exp. Cell. Res.* **221,** 520–525.
41. Noben-Trauth, N., Kohler, Q., Burki, K., et al. (1996) Efficient targeting of the IL-4 gene in a BALB/c embryonic stem cell line. *Transgenic Res.* **5,** 487–491.
42. Williams, R. L., Hilton, D. J., Pease, S., et al. (1988) Myeloid leukaemia inhibitory factor maintains the developmental potential of embryonic stem cells. *Nature* **336,** 684–687.
43. Smith, A. G., Heath, J. K., Donaldson, D. D., et al. (1988) Inhibition of pluripotential embryonic stem cell differentiation by purified polypeptides. *Nature* **336,** 688–690.
44. Nichols, J., Evans, E. P., and Smith, A. G. (1990) Establishment of germ-line-competent embryonic stem (ES) cells using differentiation inhibiting activity. *Development* **110,** 1341–1348.
45. Robertson, E. J. (1987) Embryo-derived stem cell lines, in *Teratocarcinomas and Embryonic Stem Cells. A Practical Approach.* IRL Press Limited, Oxford, UK, pp. 71–112.
46. Bradbury, M. W., Isola, L. M., and Gordon, J. W. (1990) Enzymatic amplification of a Y chromosome repeat in a single blastomere allows identification of the sex of preimplantation mouse embryos. *Proc. Natl. Acad. Sci. USA* **87,** 4053–4057.
47. Thomas, K. R. and Capecchi, M. R. (1987) Site-directed mutagenesis by gene targeting in mouse embryo-derived stem cells. *Cell* **51,** 503–512.
48. Mansour, S. L., Thomas, K. R., and Capecchi, M. R. (1988) Disruption of the proto-oncogene int-2 in mouse embryo-derived stem cells: a general strategy for targeting mutations to non-selectable genes. *Nature* **336,** 348–352.
49. Hasty, P., Rivera-Perez, J., Chang, C., et al. (1991) Target frequency and integration pattern for insertion and replacement vectors in embryonic stem cells. *Mol. Cell. Biol.* **11,** 4509–4517.
50. Hasty, P., Ramirez-Salis, R., Krumlauf, R., et al. (1991) Introduction of a subtle mutation into the Hox-2.6 locus in embryonic stem cells. *Nature* **350,** 243–246.
51. Valancius, V. and Smithies, O. (1991) Testing an in-out targeting procedure for making subtle genomic modifications in mouse embryonic stem cells. *Mol. Cell. Biol.* **11,** 1402–1408.
52. Thomas, K. R., Deng, C., and Capecchi, M. R. (1992) High-fidelity gene targeting in embryonic stem cells by using sequence replacement vectors. *Mol. Cell. Biol.* **12,** 2919–2923.
53. Sambrook, J., Fritsch, E. F., and Maniatis, T. (eds.) (1989) *Molecular Cloning: A Laboratory Manual.* Cold Spring Harbor Laboratory Press, Cold Spring Harbor, NY.

54. Kieffer, B. L. (1997) Molecular aspects of opioid receptors, in *The Pharmacology of Pain: Pain Handbook of Experimental Pharmacology* (Dickenson, A. and Besson, J. M., ed.), Springer-Verlag, Berlin, vol. 130, pp. 281–303.

55. te Riele, H., Maandag, E. R., and Berns, A. (1992) Highly efficient gene targeting in embryonic stem cells through homologous recombination with isogenic DNA constructs. *Proc. Natl. Acad. Sci. USA* **89**, 5128–5132.

56. Zhou, L., Romley, D. L., Mi, Q. S., et al. (2001) Murine inter-strain polymorphisms alter gene targeting frequencies at the mu opioid receptor locus in embryonic stem cells. *Mamm. Genome* **12**, 772–778.

57. McBurney, M. W., Sutherland, L. C., Adra, C. N., et al. (1991) The mouse Pgk-1 promoter contains an upstream activator sequence. *Nucleic Acid Res.* **19**, 5755–5761.

58. te Riele, H., Maandag, E. R., Clark, A., et al. (1990) Consecutive inactivation of both alleles of the pim-1 proto-oncogene by homologous recombination in embryonic stem cells. *Nature* **348**, 649–651.

59. Hasty, P., Rivera-Perez, J., and Bradley, A. (1991) The length of homology required for gene targeting in embryonic stem cells. *Mol. Cell. Biol.* **11**, 5586–5591.

60. Kitchen, I., Slowe, S. J., Matthes, H. W., et al. (1997) Quantitative autoradiographic mapping of μ-, δ- and κ-opioid receptors in knockout mice lacking the μ-opioid receptor gene. *Brain Res.* **778**, 73–88.

61. Slowe, S. J., Simonin, F., Kieffer, B., et al. (1999) Quantitative autoradiography of μ-, δ- and κ_1 opioid receptors in kappa-opioid receptor knockout mice. *Brain Res.* **818**, 335–345.

62. Goody, R. J., Oakley, S. M., Fillial, D., et al. (2002) Quantitative autoradiography mapping of opioid receptors in the brain of δ-opioid receptor gene knockout mice. *Br. Res.* **945**, 9–19.

63. Schwartzberg, P. L., Goff, S. P., and Robertson, E. J. (1989) Germ-line transmission of a c-abl mutation produced by targeted gene disruption in ES cells. *Science* **246**, 799–803.

64. Cosgrove, D., Gray, D., Dierich, A., et al. (1991) Mice lacking MHC class II molecules. *Cell* **66**, 1051–1066.

65. Soriano, P., et al. (1991) Targeted disruption of the c-src proto-oncogene leads to osteopetrosis in mice. *Cell* **64**, 693–702.

66. Ramirez-Solis, R., Zheng, H., Whiting, J., et al. (1993) Hoxb-4 (Hox-2.6) mutant mice show homeotic transformation of a cervical vertebra and defects in the closure of the sternal rudiments. *Cell* **73**, 279–294.

67. Bradley, A. (1987) Production and Analysis of Chimeric Mice, in *Teratocarcinomas and Embryonic Stem Cells. A Practical Approach.* IRL Press Limited, Oxford, UK, pp. 113–151.

68. Steward, C. L. (1993) Production of chimeras between embryonic stem cells and embryos, in *Guide to Techniques in Mouse Development* (Wassarman, P. M., and De Pamphlis, M. L., eds.), Academic Press, Inc., San Diego, vol. 225, pp. 823–855.

69. Lallemand, Y. and Brulet, P. (1990) An in situ assessment of the routes and extents of colonisation of the mouse embryo by embryonic stem cells and their descendants. *Development* **110**, 1241–1248.

70. Wood, S. A., Allen, N. D., Rossant, J., et al. (1993) Non-injection methods for the production of embryonic stem cell-embryo chimaeras. *Nature* **365,** 87–89.

71. Nagy, A. and Rossant, J. (1999) Production of ES-cell aggregation chimeras, in *Gene Targeting. A Practical Approach.* IRL Press, Oxford, pp. 177–205.

72. Crawley, J. N. (1999) Behavioral phenotyping of transgenic and knockout mice: experimental design and evaluation of general health, sensory functions, motor abilities and specific behavioral tests. *Brain Res.* **835,** 18–26.

73. Wilson, S. G. and Mogil, J. S. (2001) Measuring pain in the (knockout) mouse: big challenges in a small mammal. *Beh. Br. Res.* **125,** 65–73.

74. Malmberg, A. B. and Basbaum, A. I. (1998) Partial sciatic nerve injury in the mouse as a model of neuropathic pain: behavioral and neuroanatomical correlates. *Pain* **76,** 215–222.

75. Olivar, T. and Laird, J. M. A. (1999) Cyclophosphamide cystitis in mice: behavioral characterization and correlation with bladder inflammation. *Eur. J. Pain* **3,** 141–149.

76. Qiu, C., Sora, J., Ren, K., et al. (2000) Enhanced delta-opioid receptor-mediated antinociception in mu-opioid receptor-deficient mice. *Eur. J. Pharmacol.* **387,** 163–169.

77. Kerr, B. J., Gupta, Y., Pope, R., et al. (2001) Endogenous galanin potentiates spinal nociceptive processing following inflammation. *Pain* **93,** 267–277.

78. Lariviere, W. R., Chesler, E. J., and Mogil, J. S. (2001) Transgenic studies of pain and analgesia: mutation or background phenotype? *J. Pharm. Exp. Ther.* **297,** 467–473.

79. Silva, A. J., Simpson, E. N., and Takahashi, J. S. (1997) Mutant mice and neurosciences: recommandations concerning genetic background. *Neuron* **19,** 755–759.

80. Crabbe, J. C., Wahlsten, D., and Dudek, B. C. (1999) Genetics of mouse behavior: interactions with laboratory environment. *Science* **284,** 670–672.

81. Wobus, A. M., Wallukat, G., and Hescheler, J. (1991) Pluripotent mouse embryonic stem cells are able to differentiate into cardiomyocytes expressing chronotropic responses to adrenergic and cholinergic agents and Ca^{2+} channel blockers. *Differentiation* **48,** 173–182.

82. Yang, Z. M., Le, S. P., Chen, D. B., et al. (1995) Leukemia inhibitory factor, LIF receptor, and gp130 in the mouse uterus during early pregnancy. *Mol. Reprod. Dev.* **42,** 407–414.

83. van Eijk, M. J., Mandelbaum, J., Salat-Baroux J., et al. (1996) Expression of leukaemia inhibitory factor receptor subunits LIFR beta and gp130 in human oocytes and preimplantation embryos. *Mol. Hum. Reprod.* **2,** 355–360.

84. Cheng, L., Gearing, D. P., White, L. S., et al. (1994) Role of leukemia inhibitory factor and its receptor in mouse primordial germ cell growth. *Development* **120,** 3145–3153.

85. Vakakis, N., Bower, J., and Austin, L. (1995) In vitro myoblast to myotube transformations in the presence of leukemia inhibitory factor. *Neurochem. Int.* **27,** 329–335.

86. Matsui, H., Fujia, Y., Kunisada, K., et al. (1996) Leukemia inhibitory factor induces a hypertrophic response mediated by gp130 in murine cardiac myocytes. *Res. Commun. Mol. Pathol. Pharmacol.* **93,** 149–162.

87. Yamamori, T., Fukada, K., Aebersald, R., et al. (1989) The cholinergic neuronal differentiation factor from heart cells is identical to leukemia inhibitory factor. *Science* **246,** 1412–1416.
88. Li, M., Sendtner, M., and Smith, A. (1995) Essential function of LIF receptor in motor neurons. *Nature* **378,** 724–727.
89. Marshall, M. K., Doerrler, W., Feingold, K. R., et al. (1994) Leukemia inhibitory factor induces changes in lipid metabolism in cultured adipocytes. *Endocrinology* **135,** 141–147.
90. Rathjen, P. D., Toth, S., Wellis, A., et al. (1990) Differentiation inhibiting activity is produced in matrix-associated and diffusible forms that are generated by alternate promoter usage. *Cell* **62,** 1105–1114.
91. Boeuf, H., Hauss, C., Graeve, F. D., et al. (1997) Leukemia inhibitory factor-dependent transcriptional activation in embryonic stem cells. *J. Cell. Biol.* **138,** 1207–1217.

Index